T0348728

Obstetric and Gynecologic Emergencies

Editors

JOELLE BORHART
REBECCA A. BAVOLEK

EMERGENCY MEDICINE
CLINICS OF NORTH AMERICA

www.emed.theclinics.com

Consulting Editor
AMAL MATTU

May 2019 • Volume 37 • Number 2

ELSEVIER

1600 John F. Kennedy Boulevard ● Suite 1800 ● Philadelphia, Pennsylvania, 19103-2899

http://www.theclinics.com

EMERGENCY MEDICINE CLINICS OF NORTH AMERICA Volume 37, Number 2
May 2019 ISSN 0733-8627, ISBN-13: 978-0-323-67811-7

Editor: Colleen Dietzler
Developmental Editor: Casey Potter

Emergency Medicine Clinics of North America (ISSN 0733-8627) is published quarterly by Elsevier Inc., 360 Park Avenue South, New York, NY, 10010-1710. Months of issue are February, May, August, and November. Business and Editorial Offices: 1600 John F. Kennedy Boulevard, Suite 1800, Philadelphia, PA 19103-2899. Customer Service Office: 6277 Sea Harbor Drive, Orlando, FL 32887-4800. Periodicals postage paid at New York, NY, and additional mailing offices. Subscription prices are $100.00 per year (US students), $349.00 per year (US individuals), $679.00 per year (US institutions), $220.00 per year (international students), $462.00 per year (international individuals), $836.00 per year (international institutions), $220.00 per year (Canadian students), $411.00 per year (Canadian individuals), and $836.00 per year (Canadian institutions). International air speed delivery is included in all *Clinics'* subscription prices. All prices are subject to change without notice. **POSTMASTER:** Send address changes to *Emergency Medicine Clinics of North America*, Elsevier Periodicals Customer Service, 11830 Westline Industrial Drive, St. Louis, MO 63146. Customer Service (orders, claims, online, change of address): Elsevier Periodicals **Customer Service, 11830 Westline Industrial Drive, St. Louis, MO 63146. Tel: 1-800-654-2452 (U.S. and Canada); 314-453-7041 (outside U.S. and Canada). Fax: 314-453-5170. E-mail: journalscustomerservice-usa@elsevier.com (for print support)**; **journalsonlinesupport-usa@elsevier.com (for online support)**.

Reprints. For copies of 100 or more of articles in this publication, please contact the Commercial Reprints Department, Elsevier Inc., 360 Park Avenue South, New York, NY 10010-1710. Tel.: 212-633-3874; Fax: 212-633-3820; E-mail: reprints@elsevier.com.

Emergency Medicine Clinics of North America is covered in *MEDLINE/PubMed (Index Medicus), Current Contents/Clinical Medicine, EMBASE/Excerpta Medica, BIOSIS, SciSearch, CINAHL, ISI/BIOMED,* and *Research Alert.*

Contributors

CONSULTING EDITOR

AMAL MATTU, MD
Professor and Vice Chair, Department of Emergency Medicine, University of Maryland School of Medicine, Baltimore, Maryland

EDITORS

JOELLE BORHART, MD, FACEP, FAAEM
Associate Program Director, Assistant Professor of Emergency Medicine, Department of Emergency Medicine, MedStar Georgetown University Hospital and Washington Hospital Center, Washington, DC

REBECCA A. BAVOLEK, MD
Residency Program Director, Associate Clinical Professor, UCLA Emergency Medicine, Los Angeles, California

AUTHORS

Aws AL-ABDULLAH, MD
UCLA Ronald Reagan-Olive View Emergency Medicine Residency, UCLA Medical Center, Los Angeles, California

JOELLE BORHART, MD, FACEP, FAAEM
Associate Program Director, Assistant Professor of Emergency Medicine, Department of Emergency Medicine, MedStar Georgetown University Hospital and Washington Hospital Center, Washington, DC

KAYLA DEWEY, MD
Faculty, Department of Emergency Medicine, University of Rochester Medical Center, Rochester, New York

PAMELA L. DYNE, MD
Professor, Clinical Emergency Medicine, David Geffen School of Medicine at UCLA, Olive View-UCLA Medical Center, Department of Emergency Medicine, Sylmar, California

BRYN EISFELDER, MD
Affiliate, Department of Emergency Medicine, Stanford University, Palo Alto, California

STEPHANIE GUNDERSON, MD
Clinical Instructor, Department of Obstetrics & Gynecology, Washington University in St Louis, St Louis, Missouri

TYLER HAERTLEIN, MD
UCLA Ronald Reagan-Olive View Emergency Medicine Residency, UCLA Medical Center, Los Angeles, California

SUELIN M. HILBERT, MD, MPH, FACEP
Assistant Professor, Division of Emergency Medicine, Washington University in St Louis, St Louis, Missouri

NIKITA JOSHI, MD
Assistant Professor, Alameda Health Systems, Oakland, California

SARA MANNING, MD
Assistant Professor, Department of Emergency Medicine, University of Maryland School of Medicine, Baltimore, Maryland

COLLIN MICHELS, MD
Affiliate, Department of Emergency Medicine, Stanford University, Palo Alto, California

TERI ANNE MILLER, MD
UCLA Emergency Medicine Residency Program, UCLA Department of Emergency Medicine, Los Angeles, California

ADEOLU C. OGUNBODEDE, MD
Assistant Clinical Instructor, Department of Emergency Medicine, Department of Internal Medicine, University of Maryland School of Medicine, Baltimore, Maryland

JESSICA PALMER, MD
Department of Emergency Medicine, MedStar Southern Maryland Hospital Center, Clinton, Maryland

CAMIRON L. PFENNIG, MD, MHPE
Associate Professor of Emergency Medicine, Prisma Health, University of South Carolina School of Medicine Greenville, Clemson University School of Health Research, Greenville, South Carolina

ELIZABETH PONTIUS, MD, RDMS
Assistant Professor, Department of Emergency Medicine, Georgetown University School of Medicine, MedStar Georgetown University Hospital, MedStar Washington Hospital Center, Washington, DC

JEFFREY SAKAMOTO, MD
Affiliate, Department of Emergency Medicine, Stanford University, Palo Alto, California

PHILIPPA N. SOSKIN, MD, MPP, FACEP
Attending Physician, Assistant Professor, Department of Emergency Medicine, MedStar Georgetown University Hospital, MedStar Washington Hospital Center, Georgetown University School of Medicine, Washington, DC

JULIE T. VIETH, MBChB
Adjunct Clinical Assistant Professor, Department of Emergency Medicine, Clarkson University, Canton-Potsdam Hospital, Potsdam, New York; Assistant Clinical Professor, SUNY Upstate Medical University, Syracuse, New York

KATHRYN VOSS, MD
Assistant Professor, Department of Emergency Medicine, MedStar Georgetown University Hospital and Washington Hospital Center, Washington, DC

NATASHA WHEATON, MD
Assistant Clinical Professor, Associate Program Director, UCLA Ronald Reagan-Olive View Emergency Medicine Residency, UCLA Medical Center, Los Angeles, California

LINDSEY M. WHITE, MD
Chief Resident, Department of Emergency Medicine, Virginia Tech Carilion School of Medicine, Roanoke, Virginia

R. GENTRY WILKERSON, MD
Assistant Professor, Department of Emergency Medicine, University of Maryland School of Medicine, Baltimore, Maryland

CORY WITTROCK, MD
Emergency Ultrasound Fellowship Director, Medstar Georgetown University Hospital, Washington, DC

JANET S. YOUNG, MD
Associate Professor, Department of Emergency Medicine, Virginia Tech Carilion School of Medicine, Carilion Medical Center, Roanoke, Virginia

JENNIFER YU, MD, FACEP
Assistant Professor of Emergency Medicine, Attending Physician, Department of Critical Care Medicine, MedStar Washington Hospital Center, Georgetown University School of Medicine, Washington, DC

Contents

> Abnormal uterine bleeding (AUB) unrelated to pregnancy affects 20% to 30% of women at some point in life and is a common emergency department (ED) and urgent care (UC) presentation. AUB is a complex condition with extensive terminology, broad differential diagnosis, and numerous treatment options, yet few published evidence-based guidelines. In the ED or UC setting most affected patients are often more frustrated than acutely ill. These factors can make for a challenging patient encounter in the EC/UC setting. This article reviews acute and chronic AUB in the nonpregnant patient and suggests a simplified approach for its evaluation and management.

> Sexually transmitted diseases (STDs) continue to be underrecognized leading to devastating health and economic consequences. Emergency clinicians play an important role in diagnosing and managing STDs and in improving health care outcomes for both the patient and their partners. In addition, antibiotic resistance and emerging infections continue to challenge providers in clinical practice. This review focuses on the cause, history, physical examination, diagnostic studies, and treatment strategies for bacterial vaginosis, chlamydia, genital herpes, gonorrhea, human papillomavirus, granuloma inguinale, Lymphogranuloma Venereum, *Mycoplasma genitalium*, syphilis, and trichomoniasis.

> Variations in estrogen levels across a woman's lifetime lead to important changes in genital physiology and pathophysiology. Low estrogen states like menopause and the prepubertal period share important physiologic changes, including more friable, dry, and inelastic mucosa that is prone to irritation, injury, and infection. These and other factors lead to unique gynecologic pathologic conditions encountered at the extremes of age. Age-specific pathologic conditions and differences in examination techniques are discussed.

with balanced versus targeted blood products replacement is presented for low-resource versus high-resource environments. Emergency department readiness for such a patient, in combination with appropriate consultation or transfer, is essential to the effective management of late-term vaginal bleeding.

A precipitous delivery can be among the most stressful events an emergency physician encounters. The physician must assess 2 patients (mother and fetus) and be prepared to manage a variety of complications that may arise during delivery. A majority of precipitous deliveries result in good outcomes for both mother and baby, but emergency physicians must be prepared to manage feared complications, such as tight nuchal cords, shoulder dystocia, and breech presentation. An understanding of the labor process as well as advanced planning can help decrease the stress and chaos inherent to any precipitous delivery.

The period just after delivery is a high-risk period for women with associated morbidity and even mortality. There are large variations in complication rates across various groups in the United States. This article covers complications commonly encountered in the emergency department in late pregnancy and the early postpartum period. It specifically addresses postpartum depression, peripartum cardiomyopathy, and the late pregnant or postpartum patient presenting with headache or neurologic complaints. Emergency physicians should be well versed in common and life-threatening postpartum pathologies.

This article covers a high-risk time in a woman's life, the period just after delivery of her baby. There are large variations in complication rates across various groups in the United States. Many women seek care in the emergency department for routine and more serious postpartum pathologies. Emergency physicians should be well versed in common and life-threatening complications of delivery. The specific pathologies discussed in this article include lactation in the emergency department, postpartum hemorrhage, amniotic fluid embolism, endometritis, and mastitis.

The 4 categories of hypertensive disorders of pregnancy are chronic hypertension, gestational hypertension, preeclampsia-eclampsia, and chronic hypertension with superimposed preeclampsia. These disorders are among the leading causes of maternal and fetal morbidity and mortality. Proper diagnosis in the emergency department is crucial in order to initiate appropriate treatment to reduce the potential harm to the mother and the fetus. Prompt management should be undertaken when the blood pressure is greater than 160/110 mm Hg or there are other severe features such as acute kidney injury, elevated liver function tests, severe abdominal pain, pulmonary edema, and central nervous system disturbances.

Although trauma in pregnancy is rare, it is one of the most common causes of morbidity and mortality to pregnant women and fetus. Pathophysiology of trauma is generally time sensitive, and this is still true in pregnant patients, with the additional challenge of rare presentation and balancing the management of two patients concurrently. Successful resuscitation requires understanding the physiologic changes to the woman throughout the course of pregnancy. Ultimately, trauma management is best approached by prioritizing maternal resuscitation.

Cardiovascular disease has overtaken all other causes of maternal death in the United States. The physiologic changes of pregnancy place a significant amount of stress on the cardiovascular system and put pregnant women at risk for potentially catastrophic complications, such as pulmonary embolism, aortic or coronary artery dissection, myocardial infarction, and peripartum cardiomyopathy. The diagnosis of these conditions is challenging because the symptoms can mimic those experienced in normal pregnancies. There are subtle differences in the diagnosis and treatment of cardiovascular emergencies in pregnant patients that clinicians must be aware of; however, the overall management goals are similar.

Many health care providers lack familiarity with maternal physiologic changes and the distinctive underlying etiology of cardiac arrest in pregnancy. Knowledge of what changes are expected in pregnancy and an understanding of how to adapt clinical practice is essential for the care of the pregnant woman in the emergency department. Amniotic fluid embolism should be recognized as a rare cause of cardiac arrest in pregnancy, characterized by the triad of cardiovascular collapse, hypoxic respiratory failure, and coagulopathy. Cardiopulmonary resuscitation should follow standard AHA ACLS guidelines. Resuscitative hysterotomy may be attempted to restore perfusion to both mother and fetus.

EMERGENCY MEDICINE
CLINICS OF NORTH AMERICA

FORTHCOMING ISSUES

August 2019
Critical Care in the Emergency Department
John Greenwood and Tsuyoshi Mitarai,
Editors

November 2019
Genitourinary Emergencies
Ryan Spangler and Joshua Moskovitz,
Editors

February 2020
Orthopedic Emergencies
Michael C. Bond and Arun Sayal, *Editors*

RECENT ISSUES

February 2019
Ear, Nose, and Throat Emergencies
Laura J. Bontempo and Jan Shoenberger,
Editors

November 2018
Infectious Disease Emergencies
Stephen Y. Liang and Rachel Chin, *Editors*

August 2018
Hematologic and Oncologic Emergencies
Colin G. Kaide and Sarah B. Dubbs, *Editors*

SERIES OF RELATED INTEREST

Critical Care Clinics
https://www.criticalcare.theclinics.com/

THE CLINICS ARE NOW AVAILABLE ONLINE!
Access your subscription at:
www.theclinics.com

Erratum

An error was made in the November 2018 issue (Volume 36, Issue 4, p645-888) in Table 4 (pg. 825) in the article "Biothreat Agents and Emerging Infectious Disease in the Emergency Department" by Amesh A. Adalja. Under the Treatment column, the dose for Linezolid should be 600 mg instead of 6000 mg and meropenem 1 g IV q8h instead of q24.

Emerg Med Clin N Am 37 (2019) xiii
https://doi.org/10.1016/j.emc.2019.02.001
0733-8627/19/© 2019 Published by Elsevier Inc.

Foreword

Obstetric and Gynecological Emergencies

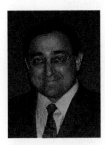

Amal Mattu, MD
Consulting Editor

Ask any emergency health care provider (HCP) which clinical scenarios are associated with the greatest level of chaos and stress in the emergency department (ED) and I'll bet they'll list childbirth at or near the top of the list. The irony here is that childbirth is such a normal and natural process, one that has been ongoing for thousands of years, that it should be a fairly stress-free process...or it should, at least, be a process that elicits less stress than "true emergencies," such as acute myocardial infarction, stroke, or sepsis. Yet nothing could be further from the truth. I personally feel more comfortable caring for just about any emergency than managing a precipitous delivery in the ED. Many of my colleagues would say the same thing.

The stress to HCPs associated with childbirth clearly comes from the fact that we are dealing with two patients rather than one, and also from the expectation of a perfect outcome. However, when the patient arrives, the threat of a pregnancy complication or a difficult delivery hangs over us like a storm cloud. Consultant help often doesn't arrive soon enough, if at all.

Complications during delivery are not the only obstetric concern we routinely face in emergency medicine. We must address postpartum complications, early-pregnancy complications, such as ectopic pregnancy, hypertensive crises, trauma in pregnancy, and increasingly common cardiovascular complications in pregnancy. Although pregnancy may be a completely natural state, it is rife with potential complications and stressors to emergency HCPs!

Fortunately, to our rescue come Guest Editors Dr Rebecca Bavolek and Dr Joelle Borhart. Drs Bavolek and Borhart have assembled an outstanding group of authors to address all of these concerns of pregnancy. But this issue of *Emergency Medicine Clinics of North America* that they have created is not simply focused on emergencies of pregnancy. The Guest Editors and authors have expanded the issue and address many non-pregnancy-related gynecologic issues as well. Early articles address

Emerg Med Clin N Am 37 (2019) xv–xvi
https://doi.org/10.1016/j.emc.2019.02.003
0733-8627/19/© 2019 Published by Elsevier Inc.

common chief complaints, such as nonpregnant vaginal bleeding and pelvic pain; they also provide updates on sexually transmitted infections. Rounding out the topics on nonpregnant patients is an excellent article on genital complaints at extremes of age.

This issue of *Emergency Medicine Clinics of North America* represents an important addition to the emergency medicine literature. Drs Bavolek, Borhart, and their authors have provided a cutting-edge curriculum in obstetrics and gynecology for the emergency HCP. Kudos to the contributors for an outstanding issue that will improve patient care and will certainly ease our stress when managing these patients!

Amal Mattu, MD
Department of Emergency Medicine
University of Maryland School of Medicine
110 South Paca Street
6th Floor, Suite 200
Baltimore, MD 21201, USA

E-mail address:
amalmattu@comcast.net

Preface

Obstetric and Gynecologic Emergencies

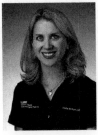
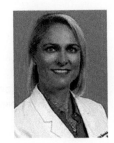

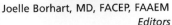

Joelle Borhart, MD, FACEP, FAAEM   Rebecca A. Bavolek, MD
Editors

Patients of all ages frequently present to the emergency department with a variety of gynecologic and obstetric complaints. These complaints can range in severity from completely benign (estrogen-withdrawal vaginal bleeding in the neonate) to potentially catastrophic (maternal cardiac arrest). Obstetric emergencies in particular can be among the most stressful events an emergency physician will face in their entire career as two lives are at stake. This issue covers the spectrum of problems encountered throughout all trimesters of pregnancy as well as the postpartum period. Gynecologic complaints across all stages of a woman's life are discussed, including the less commonly covered geriatric postmenopausal period. Articles reviewing complications of assisted reproductive technology and up-to-date management of sexually transmitted diseases for both female and male patients are also presented.

This issue is written for emergency physicians in all practice settings. Obstetric and gynecologic support services vary widely between different facilities, and emergency physicians must be prepared to initially manage any patient with a gynecologic or obstetric emergency who walks through the door. It is our hope that this issue provides useful information for daily practice as well as preparation for the rarely encountered and potentially life-threatening events.

It has been an honor to serve as guest editors for this *Emergency Medicine Clinics of North America* issue, and we are grateful to Dr Amal Mattu for the opportunity. We would also like to thank each of the authors for their contributions to this issue, as well as Casey Potter and the Elsevier editorial team for their guidance and

Emerg Med Clin N Am 37 (2019) xvii–xviii
https://doi.org/10.1016/j.emc.2019.02.002
0733-8627/19/© 2019 Published by Elsevier Inc.

support. We hope you enjoy this issue of *Emergency Medicine Clinics of North America* Gynecologic and Obstetric Emergencies!

Joelle Borhart, MD, FACEP, FAAEM
Department of Emergency Medicine
Georgetown University Hospital & Washington Hospital Center
Washington, DC 20007, USA

Rebecca A. Bavolek, MD
UCLA Emergency Medicine
924 Westwood Boulevard, Suite 300
Los Angeles, CA 90095, USA

E-mail addresses:
joelle.borhart@gmail.com (J. Borhart)
RBavolek@mednet.ucla.edu (R.A. Bavolek)

The Patient with Non–Pregnancy-Associated Vaginal Bleeding

Pamela L. Dyne, MD[a],*, Teri Anne Miller, MD[b]

KEYWORDS

- Vaginal bleeding • Abnormal uterine bleeding • Nonpregnant vaginal bleeding
- Life-threatening vaginal bleeding • Intrauterine tamponade

KEY POINTS

- The etiologies of acute AUB are classified based on the PALM-COEIN acronym: Polyp, Adenomyosis, Leiomyoma, Malignancy and hyperplasia, Coagulopathy, Ovulatory dysfunction, Endometrial, Iatrogenic, and Not otherwise classified.
- When first evaluating a patient with AUB there are 2 critical determinations to consider: (1) Is the patient pregnant? (2) Is the patient hemodynamically stable?
- Medical management is the first-line treatment for most stable patients; options include oral contraceptive pills, oral progesterone, NSAIDs, and tranexamic acid.
- The unstable patient should be resuscitated accordingly, and IV conjugated equine estrogen is considered a first-line treatment.
- Placement of an intrauterine tamponade device such as a Foley catheter or vaginal packing is a second-line maneuver for treatment of the unstable patient.

INTRODUCTION

Abnormal uterine bleeding (AUB) unrelated to pregnancy affects 20% to 30% of women at some point in their lives and is a common emergency department (ED) and urgent care (UC) presentation with major medical and social implications for women worldwide.[1,2] Despite this significance, there are few published evidence-based guidelines or emergency medicine-oriented reviews. AUB is a complex condition with extensive terminology, a broad differential diagnosis, and numerous treatment options. All of these factors can make for a challenging patient encounter in the acute care setting. This article reviews both acute and chronic

[a] UCLA-OV Emergency Medicine, Olive View-UCLA Department of Emergency Medicine, 14445 Olive View Drive, North Annex, Sylmar, CA 91342, USA; [b] UCLA-OV Emergency Medicine, UCLA Department of Emergency Medicine, 924 Westwood Boulevard, Suite 300, Los Angeles, CA 90024, USA
* Corresponding author.
E-mail address: pdyne@dhs.lacounty.gov

Emerg Med Clin N Am 37 (2019) 153–164
https://doi.org/10.1016/j.emc.2019.01.002
0733-8627/19/© 2019 Elsevier Inc. All rights reserved.

emed.theclinics.com

AUB in the nonpregnant patient, and suggests a simplified approach for evaluation and management of these patients in the ED and UC setting.

BACKGROUND

Historically the terminology used to classify uterine bleeding has been largely inconsistent and ambiguous. In an effort to standardize and simplify the terminology, the most appropriate term to describe uterine bleeding characterized by the patient to be other than an expected, regular menstrual period is AUB.[3] The use of the term "dysfunctional uterine bleeding" is no longer recommended.

To define AUB it is important to first define normal uterine bleeding. There are 4 parameters used to characterize a menstrual period: regularity, frequency, duration, and volume.[3] Normal uterine bleeding occurs every 24 to 38 days with cycle-to-cycle variation of 2 to 20 days, and duration of 4 to 8 days. Normal volume loss is 5 to 80 mL,[4] which loosely equates to one or less pad or tampon per 3-hour period (**Box 1**).[5] In general, volume is difficult to characterize and objective measures such as sanitary supplies used per day are generally unreliable.[6] Given the interpersonal variability in estimation of volume and the wide array of menstrual products from "light" to "maxi" or "heavy" pads, this is not surprising. The most practical measure is the patient's subjective characterization of her bleeding (normal, heavy, or light) and its impact on her life, as well as whether the amount she is bleeding represents a change from her baseline.[7]

When first evaluating a patient with heavy or frequent AUB, acute or chronic, there are 2 critical determinations to consider: (1) is the patient pregnant and (2) is she hemodynamically stable? Both of these drastically alter the evaluation and treatment plan. This review focuses on the evaluation and management of AUB unrelated to pregnancy.

CLASSIFICATION AND PATHOGENESIS OF ABNORMAL UTERINE BLEEDING

The mnemonic PALM-COIEN (pronounced "palm-coin") is now used to identify and help remember the known causes of AUB (**Fig. 1**).[8] This classification system was approved in 2011 by the Federation of International Gynecology and Obstetrics and is also supported by the American College of Obstetrics and Gynecology. The terms "menorrhagia," "metrorrhagia," and "menometrorrhagia" are also increasingly being abandoned because of their confusing nature and the miscommunication it promotes between providers. The modifiers "heavy" or "intermenstrual" are used to characterize the form of AUB in this classification system, and are used in this article.

Structural causes of AUB are represented in the "PALM" part of the mnemonic, and include polyps (P), adenomyosis (A), leiomyomas (L), and malignancy (M). Polyps are localized tumors of the epithelium (endocervix or endometrial). Bleeding from polyps is

---

Box 1
Normal menstrual cycle

- Occurs regularly
- Frequency: 24 to 38 days
- Cycle-to-cycle variation: 2 to 20 days
- Duration of bleeding: 4 to 8 days
- Volume: 5 to 80 mL ($\sim$1 pad per 3 hours)

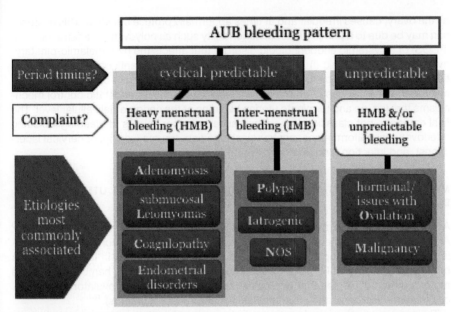

Fig. 1. Abnormal uterine bleeding pattern. Not otherwise specified (NOS): atrioventricular (AV) malformations, postsurgical bleeding, trauma (vaginal or cervical lacerations), and infection (endometritis). (*Adapted from* Munro M. Abnormal uterine bleeding. New York: Cambridge University Press; 2010.)

irregular and may be intermenstrual, that is, mid-cycle in timing.[9] Adenomyosis (A) is a disorder whereby endometrial glands and stroma invade the myometrium. The mechanism by which adenomyosis causes uterine bleeding remains unclear.[10] Leiomyomas (commonly referred to as fibroids) are common benign uterine tumors, which, depending on their location in the uterus, may cause heavy uterine bleeding. Not all leiomyomas cause bleeding; the closer the leiomyoma is located to the endometrium the more likely it will cause bleeding.[7] Malignant or premalignant lesions can cause irregular or heavy menses and are an important cause of AUB to consider at any age.[7]

Nonstructural causes of AUB are represented in the "COEIN" part of the mnemonic, and include coagulopathy (C), ovulatory dysfunction (O), endometrial (E), iatrogenic (I), and not classified (N). Disorders of hemostasis, that is, coagulopathy (C), may contribute to vaginal bleeding more than previously recognized.[7] Up to 20% of patients with heavy menstrual bleeding (HMB) may have an underlying coagulation disorder. One of the most common coagulopathies found to cause AUB is von Willebrand disease (vWD), a variant of which has been found to be the cause in up to 13% of patients.[11,12] Although vWD is the most common coagulopathy, the physician must also consider other acquired (eg, secondary to platelet dysfunction in systemic diseases such as kidney or liver failure), inherited, and iatrogenic bleeding disorders. Screening questions for bleeding disorders, especially in adolescents, such as history of easy bruising, epistaxis, gum bleeding, family history of bleeding disorders, a history of menses longer than 7 days, history of treatment for anemia, or history of excessive bleeding with tooth extraction, delivery, miscarriage, or surgery[13] can be helpful in identifying which patients should be referred to a hematologist for further workup. Ovarian dysfunction (O), that is, irregular or unpredictable release of progesterone by the ovary, causes irregular and at times abnormally profuse bleeding. This dysfunction may be due to a primary ovarian abnormality such as polycystic ovarian syndrome (PCOS) or a systemic endocrinologic disorder that affects the hypothalamic-pituitary-ovarian axis.[7] Iatrogenic (I) is a diverse category, including anticoagulants, medications that impair ovulation, breakthrough bleeding with a new birth-control medication, and intrauterine devices.[14] Endometrial (E) is a loss of the homeostatic control mechanisms that initiate and terminate uterine bleeding at the endometrial cellular level. The final category, not classified (N), encompasses all other causes of bleeding including arteriovenous malformations, postsurgical bleeding, trauma (vaginal or cervical lacerations), and infection (endometritis) (**Fig. 2**).

MANAGEMENT OF UNSTABLE PATIENTS WITH ACUTE ABNORMAL UTERINE BLEEDING

Acute AUB is defined as bleeding that requires urgent or emergent intervention.[8] Although most acute uterine hemorrhage occurs secondary to pregnancy, acute uterine bleeding in the nonpregnant state is perhaps more complex in its pathogenesis because all of the PALM-COEIN conditions can incite an acute hemorrhage.[15] The most common etiologies that can cause acute hemorrhage are ovulatory disorders, coagulation disorders, and structural lesions (submucosal fibroids).[16]

The emergency physician's main goal when managing uterine bleeding is to identify and stabilize life-threatening situations, and, once stabilized, to determine which patients require emergent gynecologic consultation. As with any bleeding patient, the initial management of an acute uterine bleed is focused on resuscitation and stabilization. There may be limited time for history taking and a focused physical examination; however, a pelvic examination should be performed to confirm the source of the bleeding and to better gauge the rate of blood loss. The physician should inspect the vaginal walls and cervix for any evidence of trauma or lacerations and roughly gauge the flow of blood from the cervix of a true uterine bleed, such as steady drip, continuous flow, and presence/size of clots in the vaginal vault. If the amount of bleeding appears to be brisk and the patient is symptomatic of volume depletion or anemia, 2 large-bore peripheral intravenous (IV) lines are immediately established, the patient is placed on the cardiac monitor, and blood or blood product transfusion is prepared. High-dose IV conjugated equine estrogen is indicated as first-line treatment of severe and potentially life-threatening bleeding.[17] Estrogen, 25 mg IV, may be dosed every 4 hours for a 24-hour period until adequate cessation of bleeding. This is often coadministered with an antiemetic to prevent nausea and vomiting. Contraindications to IV estrogen include history of pulmonary embolism or deep vein thrombosis, breast cancer, or liver disease. There are limited data regarding the risks of IV estrogen in patients with cardiovascular or thromboembolic risk factors, and caution is recommended (**Table 1**).

After obtaining hemostasis, patients are converted to either an oral contraceptive taper or a moderate-dose to high-dose progestin regimen. Emergent gynecologic consultation should be obtained for any unstable patient with acute AUB.

Surgical therapy for acute AUB is considered second line after failure of medical management. However, surgical management may be considered first line if bleeding is due to recent surgery, retained products of conception, or intrauterine lesions such as submucosal leiomyomas. The literature supporting surgical intervention is limited, and the exact treatment will be at the discretion of the consulting gynecologist, but options include intracavitary tamponade,[18] dilatation and curettage (D&C), endometrial ablation,[19] uterine artery occlusion,[20] and hysterectomy.[21]

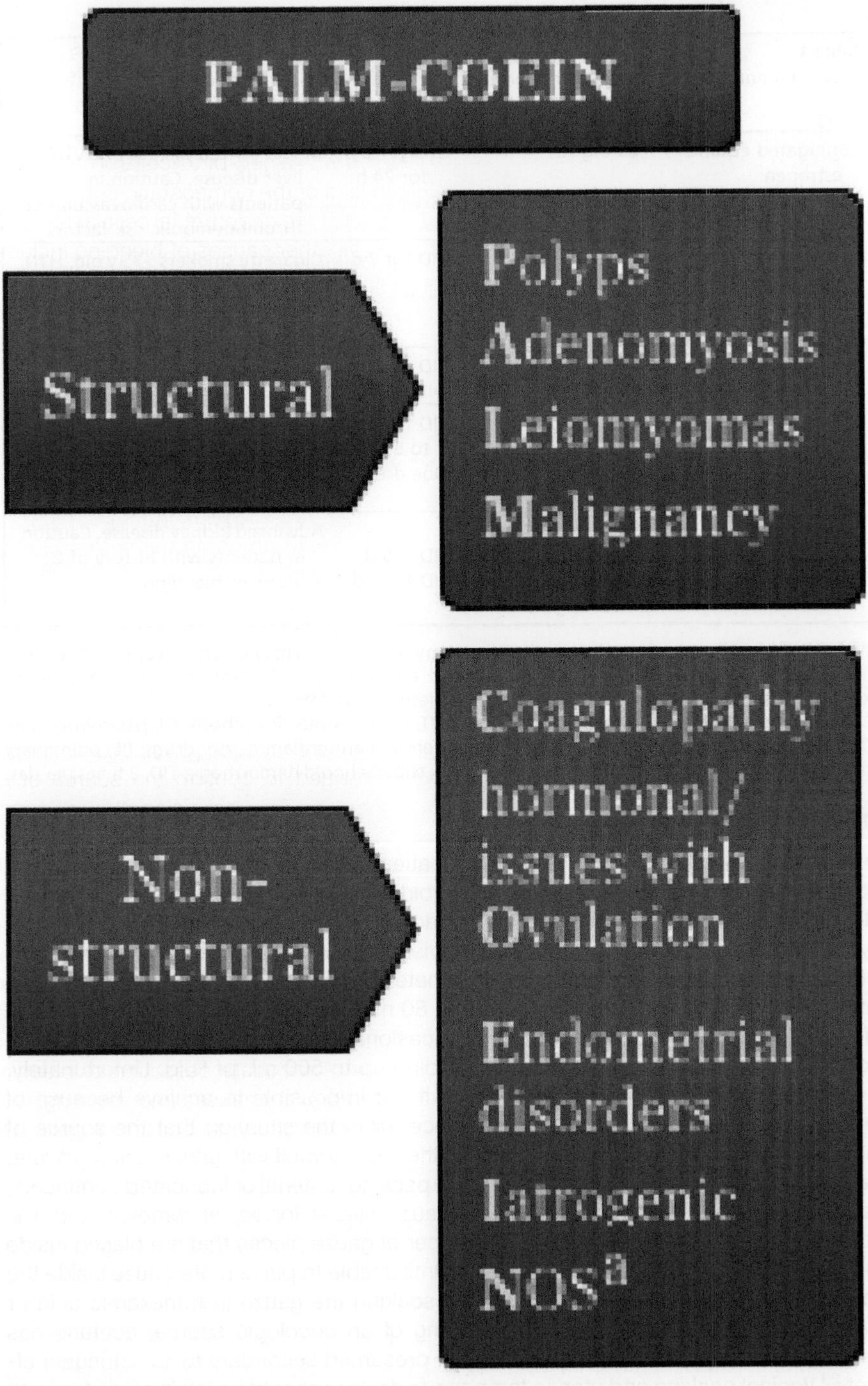

Fig. 2. PALM-COIEN pneumonic to remember causes of abnormal uterine bleeding. [a] Not otherwise specified: AV malformations, postsurgical bleeding, trauma (vaginal or cervical lacerations), and infection (endometritis). (*Adapted from* Munro MG, Critchley HO, Broder MS, et al. FIGO classification system (PALM-COEIN) for causes of abnormal uterine bleeding in nongravid women of reproductive age. Int J Gynaecol Obstet 2011;113(1):3–13.)

Table 1
Medical management options for abnormal uterine bleeding

Drug	Dose	Schedule	Contraindications
Conjugated equine estrogen	25 mg IV	Every 4–6 h for 24 h	Breast cancer, history of DVT/PE, liver disease. Caution in patients with cardiovascular or thromboembolic risk factors
Combined oral contraceptives	1 tablet	TID for 7 d	Cigarette smokers >35 y old, HTN, history of DVT/PE, breast cancer, pregnancy, ischemic heart disease, CVD, uncontrolled HTN
Medroxyprogesterone acetate	20 mg PO 10 mg PO	TID for 7 d QID × 10 d	Active or past DVT/PE, liver disease, or breast cancer
Tranexamic acid	1.3 g PO 10 mg/kg IV (max 600 mg/dose)	TID for up to 5 d One dose	Acquired impaired color vision, current or past DVT/PE, SAH Expensive
NSAIDs Ibuprofen Naproxen	 200–400 mg PO 500 mg once, then 250 mg PO	 TID × 5 d TID for 5 d	Advanced kidney disease. Caution in patients with history of GI ulcers or bleeding

This table is not all-inclusive; other medication forms and dosages may be effective. The list of contraindications is partial. The United States Food and Drug Administration's labeling contains exhaustive lists of contraindications for each of these treatments.

Abbreviations: CVD, cerebrovascular disease; DVT, deep venous thrombosis; GI, gastrointestinal; HTN, hypertension; IV, intravenous; NSAIDs, nonsteroidal anti-inflammatory drugs; PE, pulmonary embolism; PO, by mouth; QID, 4 times per day; SAH, subarachnoid hemorrhage; TID, 3 times per day.

Massive Vaginal Hemorrhage

In rare instances, the massively bleeding patient requires immediate intervention to control the bleeding within the ED to avoid hemodynamic collapse. For uterine bleeding, tamponade can be achieved by placing a Foley catheter into the uterine cavity. In this situation, a speculum is used to visualize the cervix, the cervix is swabbed with povidone-iodine solution, and the catheter is inserted approximately 6 to 8 cm into the uterus and then inflated with 30 to 80 mL of water.[22] This is the ED version of the Bakri balloon, a commercial device occasionally used by obstetricians to control postpartum bleeding that is capable of holding up to 500 mL of fluid. Unfortunately, visualization of the cervix may be difficult if not impossible to achieve because of the volume of bleeding. In this circumstance, or in the situation that the source of bleeding is within the vaginal vault, packing the vaginal vault with gauze is appropriate. Packing with commercially available vaginal packing material or lubricated continuous gauze is preferred over small, individual gauze pieces for easier removal, and it is advised to keep a written count of the number of gauze pieces that are placed inside the vaginal vault. Packing should continue until unable to place more gauze inside the vaginal vault. Adjuncts to packing include soaking the gauze in tranexamic acid or even acetone. For massive vaginal bleeding of an oncologic source, acetone has been successfully used to control bleeding, presumed secondary to its astringent effect.[23] Vaginal packing and uterine tamponade devices should be left in place for up to 24 hours. There is a theoretic risk of toxic shock syndrome and prophylactic broad-spectrum IV antibiotics are often initiated, although there is little evidence to support this practice. Emergent gynecologic consultation should be obtained for any patient who requires vaginal packing or uterine tamponade.

MANAGEMENT OF STABLE PATIENTS WITH CHRONIC ABNORMAL UTERINE BLEEDING

The keystone to the evaluation and treatment of the stable (often chronic) AUB patient is a thorough menstrual history. The ED evaluation for chronic AUB should also include the following: establish hemodynamic stability, evaluate for symptomatic anemia, perform a focused physical examination including a pelvic examination, and obtain laboratory tests including complete blood count with differential and urine pregnancy test. Because the history and physical examination findings of these patients usually do not differentiate whether the cause of their bleeding is structural or nonstructural, the vast majority of patients will also need a transvaginal ultrasound (TVUS) scan. For many stable patients with AUB the results of a TVUS scan are unlikely to change ED management and thus can be performed in an outpatient setting. Further laboratory studies such as thyroid function or coagulation studies may be added if warranted by the history. Patients may be briefly screened for an underlying disorder of hemostasis, as discussed earlier.

Suspected structural lesions and malignancy are evaluated initially with TVUS. In addition to structural lesions, color Doppler on TVUS can help detect arteriovenous malformations, a rare but important cause of AUB.[24] AVM should be considered in patients with history of instrumentation of the uterus, such as D&C. The decision as to the urgency with which TVUS is obtained, that is, whether in the ED/UC or as an outpatient with close follow-up, may be considered in concert with the patient and her primary care provider or gynecologist. Although TVUS is a very effective and safe screening tool, it can miss clinically significant polyps and may be of limited value in the setting of AUB because of intrauterine clots obscuring the endometrial lining.[25] If a patient has persistent symptoms despite a "negative" or nondiagnostic TVUS, she should be referred to a gynecologist for further evaluation, imaging, and possible endometrial biopsy, if indicated.

Medical Therapy

If the patient is stable with no clinically significant anemia, there is a variety of outpatient medical management options to consider (see **Table 1**). The goal of medical management is to help reduce the volume and duration of uterine bleeding. All patients started on medical management and discharged should be given strict ED return precautions and advised to follow up with a gynecologist within 48 to 72 hours. In addition to treatment options discussed herein, patients with anemia consistent with iron deficiency (microcytic anemia) should be started on iron supplementation. A common regimen is 324 mg of ferrous sulfate taken orally 3 times per day. Vitamin C may be started concurrently with iron to help increase absorption. Patients with significant anemia may need to be admitted for blood transfusion and urgent gynecologic evaluation.

Combination oral contraceptives

Combination oral contraceptive pill (OCP) tapers are commonly used by physicians to temporize an AUB episode, yet few studies have been conducted proving a certain formulation or efficacy. The only randomized controlled trial conducted recommends the following formulation and regimen: 35 μg of ethinyl estradiol and 1 mg of norethindrone 3 times a day for 1 week, and then daily for 3 weeks.[26] Most monophasic OCPs containing 30 to 35 μg of ethinyl estradiol and at least 1 mg of progestin (norethindrone or norethindrone acetate) are appropriate. Other OCP formulations, "tapers," and durations have been recommended and may be as effective or even more effective in temporizing bleeding, but there are insufficient data at this time. Although OCPs are generally well tolerated, it is important to consider contraindications to the estrogen in this treatment (**Box 2**).

Box 2
Contraindications to combination oral contraceptive pills

1. Previous thromboembolic event or stroke

2. History of estrogen-dependent tumor

3. Active liver disease

4. Pregnancy

5. Hypertriglyceridemia

6. Older than 35 years and smoke more than 15 cigarettes per day

7. Older than 40 years is not a contraindication, but many physicians favor progestin for this age group

8. High suspicion for malignancy (estrogen-responsive tumor)

Oral progestin

Oral progestin, such as medroxyprogesterone acetate (MPA) or norethindrone acetate (NA), is an effective therapy for HMB, and is a safe choice for patients who may have a contraindication to OCPs. As with OCPs, many different regimes have been described for oral progestin. For AUB, it is recommended that patients start at a high dose (MPA 20 mg, 3 to 6 times a day or NA, 5–15 mg daily until bleeding stops) for at least 1 to 7 days or until bleeding stops. The patient should then be transitioned to MPA, 20 to 40 mg daily, or NA, 5 to 10 mg daily, for 10 to 21 days.[26,27] In one randomized controlled trial, the median number of days for treatment of bleeding cessation for both progestin only and OCP groups was 3 days.[26] Though generally well tolerated, high-dose progestin is often associated with nausea and worsening premenstrual symptoms.

Progestin can be taken continuously or cyclically. Continuous progestin will suppress menstruation, although avoiding breakthrough bleeding with continuous suppression can be difficult. Depot formulations of progestin are associated with irregular bleeding. Cyclic progestin (10–20 mg/d days 1–14, 0 mg/d days 14–28) is used to achieve cyclic bleeding. Progestins mimic the luteal phase of menstruation, thus maintaining the uterine lining; the withdrawal of progestin causes the uterine lining to shed.

Antifibrinolytics

Tranexamic acid (TXA), an antifibrinolytic, is useful in a wide range of hemorrhagic conditions and was recently approved for use in HMB in the United States. Several studies have demonstrated that administration of TXA results in significant reduction in blood loss without increased risk for thromboembolic events.[28] TXA is an effective therapy for patients with chronic HMB,[29] and has been shown to reduce bleeding in these patients by 30% to 55%.[30,31] As with OCPs and progestin, recommended doses and duration are varied, but typically it is administered in a dose of 1.3 g 3 times a day for 3 to 5 days during menses.[32] Side effects including leg cramps and nausea are experienced by approximately one-third of patients.[33] TXA can be more expensive than other treatment options, limiting its use in common practice. TXA may also be considered when managing a severe acute episode of AUB if other temporizing measures have failed, although the risks of concomitant TXA and hormonal treatments such as high-dose IV estrogen are unclear.

Nonsteroidal anti-inflammatory medications

Nonsteroidal anti-inflammatory drugs (NSAIDs) are not only an effective analgesic but have also have been shown to decrease uterine blood loss by 20% to 50%.[30,34,35]

NSAIDs decrease prostaglandin production and thereby promote vasoconstriction in the uterus. This class of medication is most beneficial in chronic bleeding and has no proven benefit in acute bleeding. Although TXA has been shown to be significantly more effective than NSAIDs in reducing bleeding,[30] NSAIDs are a more economically accessible treatment option for most patients.

Special Considerations in Abnormal Uterine Bleeding Management

Ovulatory dysfunction
A key step in the diagnosis and management of AUB is determined by the menstrual history, that is, whether the bleeding is regular and predictable (sometimes referred to as ovulatory) or is irregular and unpredictable (sometimes referred to as anovulatory), and may be the result of ovulatory dysfunction. The distinction between ovulatory and anovulatory bleeding is important because the causes and treatments are different. Ovulatory bleeding is most commonly caused by a structural lesion (PALM), coagulopathy, or endometrial disorder. Anovulatory bleeding is often caused by malignancy or ovulatory dysfunction. In general, acute bleeding is more common in ovulatory disorders, but it can and does occur in anovulatory disorders.

Ovulatory dysfunction may result in endometrial hyperplasia caused by the effects of unopposed estrogen on the endometrium. Thus, it is important to determine which of these individuals are at increased risk for malignancy. Patients with one or more risk factors for malignancy should be referred urgently to gynecology for endometrial biopsy (**Box 3**). Oral progestin, *not* OCPs, must be used to control bleeding in patients with suspected or possible malignancy. Uterine malignancies are often hormone dependent, and combination OCPs containing estrogen are contraindicated.

Endometrial biopsy
Not all women with AUB require endometrial biopsy. Urgent gynecology referral should be considered for a select group of patients: women 45 years or older, history of chronic anovulation (history of 2 or more years of irregular and unpredictable bleeding), infertility, diabetes, obesity, family history of endometrial cancer, or history or prolonged exposure to unopposed estrogen (as seen in patients with obesity or PCOS) or tamoxifen.[36] Causes of chronic anovulation also include thyroid dysfunction, hyperprolactinemia, and certain medications that cause alterations in dopamine levels (antipsychotics and antiepileptics).

Box 3
Risks factors for endometrial cancer

Women younger than 35 years with 1 or more of the following:
1. 2 to 3 years of irregular bleeding (not cyclic)
2. Infertility
3. Nulliparity
4. Diabetes
5. Obesity
6. Family history of color or endometrial cancer
7. Tamoxifen use

Women older than 35 years with ovulatory abnormal uterine bleeding

Abnormal uterine bleeding unresponsive to medical management

Postmenopausal bleeding

Patients with ovarian dysfunction often have a systemic condition such as PCOS, disruption of the hypothalamic-pituitary-ovarian axis, hyperprolactinemia, or hypothyroidism.[37] Patients with suspected ovarian dysfunction should be referred to gynecology and/or endocrinology for further evaluation.

SUMMARY

AUB unrelated to pregnancy is a common and complex medical condition. AUB is often chronic but can also present as acute, life-threatening hemorrhage. The ED management of a nonpregnant patient presenting with AUB centers on determining the patient's hemodynamic stability and initiating measures to temporize a bleeding episode. It is critical that emergency physicians know the common causes (PALM-COIEN) and available medical and surgical therapies for this condition so that they may develop a structured and simplified diagnostic and management strategy. Most patients presenting to the ED with AUB can be safely discharged home with timely outpatient gynecologic follow-up.

REFERENCES

1. Kjerulff KH, Erickson BA, Langenberg PW. Chronic gynecological conditions reported by US women: findings from the National Health Interview Survey, 1984 to 1992. Am J Public Health 1996;86:195–9.
2. Frick KD, Clark MA, Steinwachs DM, et al. Financial and quality-of-life burden of dysfunctional uterine bleeding among women agreeing to obtain surgical treatment. Women's Health Issues 2009;19(1):70–8.
3. Fraser IS, Critchely HO, Munro MG, et al. A process defined to lead to international agreement on terminologies and definitions used to describe abnormalities of menstrual bleeding. Fertil Steril 2007;87(3):466–76.
4. Munro MG, Critchley HO, Fraser IS. The FIGO systems for nomenclature and classification of abnormal uterine bleeding in the reproductive years: who needs them? Am J Obstet Gynecol 2012;207(4):259–65.
5. Ely JW, Kennedy CM, Clark EC, et al. Abnormal uterine bleeding: a management algorithm. J Am Board Fam Med 2006;19(6):590–602.
6. Higham JM, Shaw RW. Clinical associations with objective menstrual blood volume. Eur J Obstet Gynecol Reprod Biol 1999;82(1):73–6.
7. Munro M. Abnormal uterine bleeding. New York: Cambridge University Press; 2010. p. 33–9, 43–46, 48–50.
8. Munro MG, Critchley HO, Broder MS, et al. The FIGO classification system ("PALM-COEIN") for causes of abnormal uterine bleeding in non-gravid women in the reproductive years, including guidelines for clinical investigation. Int J Gynaecol Obstet 2011;113(1):3–13.
9. Van Bogaert LJ. Clinicopathologic findings in endometrial polyps. Obstet Gynecol 1988;71(5):771–3.
10. Bergeron C, Amant F, Ferenczy A. Best pathology and physiopathology of adenomyosis. Best Pract Res Clin Obstet Gynaecol 2006;20(4):511–21.
11. Shankar M, Lee CA, Sabin CA, et al. Von Willebrand disease in women with menorrhagia: a systematic review. BJOB 2004;111(7):734–40.
12. Kadir RA, Economides DL, Sabin CA, et al. Frequency of inherited bleeding disorders in women with meonrrhagia: a systematic review. Lancet 1998;351:485–9.
13. Lusher JM. Screening and diagnosis of coagulation disorders. Am J Obstet Gynecol 1996;175(3 Pt 2):778–83.

14. Sheppard BL, Bonnar J. The effects of intrauterine contraceptive devices on the ultrastructure of the endometrium in relation to bleeding complications. Am J Obstet Gynecol 1983;146(7):829–39.
15. James AH, Kouides PA, Abdul-Kadir R, et al. Evaluation and management of acute menorrhagia in women with and without underlying bleeding disorders: consensus from an international expert panel. Eur J Obstet Gynecol Reprod Biol 2011;158(2):124–34.
16. Falcone T, Desjardins C, Bourque J, et al. Dysfunctional uterine bleeding in adolescents. J Reprod Med 1994;39(10):761–4.
17. DeVore GR, Owens O, Kase N. Use of intravenous Premarin in the treatment of dysfunctional uterine bleeding–a double-blind randomized control study. Obstet Gynecol 1982;59(3):285–91.
18. Goldrath MH. Uterine tamponade for the control of acute uterine bleeding. Am J Obstet Gynecol 1983;147(8):869–72.
19. Milad MP, Valle RF. Emergency endometrial ablation for life-threatening uterine bleeding as a result of a coagulopathy. J Am Assoc Gynecol Laparoscopists 1998;5(3):301–3.
20. Phelan JT 2nd, Broder J, Kouides PA. Near-fatal uterine hemorrhage during induction chemotherapy for acute myeloid leukemia: a case report of bilateral uterine artery embolization. Am J Hematol 2004;77(2):151–5.
21. Thakar R, Ayers S, Clarkson P, et al. Outcomes after total versus subtotal abdominal hysterectomy. N Engl J Med 2002;347(17):1318–25.
22. Georgiou C. Balloon tamponade in the management of postpartum haemorrhage: a review. BJOG 2009;116(6):748–57.
23. Pastor B. Topical acetone for control of life-threatening vaginal hemorrhage from recurrent gynecologic cancer. Eur J Gynaecol Oncol 1993;14(1):33–5.
24. Timmerman D, Van den Bosch T, Peeraer K, et al. Vascular malformations in the uterus: ultrasonographic diagnosis and conservative management. Eur J Obstet Gynecol Reprod Biol 2000;92(1):171–8.
25. Dueholm M, Lundorf E, Hansen ES, et al. Evaluation of the uterine cavity with magnetic resonance imaging, transvaginal sonography, hysterosonographic examination, and diagnostic hysteroscopy. Fertil Steril 2001;76(2):350–7.
26. Munro MG, Mainor N, Basu R, et al. Oral medroxyprogesterone acetate and combination oral contraceptives for acute uterine bleeding: a randomized controlled trial. Obstet Gynecol 2006;108(4):924–9.
27. Aksu F, Madazli R, Budak E, et al. High-dose medroxyprogesterone acetate for the treatment of dysfunctional uterine bleeding in 24 adolescents. Aust N Z J Obstet Gynaecol 1997;37(2):228–31.
28. Cooke I, Lethaby A, Farquhar C. Antifibrinolytics for heavy menstrual bleeding. Cochrane Database Syst Rev 2000;(2):CD000249.
29. American College of Obstetricians and Gynecologists. ACOG committee opinion no 557: management of acute abnormal uterine bleeding in nonpregnant reproductive-aged women. Obstet Gynecol 2013;121:891–6.
30. Lethaby A, Farquhar C, Cooke I. Antifibrinolytics for heavy menstrual bleeding. Cochrane Database Syst Rev 2000;(4):CD000249.
31. Lukes AS, Moore KA, Muse KN, et al. Tranexamic acid treatment for heavy menstrual bleeding: a randomized controlled trial. Obstet Gynecol 2010;116:865–75.
32. Wellington K, Wagstaff AJ. Tranexamic acid: a review of its use in the management of menorrhagia. Drugs 2003;63(13):1417–33.
33. Guidelines for the management of abnormal uterine bleeding. SOGC clinical practice guidelines. J Obstet Gynaecol Can 2001;23(8):704–9.

34. Lethaby A, Augood C, Duckitt K. Nonsteroidal anti-inflammatory drugs for heavy menstrual bleeding. Cochrane Database Syst Rev 2007;(4):CD000400.
35. Edland M, Andersson K, Rybo G, et al. Reduction of menstrual blood loss in women suffering from idiopathic menorrhagia with a novel antifibrinolytic (Kubi 2161). Br J Obstet Gynecol 1995;102:913–7.
36. Farquhar CM, Lethaby A, Sowter M, et al. An evaluation of risk factors for endometrial hyperplasia in premenopausal women with abnormal menstrual bleeding. Am J Obstet Gynecol 1999;181(3):525–9.
37. Krassas GE, Pontikides N, Kaltsas T, et al. Disturbances of menstruation in hypothyroidism. Clin Endocrinol (Oxf) 1999;50(5):655–9.

Sexually Transmitted Diseases in the Emergency Department

Camiron L. Pfennig, MD, MHPE

KEYWORDS

- Sexually transmitted disease • STD • Expedited partner therapy • Gonorrhea
- Chlamydia

KEY POINTS

- Sexually transmitted diseases (STDs) are common, and rates are increasing.
- Emergency physicians should feel comfortable initiating presumptive treatment for STDs based on clinical diagnosis alone.
- Gonorrhea is becoming increasingly resistant to cephalosporin monotherapy; dual therapy with ceftriaxone and azithromycin is now recommended.
- Expedited partner therapy should be considered for gonorrhea, chlamydia, and trichomoniasis and is permitted in most states.

INTRODUCTION

Sexually transmitted diseases (STDs) are common diseases caused by viruses, bacteria, and parasites transmitted primarily during sexual contact with an infected individual vaginally, anally, or orally. However, STDs can also be passed by sharing needles or vertically during delivery and breastfeeding. STDs continue to be underrecognized by the public and by health care professionals and can lead to devastating health consequences including infertility and facilitation of human immunodeficiency virus transmission.[1] In addition to the health impact, the high prevalence and increasing rates of STDs continue to be an economic drain on the health care system. Data suggest that there are an estimated 20 million new STDs being diagnosed in the United States each year leading to a direct cost of treating STDs of $16 billion annually.[2]

Symptoms of STDs can be nonspecific making clinical gestalt and diagnostic testing very helpful. However, because of the large numbers of STDs and the variety of testing available, choosing the appropriate diagnostic test can be difficult. Clinicians must consider the patient's signs and symptoms and infection prevalence as

Prisma Health, University of South Carolina School of Medicine Greenville, 701 Grove Road, Greenville, SC 29605, USA
E-mail address: cpfennig@ghs.org

Emerg Med Clin N Am 37 (2019) 165–192
https://doi.org/10.1016/j.emc.2019.01.001
0733-8627/19/© 2019 Elsevier Inc. All rights reserved.

emed.theclinics.com

well as the cost and availability of the tests. In both men and women, the history and physical examination conducted in privacy with the assistance of a chaperone will direct the indicated diagnostic testing and care plan. The Center for Disease Control and Prevention (CDC) has a publication to assist with sexual history-taking skills available at www.cdc.gov/std/treatment/SexualHistory.pdf focusing on the 5 "P"s of sexual health: partners, practices, protection from STDs, past history of STDs, and prevention of pregnancy.[3]

STDs have different manifestations that can be both systemic and localized; thus a complete physical examination is often indicated (**Table 1**). The evaluation begins with a review of the vital signs because tachycardia, hypotension, and fever should raise concern for possible pelvic inflammatory disease (PID) and/or sepsis. Despite the controversy regarding the utility of the pelvic examination in patients with vaginal bleeding or abdominal pain, the pelvic examination continues to play a vital role in the diagnosis of many STDs.[4]

Emergency physicians (EPs) are often faced with the challenges of initiating treatment for STDs based on clinical gestalt because many of the diagnostic tests have delayed turnaround times. Fortunately, there is ongoing development in point-of-care STD diagnostics with promise for the future.[5] In the interim, EPs often must initiate empirical treatment for STDs based on history, physical, and clinical suspicion (**Table 2**). In addition, chlamydia, gonorrhea, and syphilis are among the many infectious diseases that require mandatory reporting.[6] The requirements for reporting other STDs differ by state, so clinicians should be familiar with their specific reporting requirements.

Finally, EPs must also understand expedited partner therapy (EPT), the practice of treating the sex partners of persons who have received an STD diagnosis by providing prescriptions to the patient without clinical assessment of the partners.[7] The CDC maintains a Website (www.cdc.gov/std/EPT/legal/default.htm) with information about the legal status of EPT in all 50 states. Unless prohibited by law, EPs should consider routinely offering EPT to patients with chlamydia, gonorrhea, or trichomoniasis infection because the benefits of EPT in preventing STD reinfection outweigh the risks of possible adverse effects of antibiotics and the development of antibiotic resistance.[8]

This review focuses primarily on the cause, history, physical examination, diagnostic studies, and treatment strategies for bacterial vaginosis (BV), chlamydia, genital herpes, gonorrhea, human papillomavirus (HPV), granuloma inguinale, lymphogranuloma Venereum, *Mycoplasma genitalium*, syphilis, and trichomoniasis.

BACTERIAL VAGINOSIS

BV is the only disease discussed in this review that is not always an STD in that the role of sexual activity in the pathogenesis of BV is unclear. BV occurs when there is a decrease or absence of lactobacilli that help maintain the vagina's acidic pH leading to the overgrowth of anaerobic bacteria including most commonly Gardnerella vaginalis. Even though more than 50% of women with BV are asymptomatic, women presenting to the emergency department (ED) with BV most likely will present with a thin, gray/white homogeneous, vaginal discharge often described with a "fishy smell" with occasional dysuria or dypareunia.[9]

The diagnosis of BV is based on a physical examination and laboratory testing. A specimen from the vaginal wall and posterior fornix should be obtained during a speculum examination. Most EDs use a combination of laboratory-based and clinical bedside testing in the diagnosis of BV. The most widely accepted clinical criteria are Amsel criteria. If microscopy is available, the diagnosis requires that 3 of the

Table 1
Physical examination findings

	Bacterial Vaginosis	Chlamydia	Genital Herpes	Gonorrhea	Granuloma Inguinale	HPV	LGV	Mycoplasma Genitalium	Syphilis	Tricho-moniasis
Eyes		Chlamydial conjunctivitis —red eye with mucopurulent discharge Chlamydial keratitis —peripheral cornea may start to get infiltrates	Herpetic keratitis— dull ache or sharp pain in the eye, conjunctival injection; dendritic corneal ulcer	Gonococcal conjunctivitis —red eye with conjunctival discharge (whitish green); edematous and tender eyelids Gonococcal keratitis— starts at the peripheral cornea causing marginal ulcerations					Iridocyclitis, Scleritis and Keratitis (secondary) Argyll Robertson pupil (tertiary) Corneal opacities (Untreated congenital neuro-syphilis)	

(continued on next page)

Table 1 (*continued*)

	Bacterial Vaginosis	Chlamydia	Genital Herpes	Gonorrhea	Granuloma Inguinale	HPV	LGV	Mycoplasma Genitalium	Syphilis	Trichomoniasis
Ears									Sensorineural hearing loss (secondary) Deafness- Cranial nerve VIII involvement (Untreated congenital neuro-syphilis)	
Nose			Painful sores in nose						Saddle nose deformity (Untreated congenital neuro-syphilis)	

| Mouth/throat | Sore throat but typically no examination findings | Painful fluid-filled blisters on lips, gums, tongue, roof of mouth | Erythema, white spots or whitish/yellow discharge | Lesions on lips and oral mucosa | Warts in the throat; vocal changes | Chancres on lips, tongue, gums, throat. Sores- small red patches that grow into larger, open sores that can be red, yellow, or gray (Primary) Superficial mucosal erosions, usually painless, on palate, |

(continued on next page)

Table 1 (*continued*)

	Bacterial Vaginosis	Chlamydia	Genital Herpes	Gonorrhea	Granuloma Inguinale	HPV	LGV	Myco plasma Genitalium	Syphilis	Tricho-moniasis
									pharynx, larynx (secondary) Gummas in mouth (tertiary) Hutchinson incisors and perioral fissures (Untreated congenital neuro-syphilis)	
Lymph			Generalized lympha-denopathy	Cervical and inguinal	Lympha-denopathy from secondary bacterial infection	Cervical and inguinal	Localized inguinal adenopathy or buboes "Groove sign"		Regional lympha-denopathy (unilateral or bilateral) (primary) Generalized non-tender lympha-denopathy (secondary)	

System				
Cardiac	Gonococcal endocarditis—murmur, tachycardia			Diastolic murmur of aortic insufficiency (tertiary)
Pulmonary	Wheezing and crackles (newborn chlamydial pneumonia)			Diminished breath sounds from effusion (pulmonary syphilis-secondary)
Abdomen	Lower abdominal tenderness	Lower abdominal tenderness	Lesions on abdomen	Epigastric abdominal pain (gastric syphilis-tertiary) / Lower abdominal tenderness
Musculo-skeletal	Polyarthralgias with joint tenderness, decreased range of motion, and erythema		Lesions on arms, legs	Arthralgias, periostitis (secondary) Gummas on the leg just below the knee

(continued on next page)

Table 1 (continued)

	Bacterial Vaginosis	Chlamydia	Genital Herpes	Gonorrhea	Granuloma Inguinale	HPV	LGV	Mycoplasma Genitalium	Syphilis	Tricho-moniasis
Neurologic			AMS, dysphasia, ataxia, seizures, hemiparesis, cranial nerve defects, visual field loss, papilledema (herpes encephalitis)	Meningismus or decreased level of consciousness (gonococcal meningitis)					Lack of coordination (tertiary) Paralysis (tertiary) Numbness in toes, feet, legs (tertiary) Tabes dorsalis-ataxia and loss of pain sensation, proprioception, and deep tendon reflexes in joints (tertiary)	
Skin			Small red bumps, blisters (vesicles) or open sores	Maculopapular, pustular, necrotic, or vesicular rash at torso, limbs, palms,		Warts			Localized or diffuse muco-cutaneous rash marked	

			(ulcers) in the genital and anal areas					and soles (rash usually spares the face, scalp, and mouth) Hemorrhagic lesions, erythema nodosum, urticaria, erythema multiforme	by red or reddish-brown, penny-sized sores; palms and soles (secondary) Patchy hair loss (secondary) Coalescent granulomatous lesions (gummas) (tertiary)	
Psych									Personality changes (tertiary) Depression (tertiary) Psychosis (tertiary)	
Female pelvic	Thin, gray/white homogeneous, vaginal discharge with "fishy" smell	Cervical motion tenderness Cervical friability Adnexal fullness or tenderness Thin and mucoid urethral discharge	Small red bumps, blisters (vesicles), or open sores (ulcers)	Mucopurulent or purulent vaginal, urethral, or cervical discharge Vaginal bleeding Cervical friability Cervical	Elephantiasis-like swelling of the external genitalia Lesions on labia minora, mons veneris, fourchette,	Small, flesh-colored or gray warts on vulva, vagina, and cervix	Small, painless papule, pustule, nodule, or ulcer on posterior fourchette, vulva, or cervix	Urethritis Mucopurulent vaginal discharge	Small, painless sore (chancre) of cervix or labia (primary) Condylomata lata (secondary) Superficial	Thin, frothy yellowish-white discharge Strawberry cervix

(continued on next page)

Table 1 (continued)

	Bacterial Vaginosis	Chlamydia	Genital Herpes	Gonorrhea	Granuloma Inguinale	HPV	LGV	Mycoplasma Genitalium	Syphilis	Trichomoniasis
				motion tenderness Fullness and tenderness of adnexa	and/or cervix				mucosal erosions of vulva (secondary)	
Male genitals		Thin and mucoid urethral discharge Scrotal pain, tenderness, or swelling Perineal fullness (prostatitis)	Small red bumps, blisters (vesicles), or open sores (ulcers)	Mucopurulent or purulent urethral discharge Unilateral epididymal tenderness and edema	Large, painless, suppurative ulcers	Cauliflower-like growths on the penis and scrotum	Small, painless papule, pustule, nodule, or ulcer on coronal sulcus	Urethritis Watery penile discharge	Small, painless sore (chancre) Reddish-brown papular lesions on penis that coalesce into large elevated plaques (condylomata lata) (secondary) Superficial mucosal erosions of glans	Scant, thin penile discharge Balanoposthitis, epididymitis, and prostatitis

							penis (secondary)
Anus/ rectum	Mucopurulent rectal discharge	Small red bumps, blisters (vesicles), or open sores (ulcers)	Mucopurulent or purulent discharge with or without rectal bleeding Mucopurulent exudate and inflammation in the rectal mucosa	Anal ulcers	Warts found on the perianal skin or within the anal canal and lower rectum	Anorectal pain, bleeding, purulent discharge, proctitis	Anorectal chancre (primary) Condylo- mata lata (secondary) Superficial mucosal erosions of anus and rectum (secondary)

Table 2
Recommended treatments for STDs

STD	Primary Treatment for Nonpregnant Women and Men	Secondary Alternatives	Pregnant Women
Bacterial vaginosis	Metronidazole (500 mg PO bid × 7d) Metronidazole gel 0.75% (one app intravaginal daily × 5 d)	Clindamycin cream 2% (one app intravaginal QHS × 7 d) Oral clindamycin (500 mg PO bid × 7 d)	Same primary treatment and secondary alternatives
Chlamydia	Azithromycin (1 g PO × 1 dose) Doxycycline (100 mg PO bid × 7d)	Levofloxacin (500 mg PO × 7 d) Ofloxacin (300 mg bid × 7 d)	Azithromycin (1 g PO × 1 dose) Amoxicillin (500 mg tid × 7 d)
Genital Herpes	Acyclovir (400 mg PO tid × 7–10d) Acyclovir (200 mg PO 5x daily × 7–10 d) Valacyclovir (1 g PO bid × 7–10d) Famciclovir (250 mg PO tid × 7–10d)		Acyclovir (400 mg tid × 7–10d) Valacyclovir (1 g PO bid × 7–10d)
Gonorrhea	Ceftriaxone (250 mg IM/IV × 1 dose) + Azithromycin (1 g PO × 1 dose)	Cefixime (400 mg PO × 1 dose) + Azithromycin (1 g PO × 1 dose) Gemifloxacin (320 mg PO × 1 dose) + Azithromycin (2 g PO × 1 dose) Gentamicin (240 mg IM × 1 dose) + Azithromycin (2 g PO × 1 dose) Ceftriaxone (250 mg IM/IV) + Doxycycline (100 mg PO bid × 7 d)	Same primary treatment
Granuloma inguinale	Azithromycin (1 g PO once per wk)[a] Azithromycin (500 mg PO once daily for at least 3 wk)[a]	Doxycycline (100 mg PO bid for at least 3 wk)[a] Ciprofloxacin (750 mg PO bid for at least 3 wk)[a] Erythromycin base (500 mg PO 4x daily for at least 3 wk)[a]	Azithromycin (1 g PO once per wk) or Azithromycin (500 mg PO once daily for at least 3 wk)[a] Erythromycin base (500 mg PO 4x daily for at least 3 wk)[a]
Human papillomavirus	Cryotherapy Immune-based therapy surgical excision		
Lymphogranuloma venereum	Doxycycline (100 mg BID x21 d)	Azithromycin (1 g PO once weekly × 3 wk) Moxifloxacin (400 mg daily × 10 d)[64]	Erythromycin base 500 mg PO 4x daily × 21 d Azithromycin (1 g PO once weekly × 3 wk)

Mycoplasma genitalium	Azithromycin (500 mg PO × 1) + Azithromycin (250 mg PO once daily × 4 d)	Moxifloxacin (400 mg PO once daily × 7 d)	Azithromycin (500 mg PO × 1) + Azithromycin (250 mg PO once daily × 4 d)
Syphilis	Penicillin G benzathine (2.4 million units IM × 1 dose)		Same primary treatment
Neurosyphilis	Aqueous crystalline penicillin G (18–24 million units daily administered as 3–4 million units q 4 h or continuous infusion × 10–14 d) Procaine penicillin G (2.4 million units IM daily × 10–14 d) + Probenecid (500 mg PO qid × 10–14 d)	Ideally, penicillin desensitization Doxycycline (200 mg bid × 28 d) Ceftriaxone[ii] (250 mg IM/IV for 10–14 d)	Same primary treatment
Trichomoniasis	Metronidazole (2 g PO × 1 dose or 500 mg PO bid for 7 d) Tinidazole (2g PO × 1 dose)		Same primary treatment

Abbreviations: bid, 2 times per day; d, days; IM, intramuscular; IV, intravenous; PO, by mouth; qid, 4 times per day; tid, 3 times per day.

[a] Until all lesions have completely healed.

Data from Kang-Birken SK, Castel U, Prichard JG. Oral doxycycline for treatment of neurosyphilis in two patients infected with human immunodeficiency virus. Pharmacotherapy 2010;30(4):418 (Case Series; 2 patients); and Liang Z, Chen YP, Yang CS, et al. Meta-analysis of ceftriaxone compared with penicillin for the treatment of syphilis. Int J Antimicrob Agents 2016;47(1):6–11 (Meta-analysis).

following 4 Amsel criteria be met: a vaginal pH of greater than 4.5; the presence of clue cells; a milky, homogeneous vaginal discharge; and the release of a fishy odor before or after addition of 10% potassium hydroxide to the vaginal fluid.[10] The use of Amsel criteria for the diagnosis of BV is 90% sensitive and 77% specific.[11] However, Gram stain of a vaginal smear remains the gold standard for diagnosis of BV, but is primarily used in research studies and not in clinical practice. Ideally, the physician or the hospital laboratory would identify clue cells on saline wet mount, but if microscopy is not readily available, clinicians can make the diagnosis based on clinical examination of the characteristic vaginal discharge alone.

Treatment for BV is indicated in women for both symptomatic relief and reduction in the acquisition of STDs. In patients without documented allergy, metronidazole, 500 mg, twice daily for 7 days should be the first-line oral treatment.[12] Treatment with a single 2 g dose of metronidazole is no longer recommended.[3] In compliant patients preferring a vaginal gel, metronidazole gel has similar efficacy to 7 days of oral metronidazole and has been associated with less gastrointestinal complaints.[13] In patients who cannot tolerate one of the forms of metronidazole, clindamycin cream or oral clindamycin are the next best options. Even though BV-associated bacteria can be found in the male genitalia, treatment of male partners is not currently recommended, because there is no known benefit in the prevention of recurrence of BV.[14] In addition, data from clinical trials indicate that a woman's response to therapy for BV and the likelihood of relapse or recurrence are not affected by treatment of her sex partner. Therefore, routine treatment of sexual partners (male or female) is not recommended.[14]

CHLAMYDIA

Chlamydia is the most common bacterial STD and the most commonly reported disease with more than 1.5 million infections reported to the CDC in 2016. Most patients infected with chlamydia are asymptomatic, leading to increasing rates of infection especially in young women.[15] Most commonly, symptomatic women will present with cervicitis and men with urethritis. In symptomatic women with chlamydia, the most common examination finding is vaginal discharge followed by cervical ectopy or easily induced bleeding.[16] However, women with chlamydia can also present with urinary frequency, dysuria, or PID. Men can also present with epididymitis, prostatitis, and proctitis. In fact, acute unilateral epididymitis is most commonly due to a chlamydial infection especially in patients younger than 35 years. Finally, both men and women can also have chlamydial conjunctivitis and pharyngitis.

In women, nucleic acid amplification testing (NAAT) of vaginal swabs is the test of choice because this specimen provides the highest sensitivity.[17] Other secondary options include a first-catch urine or endocervical swab. The sensitivity of testing on urine (92%) in women seems to be slightly lower compared with vaginal samples (97%).[18] Despite the sensitivity and specificity equivalence of provider and self-collected vaginal swabs, EPs should strongly consider performing a speculum examination and bimanual examination in symptomatic women to aid in the diagnosis of PID and to rule out cervicovaginal lesions.[19] The test of choice for chlamydial infections in men is NAAT of first-catch urine with urethral swab as a secondary option.[20] NAAT can also be performed on conjunctival, rectal, and oropharyngeal swabs. However, it is important to check with hospital laboratories to assure the NAAT testing of rectal specimens has been approved under the Clinical Laboratory Improvement Amendment because NAATs are not Food and Drug Administration (FDA)-cleared for these specimens.[21]

Treatment for chlamydia is essential to prevent complicated sequelae, decrease the transmission to others, and achieve symptom resolution. Currently, azithromycin, 1 g, single-dose oral or doxycycline, 100 mg, orally twice daily for 7 days are first-line recommendations for nonpregnant patients with urogenital or oropharyngeal chlamydia.[22] Despite azithromycin and doxycycline demonstrating equal efficacy, the azithromycin option may be best in the ED patient in order to improve patient adherence. Single-dose azithromycin is also safe and effective in pregnant women with chlamydia. Fluoroquinolones including levofloxacin and ofloxacin should be reserved as a less-desirable alternative because they are often more expensive, require longer treatment regimens, and cannot be safely administered in adolescents or pregnant patients. EPT for chlamydia can be accomplished with single-dose azithromycin oral therapy or doxycycline.[23] In addition, EPs should also consider concurrent treatment for gonococcal infection due to the increasing prevalence of gonorrhea coinfection.[24]

GONORRHEA

Gonorrhea, the second most commonly reported communicable disease affecting about 0.8% of women and 0.6% of men, is caused by the diplococci bacterium Neisseria gonorrhoeae. There continues to be an increase in the rate of gonorrhea among persons in every age group since 2014, with 468,514 cases of gonorrhea reported in the United States in 2016. However, it is very likely that the number of cases is much greater secondary to underreporting and asymptomatic infections.

Similar to other STDs, gonorrhea infection can also be asymptomatic. In the ED, symptomatic women with gonorrhea most commonly present with signs and symptoms consistent with cervicitis, including vaginal pruritus, mucopurulent discharge, and friable cervical mucosa. However, women can also present with dysuria, urinary frequency, pelvic pain, or vaginal bleeding. Symptomatic urogenital gonococcal infections in men often present with urethritis including combination of mucopurulent discharge at urethral meatus and dysuria.[25] Other complications of gonorrhea include epididymitis, proctitis, pharyngitis, and conjunctivitis. Unfortunately, gonorrhea can also lead to disseminated infections causing purulent arthritis, tenosynovitis, dermatitis, polyarthralgias, and even more severe complications including endocarditis, meningitis, and osteomyelitis.

Growing antibiotic resistance to gonorrhea has forced changes in antibiotic recommendations over the past 10 years. Before the rising rates of antibiotic resistance to gonorrhea, ceftriaxone had been recommended first-line monotherapy treatment for gonorrhea, although concurrent treatment with azithromycin was encouraged given the high rates of chlamydia coinfection. Currently, combination therapy with ceftriaxone and azithromycin is recommended even if NAAT for *Chlamydia trachomatis* is known to be negative at the time of treatment. Dual therapy using 2 antimicrobials with different mechanisms of action is thought to improve treatment efficacy and potentially slow the spread of resistance of gonorrhea to cephalosporins. Patients should receive 250 mg intramuscular (IM) or intravenous (IV) ceftriaxone. This is increased from earlier recommendations of 125 mg secondary to the decreasing susceptibility to cephalosporins and ceftriaxone treatment failures. IV and IM routes have similar pharmacokinetic profiles with the plasma concentrations nearly identical after 24 hours; if the patient already has an IV in place there is no indication to use the IM route.[26] In addition to ceftriaxone, patients should also receive azithromycin, 1 g, in single oral dose. In patients with a cephalosporin allergy, oral gemifloxacin plus oral azithromycin or dual treatment with single doses of intramuscular gentamicin plus oral azithromycin can be prescribed.[27] In patients with an allergy or intolerance to azithromycin, doxycycline can be used if necessary. However, gonorrhea resistance to doxycycline is increasing, so azithromycin should be used whenever possible.[28] EPT for gonorrhea can be accomplished with the oral combination of single-dose cefixime and single-dose azithromycin.

GENITAL HERPES

Genital herpes is an STD caused by either herpes simplex virus type 1 (HSV-1) or herpes simplex virus type 2 (HSV-2) transmitted through an infected person with herpes lesions on mucosal surfaces, genital secretions, or oral secretions. Accurate statistics are difficult to obtain for genital herpes because it is not a reportable disease. However, it is thought that at least 1 out of every 6 people in the United States aged between 14 and 49 years have genital herpes.[29] Patients usually contract oral herpes from HSV-1 due to nonsexual contact with saliva. However, HSV-1 can then spread through oral sex leading to genital herpes. In fact, HSV-1 is increasingly associated with genital infection and has been reported to cause more genital infections than HSV-2, especially in young people and homosexual men.[30] HSV-2 is spread during sexual contact with an infected person.

HSV can cause either primary or reactivation infections, often with primary infections leading to systemic signs, longer duration of symptoms, and higher rates of complications. Primary genital herpes often involves systemic symptoms including fever and headache combined with localized symptoms including pain, itching, dysuria, and lymphadenopathy. During the primary HSV presentation, women may have herpetic vesicles on the external genitalia, labia, introitus, and anus. The EP will often see the patient after the vesicles rupture, leaving the patient with tender ulcers. In addition, patients may have inflamed vaginal mucosa, cervicitis, and dysuria leading to urinary retention. Men present with herpetic vesicles located in the glans penis, the penile shaft, the scrotum, the perianal area, and the rectum combined with dysuria and penile discharge (**Fig. 1**).

Recurrent genital herpes rarely involves constitutional symptoms, but often has a prodrome of pain, itching, and burning at the site of eruption in both men and women. Over time, recurrences generally become less frequent and less severe. Studies do show that there is a direct correlation between increased stress levels caused by stigmatization and pain from the virus and number and severity of HSV outbreaks leading to a vicious cycle.[31] Unfortunately, transmission can occur from contact with infected partners who do not have ulcers or vesicles and may not even know that they have HSV and are experiencing asymptomatic viral shedding.[32]

A clinical diagnosis may be the only immediate way to diagnose genital herpes, but follow-up laboratory testing should be obtained. Viral culture of vesicular fluid from an unroofed vesicle continues to be mainstream in many hospitals. However, NAAT are the preferred tests for detecting HSV in patients with active genital ulcers, because these tests detect HSV DNA and are both more sensitive and more rapid than viral culture.[3] Ideally, this sample would be taken from the base of the genital lesion. Unfortunately, viral shedding is intermittent, so failure to detect HSV does not always indicate the absence of HSV. Patients may be referred to their primary care physician for further evaluation and possible further serologic testing.

Genital herpes is a life-long viral infection with no cure currently available. However, antiviral medications including acyclovir, valacyclovir, and famciclovir can help prevent, shorten, and decrease the likelihood of transmission to partners. All patients with their first diagnosis of genital herpes should be treated ideally within 72 hours of

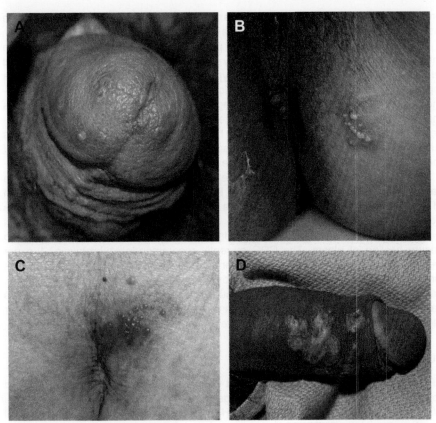

Fig. 1. Genital herpes. (*A–C*) Intact grouped vesicles and/or vesiculopustules with an erythematous base on the penis (*A*), medial buttock (*B*), and above the gluteal cleft (*C*). The buttocks represent a common location in women. (*D*) Healing ulcerations with scalloped borders on the penis. (*From* Bolognia JL, editor. Dermatology, 4th edition. Philadelphia: Elsevier; 2018; with permission.)

lesion appearance with either acyclovir, 400 mg, orally 3 times a day for 7 to 10 days; acyclovir, 200 mg, orally 5 times a day for 7 to 10 days; valacyclovir, 1 g, orally twice a day for 7 to 10 days; or famiciclovir, 250 mg, orally 3 times a day for 7 to 10 days.[33] The EP must consider the ease of administration and the cost when deciding which agent is best for the patient. Famciclovir and valacyclovir have equal efficacy when compared with acyclovir but require less frequent dosing.[3] Patients may also benefit from analgesics, sitz baths, or urinary catheter placement for severe dysuria.

Patients can present to ED with recurrent genital herpes infections or with questions about suppressive therapy to reduce the frequency of recurrences. Acyclovir, famciclovir, and valacyclovir seem equally effective for episodic treatment of genital herpes.[34] Counseling for the patient with HSV and sexual partners is critical to decrease the rate of transmission.

GRANULOMA INGUINALE

Granuloma inguinale, also called donovanosis, is caused by *Klebsiella granulomatis* endemic in India, the Caribbean, central Australia, and southern Africa.[35] For EPs practicing in the United States, it is important to obtain a careful travel and immigration history in any patients in whom granuloma inguinale is on the differential.

Patients with granuloma inguinale often present with vascular ulcerative lesions on the genitals or perineum that are generally painless and bleed easily without regional lymphadenopathy. However, there are 4 types of lesions that can occur in granuloma inguinale. Painless, suppurative ulcers typically found in skins folds are the most common. Patient may also develop a nodular inguinale lesion that is soft and erythematous that eventually ulcerates. Even though patients with granuloma inguinale typically present with genital ulcers, patients can also have oral, anal, and extragenital infections with dissemination to intraabdominal organs or bones. Elephantiasis-like swelling of the external genitalia can also occur in the later stages of granuloma inguinale.

Limited options for diagnostic testing exist for granuloma inguinale because the causative bacteria are difficult to culture. Formal diagnosis is made by visualization of Donovan bodies on microscopy from a sample obtained from the surface debris from purulent ulcers.

Multiple options for treatment are available, but all require prolonged therapy to ensure healing of ulcers. The CDC currently recommends azithromycin, 1 g per week or 500 mg daily for at least 3 weeks or until all lesions have healed. Other options include doxycycline, ciprofloxacin, erythromycin, or trimethoprim-sulfamethoxazole. Each of these treatments must be continued for at least 3 weeks or until all ulcers have healed. Close follow-up is important, because this disease can recur after several months, even in patients who were apparently fully treated.

HUMAN PAPILLOMAVIRUS

HPV is a double-stranded DNA virus that occurs at the basal cell layer of stratified squamous epithelial cells leading to changes ranging from hyperplasia to carcinoma. With more than 170 different types of HPV, most sexually active individuals will develop at least one HPV infection in their lifetime.[1] Fortunately, most infections are asymptomatic or subclinical with transient clearing within 2 years in immunocompetent persons. However, the oncogenic strains (such as HPV types 16 and 18) can lead to cervical, penile, vulvar, vaginal, anal, and oropharyngeal cancers.

On physical examination, patients may have condylomata acuminata, exophytic cauliflower-like lesions, or white plaquelike growths often referred to as genital or anal warts, on visual inspection on the external genitalia, perineum, or perianal skin. HPV does not cause discharge or dysuria, so evaluation of these symptoms should focus on other potential causes. HPV is also associated with carcinoma of the penis and is responsible for more than 95% of the cervical cancers in women.[36]

There is limited role for diagnostic testing for HPV in the ED. Genital warts are typically diagnosed by visual inspection, although biopsy may also be performed to confirm the diagnosis. Tests for oncogenic strains of HPV are typically performed in the context of cervical cancer screening. These tests are best obtained in the outpatient setting.

A variety of treatments are available for anogenital warts and cancerous and precancerous lesions, including cryotherapy, immune-based therapy, and surgical excision, with surgical excision having the highest success rate and lowest recurrence rate.[37] In addition, routine vaccination is recommended for both girls and boys at age 11 or 12 years but can occur in women through age 26 years or men through age 21 years if they were not previously vaccinated.[38] Even though administration of these treatments and vaccines is outside the ED scope, patients should be referred for follow-up and treatment. The benefit of notification and treatment of partners is less clear because of difficulties in diagnosis and treatment of HPV, but patients should be encouraged to tell their partners about the possible exposure.

LYMPHOGRANULOMA VENEREUM

Lymphogranuloma venereum (LGV), an infection of lymphatics and lymph nodes caused by serovars L1, L2, and L3 of *C trachomatis*, is found most frequently in tropical areas including Central and South America.[39] However, in the last 10 years outbreaks have appeared in North America, Europe, and Australia in the form of proctitis among men who have sex with men.[40] In the United States, the true incidence is unknown because national reporting of LGV ended in 1995.

Typically, LGV presents with painful inguinal lymphadenopathy, although patients may present with other symptoms. The primary stage is characterized by a small, painless papule, pustule, nodule, or ulcer that appears on the coronal sulcus of the man and on the posterior fourchette, vulva, or cervix of women. The initial lesions may be differentiated from herpetic lesions by the lack of pain, but differentiation from the chancre in syphilis requires serologic testing. The primary stage is usually self-limiting and patients often progress to the secondary stage, which is characterized often by unilateral lymphadenopathy. These fluctuant and suppurative lymph nodes, referred to as buboes, may either rupture or develop into hard, nonsuppurative masses. The Groove sign, a pathognomonic finding of LGV, occurs in 15% to 20% of cases when the inguinal and femoral lymph nodes are both involved and separated by the inguinal ligament.[41] In the ED, this diagnosis should be considered in any individual who presents with tender inguinal lymphadenopathy or proctitis.

Diagnosis of LGV in the ED is based on high clinical suspicion, but there are diagnostic tests available. NAAT should be performed on a specimen obtained from the primary ulcer base exudate of the anogenital lesion, the rectal mucosa, or from an aspirate from the fluctuant lymph nodes or buboes.[42] EPs are unlikely to have access to these results at the time of evaluation, so they must have a high clinical suspicion for this disease. The CDC currently recommends doxycycline, 100 mg, twice daily for 21 days, with erythromycin or azithromycin being reserved for patients who are unable to take doxycycline, including pregnant and lactating women.

Mycoplasma Genitalium

M genitalium, a slow-growing bacterium first identified in the 1980s causing urethritis in men and cervicitis and PID in women, is rapid increasingly as a cause of several STDs and is now responsible for more STDs than *Neisseria gonorrhoeae*.[43] *M genitalium* may also play a role in pathogenesis as an independent sexually transmitted pathogen or by facilitating coinfection with another pathogen. In addition, *M genitalium* has the potential to lead to an ascending infection and affect fertility.[44] Currently, there is no diagnostic test for *M genitalium* approved by the FDA for the United States. However, EPs should consider *M genitalium* in patients presenting with persistent or recurrent urethritis, cervicitis, or PID.

Treatment for suspected *M genitalium* can be difficult because this bacterium lacks a cell wall, leading to ineffectiveness of penicillin and cephalosporin agents. Patients with urethritis from suspected *M genitalium* can first be treated with an initial 500 mg dose of azithromycin followed by 250 mg daily for 4 days because this regimen has been shown to be more effective than doxycycline or 1 gm single-dose azithromycin.[45,46] However, as azithromycin resistance increases, moxifloxacin (400 mg once daily for 7 days) is emerging as the next recommended antibiotic.[47]

SYPHILIS

Syphilis is caused by the spirochete bacteria *Treponema pallidum*, and it is often referred to as "the great imitator" due to its wide variety of presentations at different stages of the disease. Nearly 24,000 cases of primary syphilis were reported in the United States in 2015 indicating a concerning 19% increase from 2014.[48] Most cases of syphilis are transmitted by sexual contact either vaginally, anogenitally, or orogenitally via microscopic abrasions of skin and mucous membranes. Rarely, syphilis is spread congenitally or from blood transfusions. The sexual transmission of syphilis occurs when there is exposure to open lesions with *T pallidum* organisms during the primary and secondary stages of infection when the primary chancre, secondary mucous patches, or condyloma lata are present. Following transmission, *T pallidum* disseminates to the lymphatics and blood stream to gain access to any organ of the body.[49]

Primary syphilis is typically characterized by the appearance of a single painless lesion known as the chancre at the site of inoculation about 3 weeks after infection (**Fig. 2**). Typically, the primary lesions occur on the genitalia with regional lymphadenopathy. Even though primary lesions may resolve spontaneously even without treatment, the disease can evolve into the secondary stage about 6 to 8 weeks later in cutaneous and mucosal locations. Sexual transmission of syphilis requires contact with the lesion so is limited to the primary and secondary stages of the disease process.

Secondary syphilis involves systemic symptoms, such as rash and lymphadenopathy. In contrast to many other rashes, the secondary syphilis rash typically involves the palms and soles of the feet (**Fig. 3**). These symptoms occur several weeks after the initial infection, which is important to consider when obtaining the patient's history.

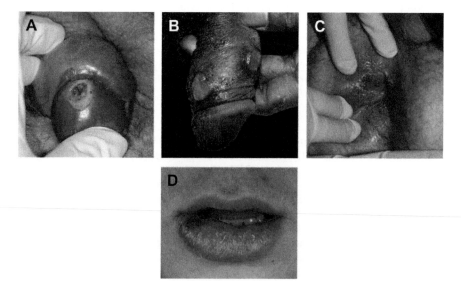

Fig. 2. Chancres of primary syphilis. The lesions are firm to palpation and are occasionally multiple. Sites of chancres can include the penis (*A, B*), perianal area (*C*), and lip (*D*). Occasionally, other sites are affected, for example, fingers. (*From* Bolognia JL, editor. Dermatology, 4th edition. Philadelphia: Elsevier; 2018; with permission.)

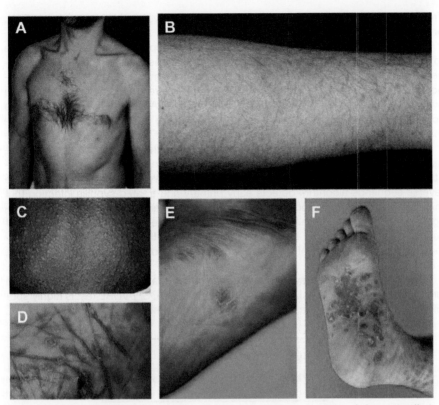

Fig. 3. Secondary syphilis. Widespread exanthem of pink papules (*A*), subtle minimally in-flamed lesions localized to the arms in an HIV-positive man (*B*), and generalized papulosquamous lesions (*C*). Lesions on the palms (*D*) and soles (*E, F*) can have a collarette of scale. (*From* Bolognia JL, editor. Dermatology, 4th edition. Philadelphia: Elsevier; 2018; with permission.)

Tertiary syphilis can lead to gummatous lesions and cardiac involvement including aortic disease that may not even appear until after 20 years of syphilis infection. Finally, many patients experience long periods of time without symptoms, which is known as latent syphilis. At any stage, the central nervous system may become infected, leading to neurosyphilis characterized by a broad array of signs and symptoms, including stroke, altered mental status, cranial nerve dysfunction, and tabes dorsalis.[50]

Unfortunately, there is no single definitive test for syphilis at all stages of the disease. There are several tests including dark-field microscopy, polymerase chain reaction, and direct fluorescent antibody testing that can directly detect *T pallidum*, but these tests are not widely available in the ED setting. In early syphilis, dark-field examination is considered to be the definitive method of detection, but ED providers must rely more on clinical manifestations and serologic testing.[51] Serologic diagnosis requires detection of both nontreponemal and treponemal antibodies. The reactivity of nontreponemal tests declines with time, whereas the reactivity of treponemal tests persists over a lifetime. Patients should be tested using a nontreponemal test, such as rapid plasma reagin test or venereal disease research laboratory (VDRL) test, as well as a treponemal test, such as fluorescent treponemal antibody absorption (FTA-ABS) test,

Treponema pallidum passive particle agglutination assay, enzyme immunoassay (EIA), or chemiluminescence immunoassay (CIA).

There are currently 2 different treatment algorithms depending on the tests available to detect syphilis. Traditionally, syphilis has been diagnosed with the use of nontreponemal screening assay followed by a treponemal confirmatory test if the initial nontreponemal test was reactive. However, there has been a recent paradigm shift with the availability of rapid treponemal assays including CIAs and EIAs with clinicians screening with a treponemal assay and then confirming with a standard nontreponemal assay.[52]

Currently the CDC recommends the traditional algorithm with reactive nontreponemal tests confirmed by treponemal testing. However, even though the traditional algorithm detects active infection, it can miss early primary and treated infection. The reverse sequence algorithm detects early primary and treated syphilis infection that might be missed with treated infection. Further studies are being conducted to investigate the reverse algorithm further because, despite the false-positive test results, it seems to offer automation, increased throughput, and the ability to detect early primary and treated syphilis infection that might be missed with treated infection (**Figs. 4** and **5**).

In the diagnosis of neurosyphilis, evaluation of cerebral spinal fluid obtained from a lumbar puncture is essential.[53] The cerebrospinal fluid (CSF)-VDRL test is highly specific for neurosyphilis but has poor sensitivity. In a patient with a negative CSF-VDRL

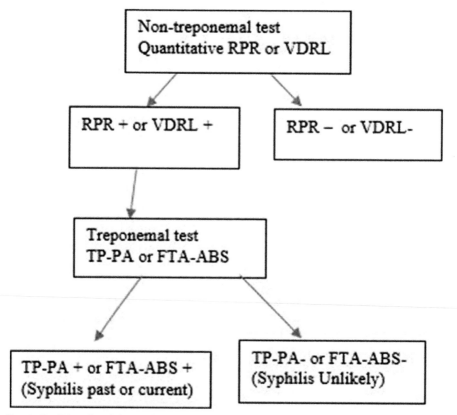

Fig. 4. Traditional syphilis serologic screening algorithm.

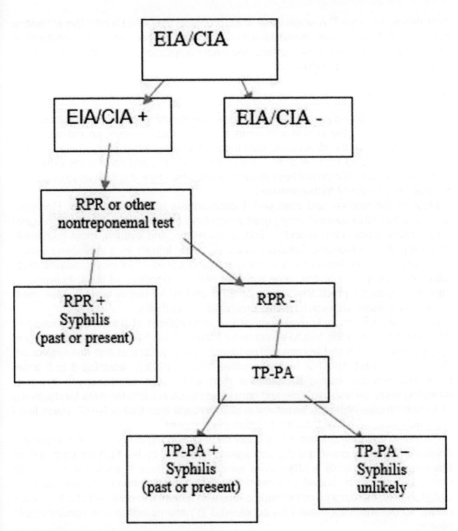

Fig. 5. Reverse sequence syphilis screening.

but high clinical suspicion for neurosyphilis, further testing with CSF FTA-ABS can be performed. Although this test has lower specificity, it is highly specific.[3]

The mainstay of treatment for syphilis is penicillin G benzathine. Current treatment guidelines recommend 2.4 million units of penicillin G benzathine IM for the treatment of primary, secondary, and early latent syphilis. The recommended regimen for neurosyphilis and ocular syphilis is aqueous crystalline penicillin G 18 to 24 million units per day, administered as 3 to 4 million units every 4 hours or continuous infusion for 10 to 14 days. Alternatively, compliant patients can receive procaine penicillin G 2.4 million units IM once daily plus probenecid, 500 mg, orally 4 times a day, both for 10 to 14 days.[54]

Patient-reported penicillin allergy is common and can represent a challenge for treatment of syphilis. For primary or secondary syphilis in compliant patients, doxycycline and tetracycline are commonly prescribed.[55] Daily ceftriaxone for 10 to 14 days may also be effective.[56] A single dose of azithromycin may also be effective at treating syphilis.[57] Data for this are limited, however, and there is a concern for resistant strains of *T pallidum*. For patients with anticipated poor compliance, desensitization for penicillin allergy should be performed.

TRICHOMONIASIS

Trichomonas vaginalis causes damage to the epithelium, leading to microulcerations most commonly in the vagina and urethra. In the United States, an estimated 3.7 million people have trichomoniasis, with many of the infected sharing similar risk factors including recent incarceration, intravenous drug use, and coinfection with BV.[58] Trichomonal infections do not have to be reported; therefore, it is difficult to determine the true prevalence of trichomoniasis.

Most of the women and men with trichomoniasis are asymptomatic. However, women with trichomoniasis may report a purulent, frothy vaginal discharge; vaginal odor; vulvovaginal irritation and itching; dyspareunia; and dysuria, most commonly peaking just after menses. Colpitis macularis, better known as a strawberry cervix, is actually only seen in about 2% to 5% of infected women.[59] However, colpitis macularis and frothy vaginal discharge together have a specificity of 99%; individually, they have positive predictive values of 90% and 62%, respectively.[60] Men most commonly present with epididymitis, prostatitis, or urethritis.

Historically, microscopic evaluation of wet preparations of genital secretions has been the most common test to evaluate for trichomonas. However, the sensitivity is very low in both men and women and no longer recommended as first-line evaluation. On the other hand, NAAT is highly sensitive (95.3%–100%), detecting 3 to 5 times more Trichomonas vaginalis infections than wet-mount microscopy.[61] Antigen-detecting tests are also available and considered to be acceptable tests for diagnosis of trichomoniasis. Although sensitivity is slightly lower than that of NAAT, these tests are much more sensitive than the traditional wet mount.

Currently, oral metronidazole (2 g orally once or 500 mg orally bid for 7 days) and tinidazole (2g orally once) are the only agents approved by the FDA for treatment of this infection. Tinidazole is often more expensive, but there is evidence to suggest that tinidazole may be superior to metronidazole in the resolution of trichomoniasis.[62] Unfortunately, there are no other medications with acceptable cure rates for trichomoniasis, so desensitization must be considered in patients with a true nitroimidazole allergy.

It is also important to discuss follow-up and partner treatment with patients diagnosed with trichomoniasis due to high reinfection rate.[63] EPT for trichomoniasis can be accomplished with metronidazole (2 g orally once or 500 mg orally bid for 7 days) or tinidazole (2 g orally).

SUMMARY

STDs continue to be a worldwide problem and rates are increasing. The scope, impact, and consequences of STDs seem to be underrecognized by the general public as well as health care providers. It is crucial that EPs recognize signs and symptoms consistent with STDs and be prepared to treat presumptively because missed diagnosis can carry both long- and short-term implications for patients and their sexual partners. In some cases when testing is not readily available, the diagnosis may be made clinically and empirical therapy started based on the CDC guidelines. The ED may also present an intervention opportunity for patients who do not regularly see a physician and use the ED as their primary health care resource.

REFERENCES

1. Satterwhite CL, Torrone E, Meites E, et al. Sexually transmitted infections among US women and men: prevalence and incidence estimates, 2008. Sex Transm Dis 2013;40(3):87–193.
2. Owusu-Edusei K, Chesson HW, Gift TL, et al. The estimated direct medical cost of selected sexually transmitted infections in the United States, 2008. Sex Transm Dis 2013;40(3):197–201.
3. A guide to taking a sexual history - centers for disease control. Atlanta (GA): US Department of Health and Human Services, CDC; 2011. Available at: www.cdc.gov/std/treatment/SexualHistory.pdf. Accessed May 22, 2018.
4. Brown J, Fleming R, Aristzabel J, et al. Does pelvic exam in the emergency department add useful information? West J Emerg Med 2011;12(2):208.
5. Cristillo AD, Bristow CC, Peeling R, et al. Point-of-care sexually transmitted infection diagnostics: Proceedings of the STAR sexually transmitted infection—clinical trial group programmatic meeting. Sex Transm Dis 2017;44(4):211–8.
6. 2017 National notifiable conditions. Centers for Disease Control and Prevention. Available at: https://wwwn.cdc.gov/nndss/conditions/notifiable/2017/. Accessed August 2, 2018.
7. Schillinger JA, Gorwitz R, Rietmeijer C, et al. The expedited partner therapy continuum: a conceptual framework to guide programmatic efforts to increase partner treatment. Sex Transm Dis 2016;43(2S):S63–75.
8. Centers for Disease Control and Prevention. Expedited partner therapy in the management of sexually transmitted diseases: review and guidance. Atlanta (GA): CDC; 2006. Available at: http://www.cdc.gov/std/treatment/eptfinalreport2006.pdf. Accessed August 27, 2017.
9. Koumans EH, Sternberg M, Bruce C, et al. The prevalence of bacterial vaginosis in the United States, 2001-2004: associations with symptoms, sexual behaviors, and reproductive health. Sex Transm Dis 2007;34:864–9.
10. Amsel R, Totten PA, Spiegel CA, et al. Nonspecific vaginitis. Diagnostic criteria and microbial and epidemiologic associations. Am J Med 1983;74:14–22.
11. Landers DV, Wiesenfeld HC, Heine RP, et al. Predictive value of the clinical diagnosis of lower genital tract infection in women. Am J Obstet Gynecol 2004;190(4):1004–10.
12. Caro-Patón T, Carvajal A, Martin de Diego I, et al. Is metronidazole teratogenic? A meta-analysis. Br J Clin Pharmacol 1997;44(2):179–82.
13. Hanson JM, McGregor JA, Hillier SL, et al. Metronidazole for bacterial vaginosis. A comparison of vaginal gel vs. oral therapy. J Reprod Med 2000;45(11):889–96.
14. Mehta SD. Systematic review of randomized trials of treatment of male sexual partners for improved bacteria vaginosis outcomes in women. Sex Transm Dis 2012;39:822–30.
15. Torrone E, Papp J, Weinstock H. Prevalence of Chlamydia trachomatis genital infection among persons aged 14-39 years - United States, 2007-2012. MMWR Morb Mortal Wkly Rep 2014;63(38):834–8.
16. Geisler WM, Chow JM, Schachter J, et al. Pelvic examination findings and Chlamydia trachomatis infection in asymptomatic young women screened with a nucleic acid amplification test. Sex Transm Dis 2007;34(6):335–8.
17. Papp JR, Schachter J, Gaydos C, et al. Recommendations for the laboratory-based detection of Chlamydia trachomatis and Neisseria gonorrhoeae—2014. MMWR Recomm Rep 2014;63(RR-02):1–19.

18. Skidmore S, Horner P, Herring A, et al. Vulvovaginal-swab or first-catch urine specimen to detect Chlamydia trachomatis in women in a community setting? J Clin Microbiol 2006;44(12):4389–94.

19. Hobbs MM, van der Pol B, Totten P, et al. From the NIH: proceedings of a workshop on the importance of self-obtained vaginal specimens for detection of sexually transmitted infections. Sex Transm Dis 2008;35(1):8–13.

20. Cook RL, Hutchison SL, Ostergaard L, et al. Systematic review: noninvasive testing for Chlamydia trachomatis and Neisseria gonorrhoeae. Ann Intern Med 2005;142(11):914–25.

21. Renault CA, Hall C, Kent CK, et al. Use of NAATs for STD diagnosis of GC and CT in non-FDA-cleared anatomic specimens. MLO Med Lab Obs 2006;38:10–24.

22. Lau CY, Qureshi AK. Azithromycin versus doxycycline for genital chlamydial infections: a meta-analysis of randomized clinical trials. Sex Transm Dis 2002;29: 497–502.

23. Hogben M. Partner notification for sexually transmitted diseases. Clin Infect Dis 2007;44(Suppl 3):S160–74.

24. Centers for Disease Control and Prevention. Expedited partner therapy in the management of sexually transmitted diseases. Atlanta, GA: US Department of Health and Human Services, 2006.

25. Sherrard J, Barlow D. Gonorrhoea in men: clinical and diagnostic aspects. Genitourin Med 1996;72(6):422–6.

26. Workowski KA, Berman S, Centers for Disease Control and Prevention (CDC). Sexually transmitted diseases treatment guidelines, 2010. MMWR Recomm Rep 2010;59(RR-12):1–110.

27. Kirkcaldy RD, Weinstock HS, Moore PC, et al. The efficacy and safety of gentamicin plus azithromycin and gemifloxacin plus azithromycin as treatment of uncomplicated gonorrhea. Clin Infect Dis 2014;59:1083–91.

28. Centers for Disease Control and Prevention (CDC). Update to CDC's Sexually transmitted diseases treatment guidelines, 2010: oral cephalosporins no longer a recommended treatment for gonococcal infections. MMWR Morb Mortal Wkly Rep 2012;61:590–4.

29. Bradley H, Markowitz L, Gibson T, et al. Seroprevalence of herpes simplex virus types 1 and 2—United States, 1999–2010. J Infect Dis 2014;209(3):325–33.

30. Bernstein DI, Bellamy AR, Hook EW III, et al. Epidemiology, clinical presentation, and antibody response to primary infection with herpes simplex virus type 1 and type 2 in young women. Clin Infect Dis 2012;56(3):344–51.

31. Merin A, Pachankis JE. The psychological impact of genital herpes stigma. J Health Psychol 2011;16(1):80–90.

32. Mertz GJ. Asymptomatic shedding of herpes simplex virus 1 and 2: implications for prevention of transmission. J Infect Dis 2008;198(8):1098–100.

33. Cernik C, Gallina K, Brodell RT. The treatment of herpes simplex infections: an evidence-based review. Arch Intern Med 2008;168(11):1137–44.

34. Chosidow O, Drouault Y, Leconte-Veyriac F, et al. Famciclovir vs. acyclovir in immunocompetent patients with recurrent genital herpes infections: a parallel-groups, randomized, double-blind clinical trial. Br J Dermatol 2001;144:818–24.

35. O'Farrell N. Donovanosis. Sex Transm Infect 2002;78:452–7.

36. Ault KA. Epidemiology and natural history of human papillomavirus infections in the female genital tract. Infect Dis Obstet Gynecol 2006;2006(Suppl):40470.

37. Lipke MM. An armamentarium of wart treatments. Clin Med Res 2006;4(4): 273–93.

38. Meites E, Kempe A, Markowitz LE. Use of a 2-dose schedule for human papillomavirus vaccination — updated recommendations of the advisory committee on immunization practices. MMWR Morb Mortal Wkly Rep 2016;65:1405–8.
39. Mabey D, Peeling RW. Lymphogranuloma venereum. Sex Transm Infect 2002;78: 90–2.
40. Ceovic R, Gulin SJ. Lymphogranuloma venereum: diagnostic and treatment challenges. Infect Drug Resist 2015;8:39–47.
41. Roest RW, Van der Meijden WI. European guideline for the management of tropical genito-ulcerative diseases. Int J STD AIDS 2001;12(3):78–83.
42. Van der Bij AK, Spaargaren J, Morré SA, et al. Diagnostic and clinical implications of anorectal lymphogranuloma venereum in men who have sex with men: a retrospective case-control study. Clin Infect Dis 2006;42(2):186–94.
43. Sethi S, Singh G, Samanta P, et al. *Mycoplasma genitalium*: an emerging sexually transmitted pathogen. Indian J Med Res 2012;136(6):942–55.
44. Alfarraj DA, Somily AM. Isolation of *Mycoplasma genitalium* from endocervical swabs of infertile women. Saudi Med J 2017;38(5):549–52.
45. Mena LA, Mroczkowski TF, Nsuami M, et al. A randomized comparison of azithromycin and doxycycline for the treatment of *Mycoplasma genitalium*-positive urethritis in men. Clin Infect Dis 2009;48:1649–54.
46. Bjornelius E, Anagrius C, Bojs G, et al. Antibiotic treatment of symptomatic *Mycoplasma genitalium* infection in Scandinavia: a controlled clinical trial. Sex Transm Infect 2008;84:72–6.
47. Jernberg E, Moghaddam A, Moi H. Azithromycin and moxifloxacin for microbiological cure of *Mycoplasma genitalium* infection: an open study. Int J STD AIDS 2008;19:676–9.
48. Syphilis - CDC fact sheet (Detailed). Centers for Disease Control and Prevention. 2017. Available at: https://www.cdc.gov/std/syphilis/stdfact-syphilis-detailed.htm. Accessed June 2, 2018.
49. Peeling RW, Hook EW III. The pathogenesis of syphilis: the Great Mimicker, revisited. J Pathol 2006;208(2):224–32.
50. Liu LL, Zheng WH, Tong ML, et al. Ischemic stroke as a primary symptom of neurosyphilis among HIV-negative emergency patients. J Neurol Sci 2012;317(1): 35–9.
51. CDC, Association of Public Health Laboratories. Laboratory diagnostic testing for Treponema pallidum, Expert Consultation Meeting Summary Report. Atlanta, GA, January 13–15, 2009.
52. Soreng K, Levy R, Fakile Y. Serologic testing for syphilis: benefits and challenges of a reverse algorithm. Clin Microbiol Newsl 2014;36(24):195–202.
53. Noy M, Rayment M, Sullivan A, et al. The utility of cerebrospinal fluid analysis in the investigation and treatment of neurosyphilis. Sex Transm Infect 2014;90(6): 451.
54. Syphilis. Centers for Disease Control and Prevention. 2016. Available at: https:// www.cdc.gov/std/tg2015/syphilis.htm. Accessed January 14, 2018.
55. Clement ME, Okeke NL, Hicks CB. Treatment of syphilis: a systematic review. JAMA 2014;312(18):1905–17.
56. Liang Z, Chen YP, Yang CS, et al. Meta-analysis of ceftriaxone compared with penicillin for the treatment of syphilis. Int J Antimicrob Agents 2016;47(1):6–11.
57. Riedner G, Rusizoka M, Todd J, et al. Single-dose azithromycin versus penicillin G benzathine for the treatment of early syphilis. N Engl J Med 2005;353(12): 1236–44.

58. Rathod SD, Krupp K, Klausner JD, et al. Bacterial vaginosis and risk for Tricho-monas vaginalis infection: a longitudinal analysis. Sex Transm Dis 2011;38(9): 882–6.

59. Schwebke JR, Burgess D. Trichomoniasis. Clin Microbiol Rev 2004;17(4):794–803.

60. Wølner-Hanssen P, Krieger JN, Stevens CE, et al. Clinical manifestations of vaginal trichomoniasis. JAMA 1989;261(4):571–6 (Prospective study; 779 patients).

61. Roth AM, Williams JA, Ly R, et al. Changing sexually transmitted infection screening protocol will result in improved case finding for Trichomonas vaginalis among high-risk female populations. Sex Transm Dis 2011;38:398–400.

62. Forna F, Gülmezoglu AM. Interventions for treating trichomoniasis in women. Cochrane Database Syst Rev 2003;(2):CD000218.

63. Kissinger P, Schmidt N, Mohammed H, et al. Patient-delivered partner treatment for Trichomonas vaginalis infection: a randomized controlled trial. Sex Transm Dis 2006;33:445–50.

64. Méchaï F, De Barbeyrac B, Aoun O, et al. Doxycycline failure in lymphogranuloma venereum. Sex Transm Infect 2010;86(4):278–9.

Genital Complaints at the Extremes of Age

Sara Manning, MD

KEYWORDS

- Vulvovaginitis • Genital trauma • Pelvic organ prolapse • Gynecologic malignancy
- Ovarian torsion

KEY POINTS

- Low-estrogen-level states like menopause and the prepubertal period are associated with thin, atrophic genital tissues with predisposition to irritation and injury.
- Genital examination of the prepubertal girl requires understanding of anatomic variations, appropriate patient positioning, and careful tissue manipulation.
- Vulvovaginitis is the most common genital complaint in the prepubertal girl and is most commonly caused by contact irritants and poor hygiene.
- Postmenopausal vaginal bleeding is the most common symptom of uterine cancer and should prompt ultrasound examination of the uterine stripe for risk assessment.
- Pelvic organ prolapse can lead to frequent urinary tract infection, urinary or bowel obstruction, nephropathy, dyspareunia, and poor self-image.

INTRODUCTION

Anatomy and physiology of pelvic and genital structures vary significantly across a woman's lifespan. Hormonal variations, most notably in estrogen, lead to changes in the genital tissues that directly affect the external appearance, ease of examination, vulnerability to injury, and pathologic processes encountered in these patients. Low estrogen states like menopause and the prepubertal period share important physiologic changes, including more friable, dry, and inelastic mucosa that is prone to irritation, injury, and infection. These and other factors lead to unique gynecologic pathologic conditions encountered at the extremes of age.

Pediatric Patients

Anatomy and physiology

The effects of maternal estrogen are commonly observed in the neonate. These effects of maternal estrogen include breast buds, nipple discharge, and genital changes. The neonate has relatively large labia, a thickened, redundant hymen, and a large

Disclosure Statement: None.
Department of Emergency Medicine, University of Maryland School of Medicine, 110 South Paca Street, 6th Floor, Suite 200, Baltimore, MD 21201, USA
E-mail address: smanning@som.umaryland.edu

Emerg Med Clin N Am 37 (2019) 193–205
https://doi.org/10.1016/j.emc.2019.01.003
0733-8627/19/© 2019 Elsevier Inc. All rights reserved.

clitoral hood. Thin vaginal secretions may be present. Vaginal bleeding may occur in the first days to week of life secondary to maternal estrogen withdrawal. This bleeding is benign and requires no intervention unless the bleeding is excessive or persists past the first weeks of life. As girls age, the estrogen effect on genital structures lessens; the labia thin and the clitoral hood recedes. Throughout infancy, the hymen typically remains relatively thick and redundant and then thins and recedes into the vaginal orifice in early childhood. Labia minora remain thin and rudimentary throughout infancy and childhood. A variety of appearances of the hymen are considered normal, including circumferential, sleevelike, and crescentic. There are a variety of congenital anomalies of the hymen that may cause symptoms or prompt parental concern for possible injury. These anomalies include imperforate, microperforate, cribriform, and septate hymens. Prepubertal mucosa is thinner, more atrophic, redder and lacks the protective secretions of estrogenized mucosa. These attributes along with the proximity to the anus predisposes prepubertal girls to irritation and infection.

Genital examination

The genital examination of the prepubertal girl differs significantly from the genital examination of the reproductive age woman. The hypoestrogenized prepubertal genitalia are less elastic and more sensitive to touch and injury. Fortunately, most gynecologic complaints in this age group can be diagnosed with simple external examination. Use of a vaginal speculum is rarely needed in this age group and should be performed under anesthesia. Girls may be positioned in a supine frog-leg position or in a prone, knee-chest position (**Fig. 1**).[1] Visualization of the urethra and vaginal orifice may be obtained through gentle labial traction. The labia majora should be grasped at the 5 and 7 o'clock position and pulled gently laterally and toward the examiner.

Genital examinations can provoke anxiety in the examiner, parent, and older child. The examiner should always explain their examination and, when appropriate, elicit the assistance of the caregiver. Children may be hesitant to allow examination, and the examiner should reinforce that only caregivers and clinicians should examine this area. The American Academy of Pediatrics (AAP) suggests that the caregiver be present for the examination of the prepubertal girl. The positioning of the caregiver should be at the choice of the patient. If sexual abuse is suspected, the AAP recommends the use of a medical chaperone.[2–4]

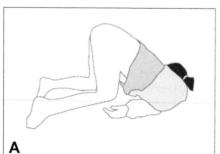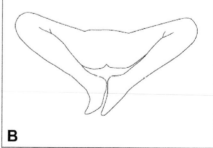

Fig. 1. Pediatric genitourinary examination positions: (*A*) prone knee-chest position; (*B*) supine frog-leg position. (*Used with permission of* EB Medicine, publisher of Emergency Medicine Practice, from: Joelle Borhart. Emergency department management of vaginal bleeding in the nonpregnant patient. Emergency Medicine Practice. 2013;15(8):1–24. © EB Medicine. www.ebmedicine.net.)

Vaginal bleeding

Apart from estrogen-withdrawal bleeding seen in the first days of life, vaginal bleeding in prepubertal girls is always abnormal and requires evaluation. Prepubertal vaginal bleeding is a concerning symptom that is usually associated with an identifiable pathologic condition.[5] These pathologic conditions range from simple vulvovaginitis to serious genital trauma, sexual abuse, and rarely, malignancy. The approach to vaginal bleeding should include a thorough history focusing on a description of the bleeding, traumatic injuries, toileting habits, access to estrogen-containing medications, urinary symptoms, and any concern for abuse.[3,5] Physical examination of the prepubertal girl with vaginal bleeding should include a general physical examination, including height, weight, signs of precocious puberty, abdominal mass, and evidence of trauma.

Vulvovaginitis

Inflammation of the vulva and vagina can be caused by infectious, chemical, or physical irritation. The majority of prepubertal vulvovaginitis is noninfectious, and it typically presents with irritation, itching, and erythema, with or without vaginal discharge and bleeding. Noninfectious vulvovaginitis is milder and gradual in onset, often presenting later than infectious cases. The microbiology of infectious vaginitis in prepubertal girls differs significantly from the postpubertal population. Bacterial vaginitis predominates with enteric and respiratory flora accounting for most cases. Fecal and oral flora are often transferred to the vagina due to poor hygiene practices. Although candidal vaginitis accounts for most vulvovaginitis in the adolescent and adult populations, it is very rare in childhood.[6] Examination may reveal erythema of the vulva and vagina, vaginal discharge, excoriations, and bleeding. Infectious vulvovaginitis is associated with more pronounced vaginal symptoms compared with the vulvar predominance of noninfectious cases. In recurrent cases or those where sexual abuse is suspected, vaginal swabs may be collected for culture or nucleic acid amplification testing. Infectious vulvovaginitis is associated with more rapid progression of symptoms, pronounced erythema, and vaginal discharge. Shigella and salmonella are associated with bloody vaginitis.[7]

Treatment of noninfectious vulvovaginitis is focused on improving hygiene practices, emphasizing front to back wiping, twice daily sitz baths, and avoidance of common irritants. Frequently cited irritants include harsh soaps, laundry detergents, bubble baths, and tight-fitting undergarments. When bacterial vaginitis is highly suspected, initial antibiotic coverage should include coverage for strep species and gram-negative organisms. Common pathogens respond well to penicillins.[8] Emphasis on improved hygiene practices should be included in both infectious and noninfectious cases.

Urethral prolapse

Weak supporting tissues of the pelvic floor, urethral hypermobility, and increased intra-abdominal pressures can lead to prolapse of the distal portion of the urethra. Urethral prolapse has a bimodal age distribution in early childhood and postmenopausal patients. Pediatric cases are most commonly observed in African American girls.[9] Urethral prolapse presents with painless bleeding and occasional mild dysuria. Examination reveals a thick, round, dark red or purple ring of tissue surrounding the urethra. Diagnosis may be aided by observed urination or catheterization through the center of the lesion.[10] Most cases are uncomplicated and resolve with application of estrogen cream and sitz baths. Rarely, significant portions of the urethra may be involved, leading to vascular strangulation and necrosis. Strangulation and necrosis can cause pain and urinary obstruction. Inability to urinate and evidence of necrosis at presentation should prompt urgent gynecologic or urologic evaluation for surgical correction.[2,3,7]

Retained foreign body

Foul smelling vaginal discharge, unexplained vaginal bleeding, and recurrent urinary tract infections should raise suspicion of retained vaginal foreign body. The most frequently observed vaginal foreign body in children is toilet tissue, but small toys, coins, bottle caps, and other household items have been reported.[11] Diagnosis is often delayed and has been associated with rare serious complications like fistula formation or perforation.[11,12] Rarely, significant symptoms can develop rapidly in the setting of caustic foreign bodies like batteries.[13] The prone knee-chest position can aid visualization. Distal foreign bodies may be carefully removed with an ear curette or moistened cotton swab.[2,7] Vaginal irrigation with warm water or saline through a small catheter inserted into the vagina can flush out more proximal foreign bodies. Most vaginal foreign bodies are radiolucent, and poorly visualized on other imaging modalities, including pelvic ultrasonography and MRI, limiting the role of imaging.[14] If foreign bodies cannot be removed with noninvasive techniques, examination and foreign body removal under anesthesia may be required.

Genital trauma

Genital trauma can occur in isolation or as part of multisystem trauma, accidentally or in the setting of sexual abuse. The rich vascular supply of genital tissues can result in significant blood loss. Perineal examination should be included in the evaluation of any multitrauma victim. If evidence of injury is encountered, examination under anesthesia may be required to assess the extent of injury.

Accidental trauma

Genital injuries are rare, accounting for less than 1% of all pediatric injuries.[15] Genital injuries occur more frequently in female children and are most commonly encountered in early childhood.[15,16] Most injuries are secondary to blunt mechanisms with straddle injuries predominating.[5,15,16] Common injury types include lacerations, abrasions, hematomas, and burns. Although most genital injuries are mild and can be managed with simple analgesia, emergency physicians should be cautious; the extent of genital injuries can be difficult to ascertain. Many suggest a low threshold for examination under anesthesia either in the operating suite or under moderate sedation in the emergency department (ED) to facilitate thorough examination.[5,16]

Small, uncomplicated lacerations can be repaired in the ED or treated with sitz baths, ice packs, and oral analgesics. Even small repairs may require moderate sedation due to sensitivity of the involved tissues and patient anxiety. Hematomas usually involve the labia, mons, and clitoris and rarely require specific treatment. Large hematomas can distort perineal structures and lead to difficulty voiding. In these cases, a Foley catheter should be placed. Most hematomas resolve with ice packs, warm sitz baths, and oral analgesics. Indications for operative management are listed in **Table 1**.

Table 1
Indications for operative exploration and repair

Lacerations	Hematomas
Length >3 cm	Very large hematomas
Lacerations through or above the hymen	Involvement of adjacent structures (vagina, mons pubis, abdominal wall)
Lacerations involving urethra or anus	Evidence of necrosis
Vaginal bleeding of unclear source	Rapid expansion
Inadequate exploration	

Penetrating injuries to the perineum or vagina can be quite severe resulting in peritoneal involvement, injury to the rectum, bladder, or reproductive tract. The unestrogenized mucosa of the preadolescent girl tears easily, and significant injury can result from relatively minor trauma. Accidental injuries can result from impalement on toys, household items, playground or sports equipment, or in the setting of blunt trauma with pelvic fracture fragments lacerating the vaginal wall.[3,15] Penetrating injuries frequently require examination under anesthesia to exclude deep structure involvement.

Nonaccidental trauma and sexual assault

The approach to genital trauma in the child should always include consideration of nonaccidental trauma. A complete discussion of sexual assault is beyond the scope of this article. The AAP and the Centers for Disease Control and Prevention both offer excellent resources for the approach to the potentially sexually abused child. In some jurisdictions, trained pediatric sexual assault examiners may be available and are best equipped to perform the examinations. Occasionally, emergency physicians will be required to examine a child should a pediatric sexual assault expert be unavailable. Verbal children should provide their own history if possible. Injury patterns that do not match the reported mechanism of injury should raise concern for abuse. Although penetrating injuries can occur through nonaccidental mechanisms, unfortunately, most penetrating vaginal injuries are the result of abuse.[3] Bruising, abrasions, and lacerations to the hymen, posterior fourchette, and lateral vaginal walls are suggestive but not diagnostic of abuse. As with suspected abuse cases in older children and adults, the lack of obvious physical signs does not exclude the possibility of abuse. In many cases of abuse there will be no abnormal genital findings. Emergency physicians are mandatory reporters and must contact Child Protective Services if any suspicion of abuse exists and ensure that the patient is going to a safe environment if being discharged; the child should be admitted to the hospital if this is uncertain.

Ovarian torsion

Ovarian torsion can be a difficult diagnosis in the pediatric patient. Although it is more common in reproductive age patients, torsion can be encountered at any age. Peaks of incidence occur at infancy and menarche.[17,18] Torsion occurs when the ovary, or more commonly the ovary and fallopian tube together, twists. Compromised venous outflow leads to edema and swelling. As swelling worsens, arterial flow is limited resulting in ischemia and necrosis. Hypermobility of the terminal ilium and cecum and longer ligamentous attachments account for the slight predominance of right-sided ovarian torsion.[18] Torsion occurs more frequently in abnormal ovaries, but up to 25% of pediatric patients with torsion have normal ovaries. In children, these abnormalities favor benign pathologic conditions, including cystic teratomas, hemorrhagic or follicular cysts, cystadenomas, or rarely, hydrosalpinx.[17,18]

Presenting complaints vary with age. Older children may describe classic symptoms of sudden onset lateralizing abdominal pain with associated nausea and vomiting. Symptoms in the preverbal child and poorly verbal toddler may include lethargy, poor feeding, and irritability. Physical examination findings include mild elevation of the temperature, abdominal tenderness with or without peritoneal signs, and an abdominal mass.[19,20] The imaging modality of choice is pelvic ultrasound. In prepubescent girls, ultrasound should be limited to the transabdominal approach. Ultrasound findings suggestive of torsion are listed in **Box 1**[17] and shown in **Figs. 2** and **3**. As with adults, a negative ultrasound, including present flow on Doppler,

> **Box 1**
> **Ultrasound findings of ovarian torsion**
>
> Unilateral ovarian enlargement
>
> Adnexal mass
>
> Abnormal Doppler flow
>
> Medialization of the ovary
>
> Uterine displacement
>
> Free fluid
>
> Whirlpool sign

does not exclude the diagnosis of torsion, and the gold standard remains direct visualization via exploratory laparoscopy.

Ovarian torsion is a surgical emergency. Rates of ovarian salvage are low but improving from 0% to 15% in the 1990s to 25% to 30% in more recent series.[19,20] In a small series documenting cases from 2005 to 2012, a detorsion rate of 95% was achieved with favorable postoperative findings on ultrasound follow-up.[20] Once the diagnosis of torsion is strongly suspected, gynecologic consult and operative intervention should not be delayed. Delayed presentation should not deter the treating physician from pursuing emergent operative management due to doubts of the organ's viability; ovaries have been successfully salvaged after prolonged symptoms.[19]

Geriatric Patients

Elderly women constitute the fastest growing segment of the American population with current female life expectancy exceeding 81 years.[21] By 2030, nearly 1 in 5 Americans will be older than the age of 65.[22] As such, an understanding of common gynecologic complaints in this age group is of increasing importance in emergency medicine practice.

Vulvar and vaginal disorders
As in the preadolescent, the postmenopausal genitalia are significantly affected by the withdrawal of circulating estrogen at the time of menopause. Tissues become thinner, less elastic, and more friable. Decreases in vaginal secretions contribute to dryness and itching. The amount of lactobacillus in the vagina decreases, and the vaginal pH increases. Urinary and stool incontinence and comorbidities like arthritis,

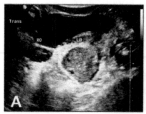 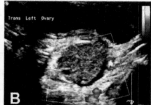 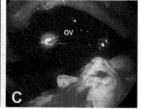

Fig. 2. Left ovarian torsion ultrasound and intraoperative image. (*A*) Left ovary (LO) enlarged and medially displaced relative to the normal right ovary (RO). (*B*) Free fluid, edema, and lack of Doppler signal. (*C*) Edematous and congested ovary (OV). (*From* Ngo AV, Otjen JP, Parisi MT, et al. Pediatric ovarian torsion: a pictorial review. Pediatr Radiol 2015;45(12):1845–55; with permission.)

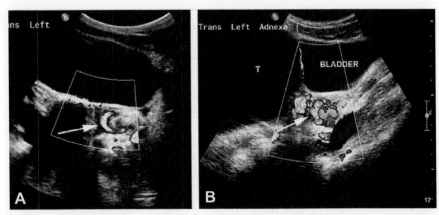

Fig. 3. (*A, B*) Whirlpool sign: specific but poorly specific. Whirlpool sign is the result of twisting vascular structures (*arrows*) at the site of torsion. This case associated with large cystic teratoma (*T*). (*From* Ngo AV, Otjen JP, Parisi MT, et al. Pediatric ovarian torsion: a pictorial review. Pediatr Radiol. 2015;45(12):1845–55; with permission.)

osteoporosis, and dementia may result in poor hygiene. Collectively, these changes increase the risk of both irritant and infectious vaginitis and recurrent urinary tract infections.[23]

Atrophic vaginitis is a common complaint among postmenopausal women. Common symptoms include pruritus, dryness, dyspareunia, burning, and bleeding. Atrophic vaginitis is the most common cause of postmenopausal bleeding. Examination will reveal thin, pale, and friable mucosa. Conservative treatments like sitz baths and careful hygiene constitute the first line of therapy. Topical estrogen therapy can reduce severity of symptoms and is available in a variety of preparations. A recent Cochrane Review suggests that topical estrogen therapy does not impart a significant risk of endometrial thickening or breast changes.[24] Infections like cervicitis, vaginitis, and pelvic inflammatory disease are more commonly encountered in younger patients but should still be considered in the postmenopausal patients. Although advanced age is associated with increased frequency of sexual dysfunction, this should not deter physicians from obtaining a sexual history in older women. Divorce or death of a long-term partner and transition to new sexual partners can increase risk of sexually transmitted disease.[22]

Vulvar and vaginal malignancies are uncommon gynecologic malignancies but can be observed on a simple external examination. Findings may include thickened, firm, asymmetric tissues with easy bleeding. Quick, reliable follow-up with gynecology should be arranged for biopsy and initiation of treatment.[25]

Postmenopausal bleeding

Although atrophic vaginitis may be the most common cause of postmenopausal vaginal bleeding, vaginal bleeding is a common symptom of gynecologic malignancies like endometrial, cervical, and rarely, ovarian cancers. As such, malignancy should be considered during any evaluation of postmenopausal vaginal bleeding. Emergency physicians should assess for symptoms, family history, and personal risk factors for various gynecologic malignancies (**Table 2**). Physical examination findings can vary widely depending on the stage of malignancy. Examinations may be entirely benign or demonstrate evidence of advanced disease with malignant effusions, ascites, cachexia, and adenopathy. Pelvic examination should be performed,

Table 2
Characteristics of gynecologic malignancies

Cancer	Incidence	Risk Factors	Symptoms
Uterine	2%–3%	Unopposed estrogen use Early menarche Late menopause Nulliparity Tamoxifen Obesity Hereditary nonpolyposis colorectal cancer (HPNCC)	Abnormal uterine bleeding (90% of cases) Abdominal or pelvic pain
Ovarian	1%–2%	Early menarche Late menopause Old age at childbirth Low parity BRCA gene mutation HPNCC	Abdominal or pelvic pain Bloating Early satiety Dysuria Vaginal bleeding
Cervical	<1%	Human papilloma virus (HPV) Early coitarche Smoking Multiple sex partners Immunosuppression Sexually transmitted infections	Vaginal bleeding Postcoital bleeding Vaginal discharge
Vaginal	Rare	HPV Late menarche Early menopause Smoking	Vaginal bleeding Pelvic pain Fistula formation
Vulvar	Rare	HPV Smoking Immunocompromise Lichen sclerosis	Pruritus Pain Dysuria Vaginal bleeding (rare)

Data from Refs.[26–29]

including speculum examination with examination of the vaginal walls and cervix. Bimanual examination may reveal fixed masses, nodularity in the cul-de-sac, and palpable ovaries. A rectovaginal examination can improve assessment of the posterior vaginal wall.

Ultrasound assessment of pelvic structures, including the endometrial stripe, is essential in the evaluation of postmenopausal bleeding. A pelvic ultrasound may be obtained as part of the ED evaluation or as an outpatient provided the patient has timely, reliable gynecologic follow-up. The American College of Obstetricians and Gynecologists (ACOG) recommends a cutoff of ≤4 mm for normal endometrial thickness. Endometrial thickness <4 mm has a negative predictive value of 99% for endometrial malignancy and requires biopsy only in the event of persistent or recurrent symptoms.[30] Women with abnormal endometrial thickness should be referred to gynecology for prompt endometrial biopsy. Ultrasound can also demonstrate worrisome findings for ovarian cancers, including complex ovarian masses, free fluid in the pelvis, and septated or thick-walled cysts. Diagnostic utility of ultrasound may be aided by contrast enhancement.[31] In hemodynamically unstable women with concern for underlying gynecologic malignancy, emergent gynecologic consultation should be obtained. Stable women with postmenopausal bleeding can safely be referred for prompt follow-up.

Pelvic organ prolapse

Pelvic organ prolapse (POP) is defined as the abnormal descent of pelvic structures due to weakening of the pelvic floor. POP is associated with incontinence, decreased self-esteem, social isolation as well as significant medical complications. Prolapse is common with more than 10% of women developing symptomatic POP.[32,33]

The pelvic floor is composed of the levator ani muscle group and coccygeus muscles, which form a broad sheet through which the urethra, vagina, and rectum pass. Weakening of these structures can occur as a result of high parity, aging, genetic predisposition, connective tissue disease, and chronically elevated intra-abdominal pressures due to obesity, constipation, or chronic obstructive pulmonary disease.[25] The location of the prolapse determines the organ involvement: cystoceles and urethral involvement prolapse through the anterior vaginal wall, rectoceles prolapse through the posterior vaginal wall, and the uterus and cervix prolapse through the vaginal apex.

Symptoms of POP include a sensation of vaginal pressure or a bulge in the vagina, difficulty voiding or defecating, splinting (digital reduction of prolapse to facilitate voiding or defecation), or recurrent urinary tract infections. Physical examination may require examination with Valsalva or even standing to elicit prolapse findings. A speculum examination may be performed with only the fixed blade to examine the anterior and posterior vaginal walls individually. POP is graded based on the distance above or below the hymen of the distal most prolapsed portion. ACOG recommends the Pelvic Organ Prolapse Quantification System (POP-Q) for assessing prolapse severity[34] (**Table 3**).

Although POP is typically a benign condition, advanced stage prolapse can cause significant complications, including hydronephrosis and obstructive uropathy, bowel obstruction, or strangulation of prolapsed organs.[35] More commonly, women report significant quality-of-life limitations, including sexual dysfunction, activity limitation, incontinence, and toileting dysfunction.[36] Treatment ranges from noninvasive approaches like Kegel exercises and pessaries to surgical correction with or without implantable mesh. Most cases of POP can be safely reduced in the ED and referred to outpatient gynecology. Advanced prolapse with evidence of obstruction of either the urinary system or bowel or evidence of pelvic organ ischemia should prompt urgent gynecologic evaluation.

Pessaries

Objects inserted into the vagina to facilitate reduction of POP have been in use for millennia. Current use is growing in popularity with most urogynecologists and ACOG recommending vaginal pessary as the first-line treatment of symptomatic

Table 3	
POP-Q staging system for pelvic organ prolapse	
Stage	**Findings**
0	No prolapse: anterior and posterior points are all −3 cm and cervix and posterior fornix are between total vaginal length and −2 cm
I	Total distal prolapse is more than 1 cm above the hymen
II	Distal most prolapse is between 1 cm above and 1 cm below the hymen
III	Distal most prolapse is more than 1 cm below the hymen but no further than 2 cm less than total vaginal length
IV	Complete procidentia or vault eversion

Data from Bump RC, Mattiasson A, Bø K, et al. The standardization of terminology of female pelvic organ prolapse and pelvic floor dysfunction. Am J Obstet Gynecol 1996;175(1):10–7.

POP over surgical intervention.[32,37] Vaginal pessaries are made of silicone-coated rubber and can be divided into 2 subtypes: support and space-occupying. The most commonly used pessary is the ring pessary. This ring pessary is a supportive pessary that fits snugly around the prolapsing cervix and is recommended for early-stage prolapse. Pessaries are sized small enough to permit easy patient insertion and removal but large enough stay in position through daily activity. Other common support pessaries include Gehrung and Hodge pessaries. Space-occupying models include the donut,. cube, and Gellhorn pessaries (**Fig. 4**).

Although routine use of pessaries is a safe practice, some complications can occur. Common complications include bleeding, excoriations, ulcerations, and impaction. These complications are relatively minor and often improve with removal of the pessary, resizing, and a course of topical estrogen. Removal of an impacted pessary can be difficult and painful. In some cases, procedural sedation or even examination under general anesthesia may be required. In extreme cases, instruments like orthopedic bone cutters or purpose designed "pessariotomes" may be required to remove the pessary in pieces.[38]

Neglected pessaries are associated with more serious complications that are occasionally life-threatening. Pessaries left in place for a prolonged period have been associated with fistula formation, erosion into the bowel or bladder, and peritonitis. These

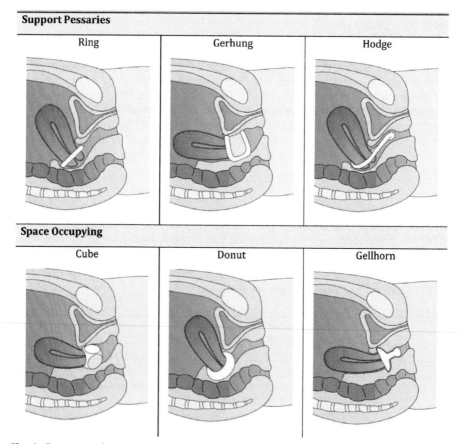

Fig. 4. Support and space-occupying pessaries.

serious complications will require emergent evaluation and operative intervention by gynecology. In addition, there have been case reports suggesting that the chronic inflammation associated with long-term pessary use may increase the risk of vaginal cancers. Patients evaluated for pessary complications should be urged to maintain routine and frequent follow-up with their gynecologist to monitor therapy.[39,40]

It should be noted that many women report embarrassment regarding POP and their use of a pessary and may not provide this history readily.[36] Focused questions regarding POP symptoms and pessary use should be considered in the evaluation of the elderly woman presenting with abdominal pain or urinary or bowel symptoms. Special consideration should be given to high-risk populations, including those with dementia, and a pelvic examination should be performed as described above.

SUMMARY

Patients at the extremes of age can present unique and challenging gynecologic pathologic conditions. Care should be taken by the emergency physician to adapt to challenges in examining unestrogenized genitalia and consider age-specific pathologic conditions.

Vulvovaginitis is a common complaint in early childhood and is usually due to contact irritation and poor hygiene. Prepubertal vaginal bleeding outside of infancy is always abnormal and should prompt a thorough history and examination to exclude rare, serious causes. Recurrent infectious vaginitis or urinary tract infection should prompt physicians to consider retained vaginal foreign body. Ovarian torsion can occur in the prepubertal female child and can be difficult to diagnose due to vague symptoms and limited utility of the physical examination. Genital trauma is rare, but often requires examination under sedation or in an operating suite to fully assess extent of injury. Although penetrating trauma can be accidental, high suspicion of abuse should be maintained.

Estrogen withdrawal at menopause leads to vaginal dryness and atrophy. Although postmenopausal bleeding is most commonly due to atrophic vaginitis, it should be considered a sign of gynecologic malignancy until proven otherwise. Ultrasound is the imaging modality of choice for assessment of the endometrial stripe and adnexal structures. POP is very common. Many cases can be treated noninvasively with Kegel exercises or vaginal pessary. Although usually benign, advanced cases of POP may be associated with obstruction of the urinary or gastrointestinal tract, recurrent infection, or necrosis. Pessary use is safe and effective, but poorly fitting or neglected pessaries can become impacted or develop serious complications requiring surgical intervention.

REFERENCES

1. Borhart J. Emergency department management of vaginal bleeding in the nonpregnant patient. Emerg Med Pract 2013;15(8):1–20.
2. Jacobs AM, Alderman EM. Gynecologic examination of the prepubertal girl. Pediatr Rev 2014;35(3):97–104.
3. Merritt DF. Evaluation of vaginal bleeding in the preadolescent child. Semin Pediatr Surg 1998;7(1):35–42.
4. Committee on Practice and Ambulatory Medicine. Use of chaperones during the physical examination of the pediatric patient. Pediatrics 2011;127(5):991–3.
5. Söderström HF, Carlsson A, Börjesson A, et al. Vaginal bleeding in prepubertal girls: etiology and clinical management. J Pediatr Adolesc Gynecol 2016;29(3): 280–5.

6. Bumbuliene Ž, Venclavičiute K, Ramašauskaite D, et al. Microbiological findings of vulvovaginitis in prepubertal girls. Postgrad Med J 2014;90(1059):8–12.

7. Sugar NF, Graham EA. Common gynecologic problems in prepubertal girls. Pediatr Rev 2006;27(6):213–23.

8. Loveless M, Myint O. Vulvovaginitis- presentation of more common problems in pediatric and adolescent gynecology. Best Pract Res Clin Obstet Gynaecol 2018;48:14–27.

9. Hillyer S, Mooppan U, Kim H, et al. Diagnosis and treatment of urethral prolapse in children: experience with 34 cases. Urology 2009;73(5):1008–11.

10. Kondamudi NP, Gupta A, Watkins A, et al. Prepubertal girl with vaginal bleeding. J Emerg Med 2014;46(6):769–71.

11. Dwiggins M, Gomez-Lobo V. Current review of prepubertal vaginal bleeding. Curr Opin Obstet Gynecol 2017;29(5):322–7.

12. Nayak S, Witchel SF, Sanfilippo JS. Vaginal foreign body: a delayed diagnosis. J Pediatr Adolesc Gynecol 2014;27(6):e127–9.

13. Semaan A, Klein T, Vahdad MR, et al. Severe vaginal burns in a 5-year-old girl due to an alkaline battery in the vagina. J Pediatr Adolesc Gynecol 2015;28(5):e147–8.

14. Kyrgios I, Emmanouilidou E, Theodoridis T, et al. An unexpected cause of vaginal bleeding: The role of pelvic radiography. BMJ Case Rep 2014;2013–4. https://doi.org/10.1136/bcr-2013-202958.

15. Casey JT, Bjurlin MA, Cheng EY. Pediatric genital injury: an analysis of the national electronic injury surveillance system. Urology 2013;82(5):1125–30.

16. Dowlut-McElroy T, Higgins J, Williams KB, et al. Patterns of treatment of accidental genital trauma in girls. J Pediatr Adolesc Gynecol 2017;31(1):19–22.

17. Ngo AV, Otjen JP, Parisi MT, et al. Pediatric ovarian torsion: a pictorial review. Pediatr Radiol 2015;45(12):1845–55.

18. Childress KJ, Dietrich JE. Pediatric ovarian torsion. Surg Clin North Am 2017;97(1):209–21.

19. Anders JF, Powell EC. Urgency of evaluation and outcome of acute ovarian torsion in pediatric patients. Arch Pediatr Adolesc Med 2005;159(6):532–5.

20. Geimanaite L, Trainavicius K. Ovarian torsion in children: management and outcomes. J Pediatr Surg 2013;48(9):1946–53.

21. Murphy SL, Xu J, Kochanek KD, et al. Deaths: final data for 2015. Natl Vital Stat Rep 2017;66(6):1–75.

22. Raglan G, Lawrence H, Schulkin J. Obstetrician/gynecologist care considerations: practice changes in disease management with an aging patient population. Women's Health (Lond) 2014;10(2):155–60.

23. Lewiss RE, Saul T, Teng J. Gynecological disorders in geriatric emergency medicine. Am J Hosp Palliat Care 2009;26(3):219–27.

24. Lethaby A, Ro A, Roberts H. Local oestrogen for vaginal atrophy in postmenopausal women. Cochrane Database Syst Rev 2016;(8). CD001500. Available at: www.cochranelibrary.com.

25. Perkins KE, King MC. Geriatric gynecology. Emerg Med Clin North Am 2012;30(4):1007–19.

26. Committee on Gynecologic Practice of American College Obstetricians and Gynecologists. Practice bulletin - endometrial cancer. Obstet Gynecol 2015;125(4):1006–26.

27. Committee on Gynecologic Practice. The role of the obstetrician – gynecologist in the early detection of epithelial ovarian cancer. Obstet Gynecol 2011;130(3):146–9.

28. Committee on Practice Bulletins. Practice bulletin 168: cervical cancer screening and prevention. Obstet Gynecol 2014;128(4):111–30.

29. Committee on Gynecologic Practice of American College Obstetricians and Gynecologists. ACOG Committee opinion no. 509: management of vulvar intraepithelial neoplasia. Obstet Gynecol 2011;118(5):1192–4.

30. Committee on Gynecologic Practice. The role of transvaginal ultrasonography in evaluating the endometrium of women with postmenopausal bleeding. Obstet Gynecol 2018;131(5):124–9.

31. Fischerova D, Burgetova A. Imaging techniques for the evaluation of ovarian cancer. Best Pract Res Clin Obstet Gynaecol 2014;28(5):697–720.

32. Committee on Practice Bulletins. Practice bulletin 185: pelvic organ prolapse. Obstet Gynecol 2017;130(5):1170–2.

33. DeLancey JOL. The hidden epidemic of pelvic floor dysfunction: achievable goals for improved prevention and treatment. Am J Obstet Gynecol 2005; 192(5):1488–95.

34. Bump RC, Mattiasson A, Bø K, et al. The standardization of terminology of female pelvic organ prolapse and pelvic floor dysfunction. Am J Obstet Gynecol 1996; 175(1):10–7.

35. Bae EJ, Kang Y, Seo JW, et al. Obstructive uropathy by total uterine prolapse leading to end-stage renal disease. Ren Fail 2012;34(6):807–9.

36. Storey S, Aston M, Price S, et al. Women's experiences with vaginal pessary use. J Adv Nurs 2009;65(11):2350–7.

37. Ding J, Chen C, Song XC, et al. Changes in prolapse and urinary symptoms after successful fitting of a ring pessary with support in women with advanced pelvic organ prolapse: a prospective study. Urology 2016;87:70–5.

38. Oliver R, Thakar R, Sultan AH. The history and usage of the vaginal pessary: a review. Eur J Obstet Gynecol Reprod Biol 2011;156(2):125–30.

39. Abdulaziz M, Stothers L, Lazare D, et al. An integrative review and severity classification of complications related to pessary use in the treatment of female pelvic organ prolapse. Can Urol Assoc J 2015;9(5–6):E400–6.

40. Roberge RJ, McCandlish MM, Dorfsman ML. Urosepsis associated with vaginal pessary use. Ann Emerg Med 1999;33(5):581–3.

Acute Pelvic Pain

Kayla Dewey, MD[a],*, Cory Wittrock, MD[b]

KEYWORDS

- Pelvic pain • Ovarian torsion • Pelvic inflammatory disease • Ovarian cyst
- Nongynecologic pain

KEY POINTS

- Acute pelvic pain can have gynecologic and nongynecologic causes.
- Determining pregnancy status is the critical first step in the management of patients with pelvic pain who are of reproductive age.
- Pelvic ultrasound is the most useful imaging test for pelvic pathologic conditions.
- Ovarian torsion can occur with normal vascular flow on Doppler ultrasound.
- Pelvic inflammatory disease can occur without risk factors for sexually transmitted infections.
- Rare but serious complications of intrauterine devices include uterine perforation.

INTRODUCTION

Pelvic pain is a frequent complaint of female patients presenting to the emergency department (ED). Abdominal pain is the most common reason behind 5% to 10% of ED visits annually; exact prevalence of visits due to pelvic pain specifically is unknown, because pelvic pain is rarely separated from abdominal pain in the various studies and available survey data.[1–3] Pelvic pain can be a challenging complaint because of the wide array of possible pathologic conditions. Determining pregnancy status is the critical first step in the management of patients with pelvic pain who are of reproductive age. In nonpregnant patients, both gynecologic and nongynecologic causes of pelvic pain must be considered. Emergency physicians should understand the initial management of nonpregnant patients who present with acute pelvic pain as well as the critical diagnoses and how to safely disposition these patients from the ED.

EMERGENCY DEPARTMENT EVALUATION

The initial ED evaluation of the patient with pelvic pain includes general overall impression, identification of vital sign abnormalities, obtaining a history, and performing a

Disclosure Statement: No disclosures.
[a] Department of Emergency Medicine, University of Rochester Medical Center, 601 Elmwood Avenue, Rochester, NY 14642, USA; [b] Medstar Georgetown University Hospital, 3800 Reservoir Road Northwest, Washington, DC 20007, USA
* Corresponding author.
E-mail address: Kayla_Dewey@urmc.rochester.edu

Emerg Med Clin N Am 37 (2019) 207–218
https://doi.org/10.1016/j.emc.2019.01.012
0733-8627/19/© 2019 Elsevier Inc. All rights reserved.

emed.theclinics.com

physical examination. Characteristics of the pain, including timing and severity, associated symptoms, such as vomiting, fever, vaginal bleeding or discharge, history of similar symptoms from known diagnoses, and risk factors play a part in establishing an initial differential.[4] Because of the multiple organ systems that contribute to or are contained within the pelvis, a broad differential must be initially considered in these patients (**Table 1**).

Pregnancy status is the single most important determination for a patient of childbearing age presenting with pelvic pain. Urine pregnancy tests are widely available and most commonly used in the ED. Establishing pregnancy status is also possible via blood tests in the form of qualitative or quantitative β-human chorionic gonadotropin (β-hCG) levels. In the unstable patient, it may be necessary to use serum tests or point-of-care ultrasound to determine if there is an obvious pregnancy or free fluid in the abdomen. In stable patients, urine or blood β-hCG testing can be performed depending on the availability of specimens and clinician preference.

Traditionally, a full pelvic examination consisting of a bimanual and speculum examination is performed as part of the ED evaluation of nonpregnant patients with pelvic pain. A bimanual examination can be helpful in identifying cervical motion tenderness, or uterine or adnexal tenderness, and is necessary to make the diagnosis of pelvic inflammatory disease (PID). Speculum examination is frequently performed, although it often does not add useful clinical information. In one study of women presenting to the ED with either acute abdominal pain or vaginal bleeding, the pelvic examination findings were unexpected and changed clinical management in only 6% of patients.[5] Sexually transmitted infections (STI), such as *Chlamydia trachomatis* and *Neisseria gonorrhoeae*, can be detected from urine antigens, making obtaining cervical samples unnecessary. If urine antigen tests are unavailable, patients may self-administer vaginal swabs to obtain samples for STI testing. The decision to perform a pelvic examination ultimately rests with the patient and the clinician. In diagnosing gynecologic emergencies, history and a focused ultrasound examination were found to be the most successful combination, whereas physical examination did not add substantial diagnostic value.[6] Laboratory tests, such as complete blood counts, chemistry panels, and urinalysis, may be helpful especially if the cause of the patient's pain is suspected to be nongynecologic.

Many patients presenting to the ED with pelvic pain will require imaging studies. Indeed, up to 65% of patients presenting with nontraumatic abdominal or pelvic pain will receive an imaging study in the ED.[7] Because the differential diagnosis for pelvic and/or lower abdominal pain in women is so broad, choosing an initial imaging modality can be difficult. Ultrasound is the initial imaging modality of choice for women

Table 1
Gynecologic versus nongynecologic causes of pelvic pain

Gynecologic Causes	Nongynecologic Causes
Ovarian torsion	Appendicitis
Ovarian cyst	Nephrolithiasis
Pelvic inflammatory disease	Hernia
Tubo-ovarian abscess	Diverticulitis
Fibroid disease	Small bowel obstruction
Dysmenorrhea/menorrhagia	Cystitis/urinary tract infection
Malpositioned IUD	Adhesions/functional abdominal pain
Endometriosis	Musculoskeletal pain

with acute pelvic pain and concern for gynecologic cause because there is high sonographic resolution of pelvic organs, and ultrasound does not confer ionizing radiation, is less expensive compared with computed tomography (CT) or MRI, and is readily available in most EDs.[8] If the suspicion for nongynecologic causes of pelvic pain is significantly higher than the gynecologic causes, CT scans offer superior diagnostic efficacy and can be performed first.[9] If the CT shows concerning pelvic findings, a follow-up ultrasound should be performed to further evaluate the pelvic structures. In one study, 22% of CT examinations performed on women of reproductive age were found to have isolated pelvic conditions.[10] If a CT is entirely negative, there is little to no utility in obtaining an immediate follow-up ultrasound.[11] Reimaging the pelvis with ultrasound is also not useful if the CT detected abnormalities in which there is a characteristic diagnostic appearance, if the finding has a clearly established origin within the myometrium, or if there is an abnormality that has a limited differential diagnosis and requires temporal observation to distinguish further.[12]

GYNECOLOGIC CAUSES OF PELVIC PAIN

When considering the gynecologic causes of pelvic pain, it is helpful to divide the causes into adnexal causes, including ovarian cysts, ovarian torsion, PID, and tubo-ovarian abscess (TOA), and uterine causes, including dysmenorrhea, fibroids, and complications of intrauterine devices (IUDs).

ADNEXAL CAUSES
Ovarian Cysts

Ovarian cysts are a common cause for pelvic pain in women, with ruptured cysts more likely in women of reproductive age.[13] Most ovarian cysts begin as physiologic follicular or corpus luteal cysts; they can cause pain when they grow rapidly, hemorrhage, or rupture. Follicular cysts occur when the nondominant follicle does not reabsorb and instead grows in size. These cysts are thin-walled, avascular, and usually unilocular. Corpus luteal cysts, if they persist beyond menstruation, are thicker, with irregular and hypervascular walls.[8] Follicular cysts are more common than corpus luteal cysts; corpus luteal cysts are more likely to be symptomatic and more likely to rupture or hemorrhage.[14] Pathologic cysts, such as endometriomas, dermoid cysts, or cystic components of benign or malignant neoplasms, can also cause pain from growth, rupture, or hemorrhage.[15] Risk of cyst rupture increases with ovulation; there is an increased risk with ovulation induction treatments and a decreased risk with use of oral contraceptive pills.[16] Patients will usually report sudden-onset, unilateral, dull, or colicky pain, and sometimes symptom onset after sexual intercourse. A bimanual examination can be performed to evaluate for adnexal tenderness and the presence of an adnexal mass. Transvaginal ultrasound is the imaging modality of choice and will be able to characterize the cyst as well as free fluid. If a cyst has ruptured, the ovary may appear normal because the rupture has decompressed the cyst; however, a moderate to large amount of free fluid is usually present.[17] Assessment of hemoglobin and hematocrit is necessary in the presence of hemorrhage, and serial testing can be helpful in the disposition decision.

Management depends largely on the degree of pain and hemorrhage, and sometimes on the type of cyst or mass. Patients with cysts without concern for torsion and without large hemorrhage can be managed conservatively as outpatients with symptom control and follow-up with a gynecologist for a repeat ultrasound in 4 to 6 weeks.[17] Patients who are hemodynamically unstable with a large degree of hemorrhage require emergent gynecology consultation because they may require laparoscopy or admission for monitoring with serial examinations.[18,19] Rarely, a dermoid cyst (mature teratoma) can rupture and sebaceous material can spill into the abdominal cavity, leading to chemical peritonitis and hemorrhagic shock. These patients will almost always require emergency surgery.[20] Similarly, if an endometrioma ruptures, the patient can experience significant hemorrhage and will likely need surgical intervention.[21]

Ovarian Torsion

Ovarian torsion is a "can't-miss" diagnosis that must be made in the ED, because early diagnosis is critical in preserving ovarian function and future fertility. Although frequently discussed, it is an uncommon cause of pelvic pain, accounting for only 3% of gynecologic emergencies.[22] Torsion occurs when the adnexa, ovary, or more rarely the fallopian tube alone, completes at least one full turn around the long axis of the infundibulopelvic ligament and the tubo-ovarian ligament.[23] This leads to stromal edema because the venous system is impaired first, followed by hemorrhagic infarction and necrosis of the adnexal structures distal to the point of torsion. The degree of vascular compromise depends on the number and severity of rotations. The ovaries have dual blood supply from the ovarian and uterine arteries, and thus, torsion can occur without complete loss of vascularity.[24]

Patients will present with pelvic or lower abdominal pain, usually unilateral, and frequently with nausea and vomiting. Premenopausal women often describe the pain as acute, sharp, intermittent, colicky, and severe. Postmenopausal women more commonly describe continuous dull abdominal pain.[25] Risk factors for adnexal torsion include previous torsion, adnexal masses or cysts, use of assisted reproductive technologies leading to ovarian hyperstimulation, polycystic ovarian syndrome, pregnancy, and previous tubal ligation.[26] Endometriosis, PID, and malignant lesions make torsion less likely because they have a role in affixing the ovary to the pelvic wall.[27] Torsion occurs more frequently on the right side compared with the left, because mass effect of the sigmoid colon is thought to prevent left adnexal twisting. Physical examination findings include localized lower abdominal/pelvic tenderness, adnexal tenderness, or mass on bimanual examination, and severe cases can result in frank peritonitis. Laboratory tests rarely add to the diagnosis beyond the initial pregnancy test, although a leukocytosis has been shown to have a modest positive predictive value for adnexal torsion.[28]

Pelvic ultrasonography is the initial study of choice for ovarian torsion. Transvaginal ultrasound and color Doppler should be used whenever possible for increased accuracy. Previous studies have cited rates of diagnostic accuracy from 74.6% to 87%.[29,30] There is a spectrum of sonographic findings, ranging from ovarian enlargement and edema to complete loss of vascular flow (**Table 2**). The presence of the "whirlpool sign," a clockwise or counterclockwise wrapping of hypoechoic vessels around a central axis, correlates closely with surgically proven torsion.[31,32] In addition, women with pathologic vascular flow were statistically significantly more likely to have surgically demonstrated torsion.[33] However, it is essential to know that the persistence of arterial flow on Doppler does not rule out adnexal torsion, because several factors can contribute to the preservation of arterial flow despite active torsion, including dual arterial supply to the ovary, intermittent and partial torsion, or isolated venous occlusion.[24] Although CT is not the ideal study for evaluation of the pelvic organs, patients with torsion may have received a CT before ultrasound because of concern for other causes of pain. Common CT findings that should raise concern for ovarian torsion include displacement of the adnexa to the contralateral side, deviation of the uterus to the side of the torsed ovary, adnexal enlargement, ovarian cysts

Table 2	
Ultrasonographic findings in ovarian torsion	
Early/Indeterminate Findings	**Late/Diagnostic Findings**
Ovary size >4 cm	"Follicular ring sign"
Hyperechoic stromal edema	"Whirlpool sign"
Peripherally displaced follicles	Venous flow impedance
Pelvic ascites	Arterial flow impedance

or masses, twist of the ovarian pedicle, infiltration of pelvic fat, and pelvic ascites.[34,35] In one study of surgery-proven cases of torsion, CT and ultrasound showed equal diagnostic performance.[36] Although a CT with concerning features for torsion should prompt increased suspicion and may incite the evaluating clinician to consult gynecology, an ultrasound may provide further evidence for the consulting team. MRI is another imaging modality option, although often limited in availability from the ED. MRI allows for the distinction between the edema of the ovary and the adjacent fallopian tube, but similar to the limitations of ultrasound, persistence of adnexal enhancement does not exclude torsion.[24,37]

Ovarian torsion is a surgical emergency, yet several studies have consistently demonstrated that the diagnosis is often missed initially. For most patients with torsion who have a delayed diagnosis, clinicians failed to consider the diagnosis at initial presentation.[22] Timely detection is key because there is a higher chance of successful detorsion, and therefore, preservation of ovarian function, the earlier the diagnosis is made. Gynecologic consultation should be obtained early in the ED course of any patient with suspected ovarian torsion. If no gynecologist is immediately available, transfer to a tertiary center for higher level of care is warranted. If the adnexa can be successfully detorsed in the operating room, there is an approximately 80% chance of normal follicular development on follow-up ultrasound.[38] Salpingo-oophorectomy may be required if the adnexa remains necrotic after detorsion. If a cyst or other adnexal mass is found and is considered to be the cause of torsion, cystectomy or cyst drainage is usually performed; this along with adnexal fixation has been shown to significantly reduce the chance of retorsion.[39] In postmenopausal patients with an adnexal mass concerning for malignancy, ultimate surgical care may be delayed because more extensive resections with biopsies may be required.[40]

Pelvic Inflammatory Disease and Tubo-Ovarian Abscess

PID is an infection of the upper genital tract in women and may include the uterus, fallopian tubes, and ovaries. Cervicitis is infection limited to the cervix; endometritis, salpingitis, and oophoritis all fall under the umbrella of PID. TOA is a complication in which infection becomes localized and contained into abscess formation. Other complications include peritonitis, pyosalpinx, and perihepatitis (Fitz-Hugh-Curtis syndrome). Long-term sequelae of PID include increased risk for ectopic pregnancy, infertility, recurrent infection, and chronic pelvic pain.[41] Most acute infections (<30 days' duration) are attributed to untreated STIs, including N gonorrhoeae and C trachomatis or bacterial vaginosis-associated microbes. The remainder of cases are attributed to respiratory or enteric organisms that have colonized the lower genital tract.[42] Although most patients have mild to moderate disease and many can be safely treated with outpatient management, serious complications can occur, such as Fitz-Hugh-Curtis syndrome (4%–6% of patients with PID) and TOA (3%–16% of patients hospitalized for PID).[41]

EMERGENCY DEPARTMENT EVALUATION

PID is largely a clinical diagnosis. PID should be suspected in any sexually active woman presenting with pelvic or lower abdominal pain. Women who are younger (<25), report a higher number of sexual partners, lack of condom use, recent STI treatment, or HIV-positive status are at increased risk.[41] Patients often present with common and nonspecific symptoms, such as pelvic pain, vaginal discharge, dysuria, and postcoital bleeding. Systemic symptoms, such as nausea, vomiting, and fevers, are less common in uncomplicated PID.[43]

Patients suspected of having PID should have a bimanual examination to evaluate for cervical motion tenderness, uterine tenderness, or adnexal tenderness. Patients with pyosalpinx or a TOA may have a palpable adnexal mass.[44] A speculum examination can be done to examine for cervical discharge and friability.[41] Laboratory tests beyond the initial pregnancy test include nucleic acid amplification tests for N gonorrhoeae/C trachomatis from either cervical or vaginal swabs or from first-void urine.[45] Cervical wet mount can be useful in detecting bacterial vaginosis and trichomoniasis. Patients who have recently completed an antibiotic course for gonorrhea or chlamydia should have a cervical culture sent in order to identify potentially antibiotic-resistant organisms.[41]

Pelvic ultrasonography is often obtained in patients with suspicion for PID in order to evaluate for other potential causes of pain as well as to evaluate for complications of PID. Patients with mild PID will usually have normal ultrasounds. However, ultrasound can have some findings indicative of PID, including thick tubal walls and the cogwheel sign.[46] Other nonspecific findings, including incomplete septations, polycystic ovaries, adnexal masses, free fluid, and hydrosalpinx, are not helpful in differentiating between patients with PID versus those without.[41] CT and MRI can also be used but have low sensitivity in mild to moderate PID. MRI has superior resolution when compared with CT in identifying tubal thickening.[47]

Current guidelines from the Centers for Disease Control and Prevention recommend that presumptive therapy for PID be initiated in sexually active women with unexplained pelvic pain and one or more of the following: cervical motion tenderness, uterine tenderness, or adnexal tenderness. Although this may seem overly expansive, these criteria have a sensitivity of greater than 95%.[48] Additional criteria can support the diagnosis of PID but are not required to initiate treatment (**Table 3**). Given that the consequences of untreated PID include future infertility, this broad definition helps to minimize the rates of misdiagnosis.

Once PID has been clinically diagnosed, treatment and disposition depend on degree of severity. Patients with mild to moderately severe PID can receive intramuscular and oral antibiotics (**Table 4**) and be safely discharged, with the instructions to abstain from

Table 3 Diagnosis of pelvic inflammatory disease	
Unexplained pelvic or lower abdominal pain plus one or more minimum criteria on examination	
Minimum criteria:	Additional criteria, not required:
• Cervical motion tenderness • Uterine tenderness • Adnexal tenderness	• Oral temperature >101°F (38.3°C) • Abnormal cervical discharge or cervical friability • Presence of white blood cells on microscopy of vaginal fluid • Elevated erythrocyte sedimentation rate • Elevated C-reactive protein • Cervical infection with N gonorrhoeae or C trachomatis

Table 4
Antibiotic regimens for pelvic inflammatory disease

Mild to Moderate PID	Severe PID	TOA
Ceftriaxone 250 mg intramuscularly × 1	Cefotetan 2 g IV q12h or Cefoxitin 2 g IV q6h	Same as for severe PID
AND	AND	AND
Doxycycline 100 mg po bid × 14 d	Doxycycline 100 mg orally or IV q12h	Clindamycin, metronidazole, or ampicillin/sulbactam

sexual intercourse until treatment is complete and until their partner or partners have been treated. It is important to note that although cervicitis may be treated with a single dose of intramuscular ceftriaxone and a single dose of oral azithromycin, this treatment regimen is not sufficient for PID. Patients with severe disease should be admitted for intravenous (IV) antibiotics and further monitoring; this includes patients who have hemodynamic instability, peritonitis, severe systemic symptoms, concern for treatment failure of oral antibiotics, and inability to tolerate oral antibiotics.[42] Patients with a TOA should be observed for at least 24 hours to ensure clinical stability and improvement.[48] If there is evidence of TOA rupture, urgent gynecologic consult is needed for operative management. Antibiotic regimens should be broadened to include coverage of anaerobic organisms in patients with TOA because of their higher prevalence (see **Table 4**). Special consideration should be made in patients with an IUD and PID; in most cases, the IUD is left in place with no difference in patient outcomes.[49]

UTERINE CAUSES

Acute pelvic pain can also be due to pathologic conditions localized to the uterus. Dysmenorrhea, or painful cramps that coincide with menstruation, is one of the most common causes of pelvic pain in women of reproductive age.[50] Primary dysmenorrhea is pain in the absence of recognizable pelvic pathologic condition, whereas secondary dysmenorrhea is from an identified cause. Primary dysmenorrhea usually occurs in adolescents and younger women, whereas endometriosis is the most common cause of secondary dysmenorrhea. Symptoms may include menorrhagia, dyspareunia, postcoital bleeding, and infertility.[51] Most patients with dysmenorrhea can be safely discharged from the ED with symptom control and outpatient gynecology follow-up. Nonsteroidal anti-inflammatory drugs, such as ibuprofen and naproxen, are first-line treatments for pain control. Hormonal contraceptives are commonly recommended, although there are no large studies to suggest efficacy.[52] These contraceptives may be initiated from the ED if the clinician desires and if the patient has adequate follow-up care.

Fibroids are another common cause of pelvic pain and are found in up to 70% to 80% of women by age 50.[53] Patients with uterine fibroids may be asymptomatic with incidentally found fibroids, or they may be chronically or acutely symptomatic. Twenty percent to 50% of women with symptomatic fibroids report a significant impact on their quality of life.[54] Uterine fibroids are the most common gynecologic tumor; they are benign and arise from the uterine smooth muscle tissue or myometrium. Fibroids, or myomas, can be solitary or multiple and vary in size, location, and vascularity. Subserosal fibroids project outside the uterus; intramural are contained within the myometrium, and submucosal project into the cavity of the uterus.[54] Fibroids are a common source of menorrhagia, but they rarely cause acute pelvic pain unless they have degenerated, have torsed, or are associated with adenomyosis or endometriosis. Larger fibroids may impact neighboring anatomic structures and cause pelvic pressure, and bowel and urinary symptoms. Acute torsion of a subserosal fibroid around its vascular pedicle can cause ischemia and peritonitis; although this is very rare, it is a surgical emergency requiring gynecologic consultation.[55,56] In the absence of a surgical emergency or vaginal bleeding requiring observation or transfusion, patients with symptomatic fibroids can safely be discharged from the ED with close gynecology follow-up.

Another rare but important cause of pelvic pain is complications of IUDs. As the use of IUDs has increased in recent years, so too has the need for the emergency clinician to understand possible complications and side effects. Patients can present with postinsertion bleeding and uterine cramping, which can be safely managed conservatively if there is no evidence of severe bleeding or uterine perforation. Perforation is rare, occurring in 1 to 2/1000 patients, usually immediately postinsertion with one-third occurring 12 months after insertion.[57,58] Lactation and recent delivery are independent cofactors for increased risk of perforation following IUD insertion.[59] Rarely, IUDs can be spontaneously expelled from the uterus. To evaluate for perforation or IUD expulsion, a speculum examination can be performed to visualize IUD strings in the cervical os. If the strings are not visualized or appear unusually short, an ultrasound can be performed to identify IUD position. If ultrasound confirms correct IUD position, no further action is necessary. If the IUD is not visualized in the uterus on ultrasound, a kidney, ureter, bladder (KUB) radiograph can be obtained. If the KUB does not show the IUD, it can be assumed that the IUD was expelled. If the KUB shows an intraperitoneal IUD, gynecology should be consulted for surgical removal. Rarely, patients present with hemodynamic instability and peritonitis. These patients should be emergently evaluated for laparoscopy. Expert consultation is recommended for all patients with confirmed or suspected uterine perforation.

NONGYNECOLOGIC CAUSES

Appendicitis is the most common cause of abdominal pain that requires surgery, and the presentation can often mimic that of right adnexal torsion.[24] In young women in which the two diagnoses are equally suspected, initial imaging with ultrasonography is recommended to help identify adnexal pathologic conditions early, preserve fertility if torsion is confirmed, and avoid radiation from CT. As outlined in earlier discussion, many patients with suspicion for nongynecologic causes receive CT imaging first, which can identify some pelvic pathologic conditions that may be the source of the patient's pain. Other causes in addition to appendicitis that should be considered include nephrolithiasis, diverticulitis, cystitis/pyelonephritis, hernias, small bowel obstruction, musculoskeletal pain, functional abdominal pain, and pain from adhesions of prior surgeries (see **Table 1**). It is important to remember that abdominal and pelvic pathologic conditions often have poorly localizing symptoms, and it may be necessary to pursue further imaging or testing if the initial workup is unrevealing.

SUMMARY

Acute pelvic pain in women is often related to the pelvic organs, but it can be difficult to distinguish between gynecologic and nongynecologic causes on initial history and examination only. Advanced imaging with pelvic ultrasound and CT imaging can help delineate the cause. Determining pregnancy status is the critical first step in the management of patients with pelvic pain who are of reproductive age. Ovarian torsion is a serious cause of acute pelvic pain and can occur with normal vascular flow on Doppler ultrasound. PID can be difficult to diagnose, and clinicians should have a low threshold for initiating presumptive treatment to avoid serious long-term sequela, such as infertility. Many pelvic conditions, such as ovarian cysts, fibroids, and dysmenorrhea, can safely be managed conservatively as outpatients. Rare but serious complications of IUDs include uterine perforation and device expulsion. Emergency clinicians must be well versed in the approach to pelvic pain and prepared to manage the various complications that can arise.

REFERENCES

1. Mura P, Serra E, Marinangeli F, et al. Prospective study on prevalence, intensity, type, and therapy of acute pain in a second-level urban emergency department. J Pain Res 2017;10:2781–8.
2. Cervellin G, Mora R, Ticinesi A, et al. Epidemiology and outcomes of acute abdominal pain in a large urban Emergency Department: retrospective analysis of 5,340 cases. Ann Transl Med 2016;4(19):362.
3. Kamin RA, Nowicki TA, Courtney DS, et al. Pearls and pitfalls in the emergency department evaluation of abdominal pain. Emerg Med Clin North Am 2003; 21(1):61–72, vi.
4. Fauconnier A, Dallongeville E, Huchon C, et al. Measurement of acute pelvic pain intensity in gynecology: a comparison of five methods. Obstet Gynecol 2009; 113(2 Pt 1):260–9.
5. Brown J, Fleming R, Aristzabel J, et al. Does pelvic exam in the emergency department add useful information? West J Emerg Med 2011;12(2):208–12.
6. Varas C, Ravit M, Mimoun C, et al. Optimal combination of non-invasive tools for the early detection of potentially life-threatening emergencies in gynecology. PLoS One 2016;11(9):e0162301.
7. Nagurney JT, Brown DF, Chang Y, et al. Use of diagnostic testing in the emergency department for patients presenting with non-traumatic abdominal pain. J Emerg Med 2003;25(4):363–71.
8. Dupuis CS, Kim YH. Ultrasonography of adnexal causes of acute pelvic pain in pre-menopausal non-pregnant women. Ultrasonography 2015;34(4):258–67.
9. Pages-Bouic E, Millet I, Curros-Doyon F, et al. Acute pelvic pain in females in septic and aseptic contexts. Diagn Interv Imaging 2015;96(10):985–95.
10. Asch E, Shah S, Kang T, et al. Use of pelvic computed tomography and sonography in women of reproductive age in the emergency department. J Ultrasound Med 2013;32(7):1181–7.
11. Gao Y, Lee K, Camacho M. Utility of pelvic ultrasound following negative abdominal and pelvic CT in the emergency room. Clin Radiol 2013;68(11):e586–92.
12. Patel MD, Dubinsky TJ. Reimaging the female pelvis with ultrasound after CT: general principles. Ultrasound Q 2007;23(3):177–87.
13. Raziel A, RonEl R, Pansky M, et al. Current management of ruptured corpus luteum. Eur J Obstet Gynecol Reprod Biol 1993;50:77.
14. Vandermeer FQ, Wong-You-Cheong JJ. Imaging of acute pelvic pain. Clin Obstet Gynecol 2009;52:2–20.
15. Bottomley C, Bourne T. Diagnosis and management of ovarian cyst accidents. Best Pract Res Clin Obstet Gynaecol 2009;23(5):711–24.
16. Milsom I, Korver T. Ovulation incidence with oral contraceptives: a literature review. J Fam Plann Reprod Health Care 2008;34:237.
17. McWilliams GD, Hill MJ, Dietrich CS. Gynecologic emergencies. Surg Clin North Am 2008;88(2):265–83.

18. Fiaschetti V, Ricci A, Scarano AL, et al. Hemoperitoneum from corpus luteal cyst rupture: a practical approach in emergency room. Case Rep Emerg Med 2014; 2014:252657.

19. Kim JH, Lee SM, Lee JH, et al. Successful conservative management of ruptured ovarian cysts with hemoperitoneum in healthy women. PLoS One 2014;9(3): e91171.

20. Koshiba H. Severe chemical peritonitis caused by spontaneous rupture of an ovarian mature cystic teratoma: a case report. J Reprod Med 2007;52:965.

21. Ye M, Huang L, Wang Y. A massive haemorrhage caused by rupture of cystic cervical endometriosis. J Obstet Gynaecol 2012;32:498.

22. Houry D, Abbott JT. Ovarian torsion: a fifteen-year review. Ann Emerg Med 2001; 38(2):156–9.

23. Huchon C, Fauconnier A. Adnexal torsion: a literature review. Eur J Obstet Gynecol Reprod Biol 2010;150(1):8–12.

24. Ssi-Yan-Kai G, Rivain AL, Trichot C, et al. What every radiologist should know about adnexal torsion. Emerg Radiol 2018;25(1):51–9.

25. Cohen A, Solomon N, Almog B, et al. Adnexal torsion in postmenopausal women: clinical presentation and risk of ovarian malignancy. J Minim Invasive Gynecol 2017;24(1):94–7.

26. Asfour V, Varma R, Menon P. Clinical risk factors for ovarian torsion. J Obstet Gynaecol 2015;35(7):721–5.

27. Sommerville M, Grimes DA, Koonings PP, et al. Ovarian neoplasms and the risk of adnexal torsion. Am J Obstet Gynecol 1991;164(2):577–8.

28. Melcer Y, Maymon R, Pekar-Zlotin M, et al. Does she have adnexal torsion? Prediction of adnexal torsion in reproductive age women. Arch Gynecol Obstet 2018; 297(3):685–90.

29. Mashiach R, Melamed N, Gilad N, et al. Sonographic diagnosis of ovarian torsion: accuracy and predictive factors. J Ultrasound Med 2011;30(9):1205–10.

30. Lee EJ, Kwon HC, Joo HJ, et al. Diagnosis of ovarian torsion with color Doppler sonography: depiction of twisted vascular pedicle. J Ultrasound Med 1998;17(2): 83–9.

31. Valsky DV, Esh-Broder E, Cohen SM, et al. Added value of the gray-scale whirlpool sign in the diagnosis of adnexal torsion. Ultrasound Obstet Gynecol 2010; 36(5):630–4.

32. Vijayaraghavan SB. Sonographic whirlpool sign in ovarian torsion. J Ultrasound Med 2004;23(12):1643–9.

33. Bar-On S, Mashiach R, Stockheim D, et al. Emergency laparoscopy for suspected ovarian torsion: are we too hasty to operate? Fertil Steril 2010;93(6): 2012–5.

34. Hiller N, Appelbaum L, Simanovsky N, et al. CT features of adnexal torsion. AJR Am J Roentgenol 2007;189(1):124–9.

35. Mandoul C, Verheyden C, Curros-Doyon F, et al. Diagnostic performance of CT signs for predicting adnexal torsion in women presenting with an adnexal mass and abdominal pain: a case-control study. Eur J Radiol 2018;98:75–81.

36. Swenson DW, Lourenco AP, Beaudoin FL, et al. Ovarian torsion: case-control study comparing the sensitivity and specificity of ultrasonography and computed tomography for diagnosis in the emergency department. Eur J Radiol 2014;83(4): 733–8.

37. Béranger-Gibert S, Sakly H, Ballester M, et al. Diagnostic value of MR imaging in the diagnosis of adnexal torsion. Radiology 2016;279(2):461–70.

38. Huang C, Hong MK, Ding DC. A review of ovary torsion. Ci Ji Yi Xue Za Zhi 2017; 29(3):143–7.
39. Tsafrir Z, Hasson J, Levin I, et al. Adnexal torsion: cystectomy and ovarian fixation are equally important in preventing recurrence. Eur J Obstet Gynecol Reprod Biol 2012;162(2):203–5.
40. Becker JH, de Graaff J, Vos MC, et al. Torsion of the ovary: a known but frequently missed diagnosis. Eur J Emerg Med 2009;16(3):124–6.
41. Bugg CW, Taira T, Zaurova M. Pelvic inflammatory disease: diagnosis and treatment in the emergency department. Emerg Med Pract 2016;18(12):1–20.
42. Brunham RC, Gottlieb SL, Paavonen J. Pelvic inflammatory disease. N Engl J Med 2015;372(21):2039–48.
43. Chappell CA, Wiesenfeld HC. Pathogenesis, diagnosis, and management of severe pelvic inflammatory disease and tuboovarian abscess. Clin Obstet Gynecol 2012;55(4):893–903.
44. Kim HY, Yang JI, Moon C. Comparison of severe pelvic inflammatory disease, pyosalpinx and tubo-ovarian abscess. J Obstet Gynaecol Res 2015;41(5):742–6.
45. Chernesky M, Jang D, Gilchrist J, et al. Head-to-head comparison of second-generation nucleic acid amplification tests for detection of *Chlamydia trachomatis* and *Neisseria gonorrhoeae* on urine samples from female subjects and self-collected vaginal swabs. J Clin Microbiol 2014;52(7):2305–10.
46. Polena V, Huchon C, Varas Ramos C, et al. Non-invasive tools for the diagnosis of potentially life-threatening gynaecological emergencies: a systematic review. PLoS One 2015;10(2):e0114189.
47. Li W, Zhang Y, Cui Y, et al. Pelvic inflammatory disease: evaluation of diagnostic accuracy with conventional MR with added diffusion-weighted imaging. Abdom Imaging 2013;38(1):193–200.
48. Workowski KA, Bolan GA. Sexually transmitted diseases treatment guidelines, 2015. MMWR Recomm Rep 2015;64(3):1–137.
49. Tepper NK, Steenland MW, Gaffield ME, et al. Retention of intrauterine devices in women who acquire pelvic inflammatory disease: a systematic review. Contraception 2013;87(5):655–60.
50. Latthe P, Latthe M, Say L, et al. WHO systematic review of prevalence of chronic pelvic pain: a neglected reproductive health morbidity. BMC Public Health 2006; 6:177.
51. Osayande AS, Mehulic S. Diagnosis and initial management of dysmenorrhea. Am Fam Physician 2014;89(5):341–6.
52. Wong CL, Farquhar C, Roberts H, et al. Oral contraceptive pill for primary dysmenorrhoea. Cochrane Database Syst Rev 2009;(4):CD002120.
53. Day Baird D, Dunson DB, Hill MC, et al. High cumulative incidence of uterine leiomyoma in black and white women: ultrasound evidence. Am J Obstet Gynecol 2003;188:100–7.
54. Vilos GA, Allaire C, Laberge PY, et al. The management of uterine leiomyomas. J Obstet Gynaecol Can 2015;37(2):157–78.
55. Imai A, Ichigo S, Takagi H, et al. Pelvic tumors with normal-appearing shapes of ovaries and uterus presenting as an emergency (Review). Oncol Lett 2012;4(1): 10–4.
56. Charles K, Raoul K, Idrissa G, et al. Torsion of uterine fibroid: a rare cause of acute pelvic pain: about one case. Gynecol Obstet Case Rep 2017;3(3):56.
57. Heinemann K, Reed S, Moehner S, et al. Risk of uterine perforation with levonorgestrel-releasing and copper intrauterine devices in the European Active Surveillance Study on Intrauterine Devices. Contraception 2015;91(4):274–9.

58. Barnett C, Moehner S, Do Minh T, et al. Perforation risk and intra-uterine devices: results of the EURAS-IUD 5-year extension study. Eur J Contracept Reprod Health Care 2017;22(6):424–8.
59. Heinemann K, Barnett C, Reed S, et al. IUD use among parous women and risk of uterine perforation: a secondary analysis. Contraception 2017;95(6):605–7.

Complications in Early Pregnancy

Elizabeth Pontius, MD, RDMS[a], Julie T. Vieth, MBChB[b],*

KEYWORDS

- Nausea and vomiting in pregnancy • Hyperemesis gravidarum
- Spontaneous miscarriage • Threatened miscarriage • Ectopic pregnancy
- Pregnancy of unknown location

KEY POINTS

- Nausea and vomiting in pregnancy are common and can be managed with oral medications but may require intravenous medications or fluids.
- When a patient presents with vaginal bleeding in early pregnancy, ectopic pregnancy must be ruled out.
- All patients presenting with vaginal bleeding or abdominal pain should have a pelvic ultrasound to evaluate for ectopic pregnancy regardless of β-hCG level.
- If an intrauterine pregnancy is established, threatened miscarriage should be considered.
- If neither ectopic pregnancy, nor intrauterine pregnancy is established, patients should be managed as a pregnancy of unknown location with serial ultrasound and β-hCG measurements.

INTRODUCTION

The first trimester of pregnancy can be a difficult time for many women. Many women suffer from nausea and vomiting, which can range from mild discomfort, managed by dietary modifications and/or oral medications, to severe, leading to significant dehydration and requiring intravenous fluids and medications. Women also may experience vaginal bleeding early in pregnancy, and ectopic pregnancy must be ruled out. If a viable intrauterine pregnancy (IUP) is identified, miscarriage is still possible. If neither an IUP nor ectopic pregnancy can be established, pregnancy of unknown location (PUL) is diagnosed. Patients with PUL should return for serial evaluations until either an IUP, ectopic pregnancy, or failed pregnancy is diagnosed.

The authors have no financial disclosures.
[a] Department of Emergency Medicine, Georgetown University School of Medicine, MedStar Georgetown University Hospital, MedStar Washington Hospital Center, 110 Irving Street, Northwest, NA 1177, Washington, DC 20010, USA; [b] Department of Emergency Medicine, Canton-Potsdam Hospital, 50 Leroy Street, Potsdam, NY 13676, USA
* Corresponding author.
E-mail address: viethjt@gmail.com

Emerg Med Clin N Am 37 (2019) 219–237
https://doi.org/10.1016/j.emc.2019.01.004
0733-8627/19/© 2019 Elsevier Inc. All rights reserved.

NAUSEA AND VOMITING IN EARLY PREGNANCY
Background and Definitions

Nausea and vomiting of pregnancy (NVP) is extremely common, affecting approximately 50% to 80% of pregnant women. Despite the colloquial term "morning sickness," NVP affects women at all times of day and night. Approximately one-third of those affected with NVP will require medical intervention and NVP is the most frequent reason for hospital admission during the first 20 weeks of pregnancy.[1,2] Although some consider NVP to be a "normal" part of pregnancy, for many women it affects quality of life, contributes to higher rates of depression, can strain family relationships, and was estimated to have had an economic burden of $1.77 billion in 2012 in the United States.[3,4]

NVP typically begins between 6 and 9 weeks' gestation, peaks at approximately 12 weeks, and in 50% of women, symptoms will abate by 14 weeks.[5] By 22 weeks, 90% of women will have resolution of their symptoms.[6]

At the most severe end of the spectrum of NVP is the condition known as hyperemesis gravidarum (HG). HG is estimated to affect 0.3% to 3.0% of pregnant women.[7] Generally, HG is a clinical diagnosis.[7,8] Patients with HG have intractable vomiting, evidence of starvation (ketonuria, dehydration, or electrolyte imbalance), or weight loss of 5% or more.[7,9,10] There is no single test to diagnose HG.[11]

Etiology and Risk Factors

The cause of NVP is debatable and likely multifactorial, including genetic, gastrointestinal, and hormonal factors. Women with a first-degree female relative with the condition are more likely to have NVP. Hormones possibly contributing to NVP and HG include human chorionic gonadotropin (hCG), estrogen, progesterone, serotonin, and thyroid hormone. However, the actual role of hormones in the development of NVP is unclear.[3] Women with multiple gestation, gestational trophoblastic disease, a fetus with triploidy including trisomy 21, and hydrops fetalis are associated with higher rates of HG.[12]

Complications and Long-Term Outcomes

Mild NVP is associated with good fetal outcomes and with lower rates of miscarriage in the first trimester. Unlike mild NVP, HG does have significant morbidity and can lead to adverse birth outcomes.[3] Rare but serious maternal complications of HG include Wernicke encephalopathy, acute renal failure, liver function abnormalities, splenic avulsion, esophageal rupture, and pneumothorax.[13]

Emergency Department Evaluation

For patients presenting to the emergency department (ED) with nausea and vomiting, a large differential diagnosis must be considered (**Box 1**). Nausea or vomiting that starts after 9 weeks' gestation, abdominal pain, diarrhea, or fever all point toward diagnoses other than NVP or HG and should be investigated accordingly.[9] Laboratory tests for NVP might include serum electrolytes, liver function tests, and urinalysis, both for infectious markers as well as ketones. A pelvic ultrasound can be considered to rule out molar pregnancy and a multiple-gestation pregnancy.[2,9,14] Several lifestyle and dietary modifications are suggested for NVP, but there are few data to support these recommendations (**Box 2**). Approximately 10% to 15% of women will not respond to these changes and will go on to need prescribed medications.[9,15] The American College of Obstetricians and Gynecologists (ACOG) advises that early treatment of NVP should be offered to help prevent progression to HG.[7]

Box 1
Differential diagnosis of pregnant patients with nausea and vomiting

Gastrointestinal conditions
- Gastroenteritis
- Gastroparesis
- Achalasia
- Biliary tract disease
- Hepatitis
- Intestinal obstruction
- Peptic ulcer disease
- Pancreatitis
- Appendicitis

Conditions of the genitourinary tract
- Pyelonephritis
- Uremia
- Ovarian torsion
- Kidney stones
- Degenerating uterine leiomyoma

Metabolic conditions
- Diabetic ketoacidosis
- Porphyria
- Addison disease
- Hyperthyroidism
- Hyperparathyroidism

Neurologic disorders
- Pseudotumor cerebri
- Vestibular lesions
- Migraine headaches
- Tumors of the central nervous system
- Lymphocytic hypophysitis

Miscellaneous conditions
- Drug toxicity or intolerance
- Psychological conditions

Pregnancy-related conditions
- Acute fatty liver of pregnancy
- Preeclampsia

Reprinted with permission from the American College of Obstetricians and Gynecologists. From Goodwin TM. Hyperemesis gravidarum. Obstetrics and Gynecology Clinics of North America 2008;35(3):401–17, *with permission from* the Foreign Policy Research Institute.

Box 2
Lifestyle and dietary modifications for the treatment of nausea and vomiting of pregnancy

Lifestyle Modifications	Dietary Modifications
<ul><li>Avoid sensory stimuli (odors, heat, humidity, noise, flickering lights)</li><li>Increased rest</li><li>Avoid brushing teeth immediately after meals</li><li>Allow food to digest before lying down</li></ul>	<ul><li>Frequent small meals to avoid empty and full stomach</li><li>Avoidance of spicy or high-fat foods</li><li>Eliminate iron-containing prenatal vitamin (unless anemic); substitute folic acid</li><li>High-protein snacks</li><li>Crackers before rising in the morning</li><li>Maintain adequate hydration</li></ul>

Data from Tian R, MacGibbon K, Martin B, et al. Analysis of pre- and post-pregnancy issues in women with hyperemesis gravidarum. Auton Neurosci 2017;202:73–8; and Anderka M, Mitchell AA, Louik C, et al. Medications used to treat nausea and vomiting of pregnancy and the risk of selected birth defects. Birth Defects Res A Clin Mol Teratol 2012;94(1):22–30.

Treatment of patients with NVP and HG begins with volume replacement. Oral rehydration may be sufficient to restore euvolemic status for patients with mild symptoms. Patients with HG will likely need intravenous fluids. Both normal saline and 5% dextrose with normal saline have been shown to be effective.[5,8] In the rare case in which Wernicke encephalopathy is suspected, 100 mg of intravenous thiamine should be administered before any dextrose-containing solution.[16]

While patients are being rehydrated, interventions to treat the nausea and vomiting also should be implemented. Multiple medication choices exist for ED use and others are available for home use. Almost all medications used for NVP are prescribed off-label, with the exception of the combination medication pyridoxine plus doxylamine.

Vitamin B6, or pyridoxine hydrochloride, a water-soluble vitamin, is considered first-line pharmacologic treatment for NVP when nonpharmacologic options have failed. This can be given alone (10 mg to 25 mg by mouth) up to 75 mg per day and has been shown to be effective in the treatment of NVP.[8] It also can be given in combination with doxylamine (10 mg to 20 mg by mouth). The combination product comes as two versions in the United States and is available only by prescription, with some insurance companies limiting coverage. Diclegis is a delayed-release version in the United States sold as 10 mg of doxylamine and 10 mg of pyridoxine to be started at bedtime. Bonjesta is an extended-release version sold as 20 mg of each component with half the dose released immediately and half the dose released in an extended fashion. These are the only medications currently on the market specifically approved by the Food and Drug Administration for the treatment of NVP.[17] Multiple cohort and case-control studies have demonstrated its effectiveness and fetal safety.[6] A double-blind, multicenter, placebo-controlled randomized controlled trial (RCT) showed that pyridoxine/doxylamine was not associated with any increased risk in adverse events compared with placebo.[18] The same study population was used to determine effectiveness, and patients taking pyridoxine/doxylamine had significant improvement in NVP symptoms compared with placebo.[19] Side effects listed include somnolence, headache, dizziness, and dry mouth.[6]

If pyridoxine/doxylamine is not controlling symptoms, ACOG recommends trying either an antihistamine, dimenhydrinate or diphenhydramine, or a dopamine antagonist, such as prochlorperazine, promethazine, or metoclopramide. The antihistamines act on the trigger zone chemoreceptors. Multiple studies have demonstrated both their efficacy in NVP as well as safety in pregnancy.[3,20] Antihistamines can cause dry mouth and drowsiness so many patients will tolerate these medications only at night.

The dopamine antagonists can all be used in pregnancy as second- or third-line therapies. No single agent dominates in efficacy, and all have demonstrated good safety profiles with a low risk of fetal adverse effects.[5,20–22] Promethazine trends toward causing more drowsiness than prochlorperazine and metoclopramide. Dosing regimens are included in **Table 1**. If using multiple medications, the risks of complications must be considered, especially as extrapyramidal side effects, prolonged QT, and the possibility of neuroleptic malignant syndrome is increased when combining medications.

Ondansetron, a serotonin receptor antagonist, is the most commonly used antiemetic for NVP in the United States.[23] Ondansetron has been shown to be as effective, and perhaps more effective, as other antiemetics, including pyridoxine, but is often better tolerated, as there is less sedation.[24] Ondansetron can be given by mouth, via the intravenous route, or as an oral dissolvable tablet. Prolonged QT is a maternal risk and caution should be used when ondansetron is administered with other

Table 1
Medications for nausea and vomiting in pregnancy

Class/Medications	Former FDA Category[a]	Treatment Regimen	Clinical Considerations
Pyridoxine	A	25 mg PO every 6 h	Available OTC as vitamin B6
Antihistamines			
Dimenhydrinate	B	50 mg PO every 6 h	Available OTC
Diphenhydramine	B	25 mg PO/IV every 6 h	Available OTC
Phenothiazines			
Prochlorperazine	C	10 mg PO/IV every 6 h	
Promethazine	C	25 mg PO/PR/IV every 6 h	
Dopamine antagonists			
Metoclopramide	B	10 mg PO/IV/IM every 6 h	May cause tardive dyskinesia, acute dystonia; limit to <3 mo total use
Serotonin 5H3 antagonists			
Ondansetron	B	4–8 mg PO/ODT/IV every 8 h	Potential maternal QT prolongation
Combination			
Pyridoxine with doxylamine	A	Pyridoxine 25 mg + doxylamine 12.5 mg every 6 h	OTC as vitamin B6 and doxylamine may be less effective and more sedating than Diclegis
Diclegis	A	Pyridoxine 10 mg + doxylamine 10 mg PO; 2 tabs at bedtime	Delayed release; up to 4 tabs daily Not always covered by insurance
Bonjesta	A	Pyridoxine 20 mg + doxylamine 20 mg PO; 1 tab at bedtime	Extended release 10 mg/10 mg released immediately Up to 2 tabs daily
Steroids			
Methylprednisone	C	16 mg PO/IV every 8 h	Limit before 10 wk Last line (discuss with OB) and taper over 2 wk after 3 d if working; stop if not working

Abbreviations: FDA, food and drug administration; IM, intramuscular; IV, intravenous; OB, obstetrician; ODT, oral dissolvable tablet; OTC, over the counter; PO, by mouth; PR, per rectal; serotonin 5H3 antagonists, serotonin 5-hydroxytryptamine type 3 receptor antagonists.
 [a] The FDA eliminated the drug risk categorization of medications (formerly A, B, C, D, X) in 2014. Drugs manufactured before 2001 do not apply to this ruling. Current labeling now includes pregnancy exposure registry, risk summary, clinical considerations, and data.[29]

medications also known to potentially prolong the QT interval. An electrocardiogram can be obtained before usage if there is concern.

Recently, ondansetron has received intense scrutiny in the medical literature as well as in the layperson press out of concern it may cause fetal anomalies; specifically, cardiac malformations and cleft palate. The first study demonstrating an association between ondansetron use in the first trimester and cleft palate was by Anderka and colleagues[25] in 2012. A 20% prevalence of cleft palate was observed in infants exposed to ondansetron (n = 55) compared with 11% prevalence (n = 4479) in those not exposed. However, exposure was based on maternal recall and the number of exposures with such a high prevalence rate was not shown in a repeat study published 1 year later by Pasternak and colleagues.[26] Other smaller studies also have failed to show this association.[3]

The retrospective analysis by Pasternak and colleagues[26] of 6165 patients (1233 exposed to ondansetron) within the Danish National Birth Registry showed a 2.9% occurrence of any major birth defect in both groups (adjusted prevalence odds ratio [OR] 1.12, confidence interval [CI] 0.69–1.82), which included cardiac defects. The exposure group had zero cases of cleft palate. There was also no increased risk for spontaneous miscarriage, stillbirth, preterm delivery, delivery of a small-for-gestational-age infant, or delivery of a low-birth-weight infant in the exposed group.[26]

Andersen and colleagues,[27] also in 2013, used the same registry data but expanded the cohort to include an additional 7 years of data. In actuality, this added only an additional 15 women to the ondansetron exposure group. The results were published in abstract form only but were widely publicized as demonstrating a higher incidence of cardiac malformations in infants who had been exposed to ondansetron in utero. This was followed by a 2014 large retrospective analysis by Danielsson and colleagues[28] using the Swedish Medical Birth Register that initially reported that no significant difference in the rate of major birth defects was seen between the group exposed to ondansetron and the unexposed group (OR 0.95, 95% CI 0.72–1.26). These data were adjusted for confounders and an increased risk of primarily septal defects was noted (OR 1.62, 95% CI 1.04–2.14).

In 2016, one more large retrospective analysis was published by Fejzo and colleagues,[29] which compared outcomes for women in the United States with HG treated with ondansetron with women with HG treated without ondansetron (68% treated with other medications), and a control group of women without HG. Major birth defects, including heart defects and cleft lip/palette, were similar in the HG ondansetron group compared with the control group.

Overall, there is insufficient evidence to suggest that ondansetron should be avoided in pregnancy. The benefits of treating NVP and HG with any of the discussed medications, including ondansetron, likely outweigh the maternal and fetal risks of untreated disease. If patients have concerns given the lay press regarding ondansetron, they can be counseled on these possible very low rates of congenital defects.

Steroids are one of the last-line treatment options for NVP or HG and their use remains controversial. Three studies have shown an association between methylprednisone and oral clefts when used in the first trimester.[21] Steroids may be of some benefit in cases of refractory HG, but the decision to use steroids as a last resort should be made in conjunction with an obstetrician.[7]

Alternative treatments

Ginger has been extensively studied and has been compared with placebo in 8 studies. Its mechanism of action as an antiemetic is unknown, but it does possess weak cholinergic activities.[30] Multiple studies, including several RCTs, have shown ginger to improve nausea in pregnancy, but not vomiting. Current research suggests that ginger is likely very safe in pregnancy and usage has not been shown to increase adverse maternal or fetal outcomes, including miscarriage.[8,31] Dosing regimens vary, but commonly, ginger is taken as 250-mg capsules 4 times daily. One notable side effect is reflux, and care should be taken when using any herbal supplement with prescribed medications, as not all potential interactions are known.

VAGINAL BLEEDING AND PAIN IN EARLY PREGNANCY

Vaginal bleeding in pregnancy is a concerning symptom for pregnant patients, and there are many causes ranging from benign to life threatening. Any woman of childbearing age presenting with a positive pregnancy test and with vaginal bleeding and/or abdominal pain should be assumed to have an ectopic pregnancy until proven otherwise.[32–35] The approach to a patient with vaginal bleeding in early pregnancy includes assessment of hemodynamic stability, resuscitation if needed, physical examination, ultrasound evaluation, and determination of Rh status.

Initial Evaluation

Patients presenting with vaginal bleeding and/or pain in early pregnancy should be assessed for signs of significant hemorrhage, including hemodynamic instability. Unstable patients should be resuscitated with intravenous fluids and O-negative blood if type-specific blood is not immediately available.[32,33,35,36] In hemodynamically stable patients, a full gynecologic and obstetric history should be acquired, including the last known normal menstrual period (LMP) to facilitate dating of the current pregnancy. In addition, the emergency physician should inquire as to the duration and amount of vaginal bleeding and whether pain is present. The physical examination may include a chaperoned pelvic examination to visually inspect the vaginal vault and cervix for obvious lesions that might be the source of hemorrhage, and an estimation of ongoing hemorrhage. Non–pregnancy-related causes of vaginal bleeding include vaginal or cervical lesions, which are often related to sexually transmitted diseases (human papilloma and herpes simplex viruses) or trauma. Vaginal wall lesions can be highly vascular and a source of heavy bleeding.[37]

Anti-D Immunoglobulin

If the Rh status of the woman is negative, then any vaginal bleeding is usually treated with anti-D immunoglobulin (RhIG). RhIG should be given in all Rh-negative women undergoing surgical treatment for miscarriage and in any ectopic pregnancy.[38] ACOG states that as the risk of allo-immunization is low in early first-trimester spontaneous miscarriage treated nonsurgically, but RhIG treatment should be considered based on expert opinion and extrapolation of third-trimester fetomaternal hemorrhage.[39,40] Dosing varies from 50 µg to 120 µg if given before 12 weeks; 300 µg is given if after 12 weeks. There is no harm is administering the more readily available 300-µg dose before 12 weeks. In the case of threatened miscarriage without vaginal bleeding, there is inconsistent evidence to support the administration of RhIG and no formal recommendation is given.[38]

MISCARRIAGE

Miscarriage is any pregnancy loss that occurs before 20 weeks. Early pregnancy loss refers to either a nonviable IUP or a developing embryo or fetus without fetal cardiac activity before 13 weeks' gestation. Although the terms are often used interchangeably, this section focuses only on miscarriage within the first trimester (12–13 weeks), as the management for second-trimester pregnancy loss may be different.[41] There are 5 types of miscarriage: threatened, inevitable, complete, incomplete, and missed **(Table 2)**.[36,42,43]

Miscarriage is the most common complication of pregnancy, with 1 in 3 women experiencing a miscarriage during the reproductive years.[44–46] Approximately 12% to 14% of all recognized pregnancies end in a spontaneous miscarriage before 20 weeks.[47] Of those, 80% will occur before 13 weeks and 50% to 80% are due to

Table 2
Early pregnancy complications

Term	Definition
Early pregnancy loss	Spontaneous pregnancy demise or a nonviable IUP before 13-wk GA
Miscarriage	IUP demise before 20-wk GA confirmed by ultrasound or histology; also called spontaneous miscarriage or spontaneous abortion
Threatened miscarriage	Vaginal bleeding present without findings consistent with spontaneous miscarriage and a closed os
Incomplete miscarriage	Vaginal bleeding ± pain, an open os, and products of conception found within the cervical canal
Complete miscarriage	Products of conception expelled from the uterus, os has closed, and vaginal bleeding ± pain usually improved
Inevitable miscarriage	Vaginal bleeding with an open os
Missed miscarriage	Fetal or embryonic demise without passage of the uterine contents; no vaginal bleeding and os closed
Ectopic pregnancy	Ultrasonic or surgical visualization of a pregnancy outside of the endometrial cavity

Abbreviations: GA, gestational age; IUP, intrauterine pregnancy.

chromosomal abnormalities.[41,44,48] Maternal age is an independent risk factor for miscarriage.[48] Rates greater than 90% are reported for women 45 years or older, but as low as 15% or less for women younger than 34 years.[49] Additional risk factors include previous miscarriage, obesity, poorly controlled type 1 diabetes, thyroid disease, the use of cocaine and alcohol, structural abnormalities of the uterus, inherited thrombophilias, and antiphospholipid syndrome.[50–52]

An anembryonic pregnancy, previously called a "blighted ovum," is one that occurs without the development of a yolk sac or fetal pole. Many women who have an anembryonic pregnancy will not know they are pregnant, as the vaginal bleeding can occur shortly after the normal menses cycle is due.[53,54] However, when an ultrasound is obtained, only an empty intrauterine hypoechoic sac is seen. When the typical progression of ultrasound findings in normal pregnancy are not seen, and a definite ectopic pregnancy is also not seen, eventually, the diagnosis of anembryonic pregnancy, now called "early pregnancy failure" is made.[55] The specific ultrasonographic findings that support this diagnosis are included in **Table 3**. Most often, unless the patient presents for repeat visits, a gynecologist will make this diagnosis.

When evaluating a pregnant woman with a possible miscarriage, the emergency physician must be familiar with management options that, in consultation with a gynecologist, may be offered to the patient. Ultrasound will help confirm either an IUP versus ectopic pregnancy, and a viable versus nonviable or failed pregnancy (see **Table 3**). When ultrasound is nondiagnostic, repeat testing over the following 7 to 14 days can confirm the diagnosis.[48]

Clinical Findings

Miscarriage usually presents as vaginal bleeding in pregnancy and/or lower abdominal pain. The prevalence of vaginal bleeding in early pregnancy is highest from 5 to 8 weeks' gestation, which coincides with the development of the hormonally dependent placenta.[56,57] Not all first-trimester bleeding is due to miscarriage, and many women will go on to have normal pregnancies. Although light bleeding or spotting does not seem to be associated with an increased risk of miscarriage,

Table 3
Guidelines for transvaginal ultrasonographic diagnosis of pregnancy failure in a woman with an intrauterine pregnancy of uncertain viability[a]

Findings Diagnostic of Pregnancy Failure	Findings Suspicious for, but Not Diagnostic of, Pregnancy Failure
CRL of ≥7 mm and no heartbeat	CRL of <7 mm and no heartbeat
MSD of ≥25 mm and no embryo	MSD of 16–24 mm and no embryo
Absence of embryo with heartbeat ≥2 wk after a scan that showed a gestational sac without a yolk sac	Absence of embryo with heartbeat 7–13 d after a scan that showed a gestational sac without a yolk sac
Absence of embryo with heartbeat ≥11 d after a scan that showed a gestational sac with a yolk sac	Absence of embryo with heartbeat 7–10 d after a scan that showed a gestational sac with a yolk sac
	Absence of embryo ≥6 wk after LMP
	Empty amnion (amnion seen adjacent to yolk sac, with no visible embryo)
	Enlarged yolk sac (>7 mm)
	Small gestational sac size in relation to the embryo (MSD − CRL <5 mm)

Abbreviations: CRL, indicates crown-rump length; LMP, last menstrual period; MSD, mean sac diameter.
[a] Criteria are from the Society of Radiologists in Ultrasound Multispecialty Consensus Conference on Early First Trimester Diagnosis of Miscarriage and Exclusion of a Viable Intrauterine Pregnancy, October 2012.
Adapted from Doubilet PM, Benson CB, Bourne T, et al. Diagnostic criteria for nonviable pregnancy early in the first trimester. Ultrasound Q 2014;30:3–9; with permission.

heavy bleeding (defined as similar to or greater than that seen during a normal menses), especially with pain, carries an increased risk of a first-trimester miscarriage (adjusted OR 2.84, 95% CI 1.93–4.56).[56] First-trimester bleeding does increase the risk of complications later in the pregnancy, including preterm delivery, premature rupture of membranes, and placental abruption, but not stillbirth.[58,59]

Very early in the pregnancy, some women will have implantation bleeding. This usually occurs approximately 4 weeks after the LMP and is a small amount, typically pink or brown in color. This is due to the embryo being embedded in the endometrial wall. The bleeding is typically of short duration, and occurs without cramping or pain. Although implantation bleeding is benign, it is a diagnosis of exclusion.[37]

Emergency Department Evaluation

The diagnosis of miscarriage requires a history and physical examination, laboratory investigations, and imaging. There is significant debate regarding the utility of the pelvic examination for women with bleeding in early pregnancy. Several investigators have argued that the pelvic examination has a limited role and does not often add to the management of these patients, especially if an IUP was noted on ultrasound.[60–63] Pelvic examination may be warranted if there is suspicion for clot or products of conception within the cervical os, as this can prevent the os from closing and cause continued bleeding. Clot or tissue retained within the os should be gently removed with forceps. It can be difficult to differentiate between clot and products of conception; if there is doubt, a sample can be sent to pathology.[37]

Laboratory tests include a complete blood count for a baseline hemoglobin level, blood type with Rh status, with a cross-match for life-threatening hemorrhage. The quantitative β-hCG is not particularly useful in miscarriage if the patient has a previously documented IUP with cardiac activity, but it may be used in follow-up to ensure levels return to zero during the treatment phase.[37]

Ultrasound, either performed and interpreted by the emergency physician or performed by a sonographer with radiologist interpretation, should be completed. Embryonic or fetal growth, cardiac activity, and any anatomic abnormalities (ie, subchorionic hemorrhage) should be noted. In general, a fetal heart rate (FHR) of less than 80 is almost always associated with a future miscarriage. A normal FHR of 120 to 160 beats per minute is reassuring. In fact, a woman with vaginal bleeding but a reassuring ultrasound with a normal FHR has significantly decreased odds of progressing to a complete miscarriage.[64] A crown-rump length (CRL) of ≥7 mm without cardiac activity is consistent with a failed pregnancy (see **Table 3**).[55]

Approximately 18% of women with first-trimester vaginal bleeding and an IUP will be diagnosed with a subchorionic hemorrhage. If the hematoma seen is less than 25% of the gestational sac area, then the prognosis for the pregnancy generally is good.[36] However, subchorionic hematomas are associated with an increased risk of miscarriage, as well as late pregnancy loss and complications.[65]

Management

The management of a threatened miscarriage is largely supportive with anticipatory guidance. The patient should be counseled that a spontaneous miscarriage may still occur. She also will need timely gynecologic follow-up, ED return precautions, including heavy vaginal bleeding, fever, dizziness, syncope, or pain. "Pelvic rest" can be considered, but the implementation of pelvic rest has not been shown to improve pregnancy outcomes. However, patients may incorrectly associate a pregnancy loss with sexual activity.[45,53] Pelvic rest is a benign recommendation that may decrease the emotional impact should a threatened miscarriage become a spontaneous miscarriage. There is no role for bed rest in the patient with a threatened miscarriage.[66]

Traditionally, surgical curettage was routinely performed for women with missed, inevitable, or incomplete miscarriages. Now, treatment may include expectant (conservative) management, medical, or surgical interventions. A recent Cochrane review found no significant difference in outcomes for women treated with expectant versus medical treatment, nor between medical and surgical treatment.[67] Fertility and pregnancy outcomes of future pregnancies were no different between treatment groups.[68] The miscarriage treatment trial (MIST) showed that gynecologic infection occurred 2% to 3% of the time, irrespective of the type of treatment chosen.[69]

Expectant management, the "wait and see" approach, results in complete expulsion of uterine contents in 75% of women within 1 week.[70] It may take some women several weeks for this happen and there is no limit to how long it is safe to wait in the absence of hemorrhage or infection.[53] Expectant management is more successful for an incomplete miscarriage compared with a missed miscarriage or anembryonic pregnancy. The cost of expectant management is lower than surgical options; however, women have more days of bleeding and a higher likelihood of needing unplanned surgery.[42] Women who elect for expectant management should be prescribed pain medications and given anticipatory guidance. In addition, they should be cautioned that surgical intervention may be necessary if complete expulsion does not occur.[41]

Medical management includes misoprostol, a prostaglandin analog. Misoprostol is a uterine stimulant and thus contractions expulse the uterine contents. It can be given by mouth, sublingually, rectally, or intravaginally. ACOG recommends a first dose of

800 μg to be given intravaginal.[41] Mifepristone, a progesterone antagonist, is more commonly used in first-trimester medically assisted abortions, but also may be used in conjunction with misoprostol in the setting of an incomplete miscarriage to promote expulsion of placental tissue.[67] Until 2018, there was no evidence that using both medications is more effective than misoprostol alone, and the combination of misoprostol plus mifepristone is not currently recommended by ACOG.[38,41] However, in June 2018, Schreiber and colleagues[71] published their study of 300 women with either a missed miscarriage or early failed pregnancy who were randomized to either 800 μg of misoprostol alone or pretreatment with 200 mg of mifepristone followed by the 800 μg of misoprostol. Women who were pretreated with mifepristone had complete expulsion of uterine contents 83.4% of the time (95% CI 76.8–89.3) compared with 67.1% of the time in the misoprostol alone group (95% CI 59.0–74.6). The rate of complications was similar between the 2 groups, including the need for blood transfusion and pelvic infection. Approximately 1% of women taking misoprostol will need emergency surgery for heavy bleeding.[44] Medical management should be initiated in conjunction with a gynecologist.

Surgical options include vacuum aspiration or dilation and curettage (D&C); the latter is the recommended treatment for all unstable patients. Vacuum aspiration can be done in an office setting or may be offered by gynecology in the ED. D&C was once considered the standard for all women with an incomplete or missed miscarriage, and is associated with shortest duration of bleeding. Surgical complications, including uterine perforation, cervical laceration, hemorrhage, and intrauterine adhesions (Asherman syndrome), occur 2% to 8% of the time.[44]

Emotional support is essential for both the patient and her partner. Only 45% of women (and partners) who experienced a miscarriage felt they received adequate emotional support from the medical community.[45] Emotions ranging from denial, shock, anger, blame and jealousy, sleep disturbance, social withdrawal, and marital disturbance have been described after pregnancy loss. Studies have shown that 30% to 50% of women display symptoms of anxiety and 10% to 15% have depressive symptoms after a miscarriage.[72] Patients and partners should be counseled that many of these emotions are expected, but if they are becoming severe or interfering with daily activities, then psychological help may be needed.[73] Patients or partners may ask how long they should wait before trying to conceive again. The most recent ACOG practice bulletin from 2015 states, "Small observational studies show no benefit to delayed conception after early pregnancy loss." Some investigators counsel that vaginal intercourse should be delayed until 1 to 2 weeks after the complete passage of pregnancy tissue to help prevent infection. However, there also are no data to support this recommendation.[41]

ECTOPIC PREGNANCY

Ectopic pregnancy is defined as any pregnancy occurring outside of the uterine cavity. Approximately 1.5% to 2.0% of pregnancies in the United States are ectopic; however, in patients presenting to the ED with first-trimester bleeding and/or pain, the rate of ectopic pregnancy varies from 6% to 16%. Ninety-six percent of ectopic pregnancies occur in the fallopian tube, with rare occurrences in the cornual region of the uterus (2%–4%), cervix, ovary, abdominal cavity, or cesarean scar (<1% each).[32–36] Heterotopic pregnancies, or simultaneously occurring intrauterine and ectopic pregnancies, were initially thought to occur spontaneously in 1 in 30,000 pregnancies; current estimates are 1 in 4000 pregnancies spontaneously, and 1 in 100 patients undergoing assisted reproductive techniques.[32–34,36,74]

Ectopic pregnancy is the leading cause of pregnancy-related death in the first trimester. Six percent to 9% of pregnancy-related deaths in the United States are due to ectopic pregnancy.[32–35] Misdiagnosis is common, as 40% to 50% of women receive a different diagnosis during their initial ED evaluation.[32,75,76] Risk factors for ectopic pregnancy include prior ectopic pregnancy, history of pelvic inflammatory disease, current intrauterine device use, any tubal surgery, in utero exposure to diethylstilbestrol, and smoking.[32–34,36,75,77] However, approximately half of patients diagnosed with ectopic pregnancy have none of these risk factors.[32,33,35,75]

Clinical Findings

Although most patients present with pain, the absence of pain should not eliminate the diagnosis of ectopic pregnancy from the differential.[32] Vaginal bleeding occurs in 50% to 80% of ectopic pregnancies, can vary from minimal to profound, and can include the passage of tissue.[32,33,35,76] Hypotension and tachycardia can both be seen, particularly if the ectopic pregnancy has ruptured, but patients commonly have normal vital signs.[32,35,36] Physical examination may reveal peritoneal signs, abdominal and pelvic tenderness, cervical motion tenderness, or an adnexal mass, but the absence of any of these findings does not rule out ectopic pregnancy.[32,35] Any pregnant patient presenting with hemodynamic instability, a low hematocrit, or an acute abdomen merits emergent gynecologic consultation for possible ruptured ectopic pregnancy and surgical management.

Laboratory Testing

Blood should be sent for hematocrit, blood type, and Rh-status, and a quantitative β-hCG.[32,33,35,36] The β-hCG can help the emergency physician assess the probability of ectopic pregnancy. In a normal pregnancy, β-hCG should double every 1.4 to 2.1 days until peaking at more than 100,000 mIU/mL. Although a single β-hCG level can diagnose pregnancy, it is less useful to distinguish between a normal IUP and ectopic pregnancy. Once the β-hCG level is greater than 1500 to 3510 mIU/mL, an IUP, if present, should be consistently seen on transvaginal ultrasound.[32,33,35] However, ectopic pregnancies can be seen with β-hCG levels well below this "discriminatory zone," and a single β-hCG value should not be used to rule out ectopic pregnancy.[32,35,75] In fact, up to 7% of all ruptured ectopic pregnancies occur with β-hCG levels less than 100 mIU/mL, and 50% of patients with clear ectopic pregnancies on ultrasonography have a β-hCG less than 2000 mIU/mL.[32,34,35]

Ultrasonography

In stable patients presenting with vaginal bleeding or abdominal pain, ultrasonography should be the next step in evaluation. The 2017 clinical policy of the American College of Emergency Physicians is to obtain a pelvic ultrasound for any pregnant patient with abdominal pain or vaginal bleeding regardless of β-hCG level.[78] Identification of a gestational sac with yolk sac or fetal pole outside the endometrial cavity defines ectopic pregnancy.[32,36,79] Other findings suggestive, but not diagnostic, of ectopic pregnancy include the following:

1. A β-hCG level above the discriminatory zone with an empty uterus
2. An adnexal mass separate from the ovary that is anything other than a simple cyst, such as
   a. An inhomogeneous mass (the "blob" sign), or
   b. An extrauterine saclike structure (the "bagel" sign)

3. Any echogenic fluid in the cul-de-sac
4. A moderate to large amount of fluid in the cul-de-sac[32,79–81]

If the pelvic ultrasound shows a definite ectopic pregnancy, or findings highly suggestive of ectopic pregnancy, emergent gynecologic consultation is warranted. Approximately 26% of patients with ectopic pregnancy have an initially "normal" transvaginal pelvic ultrasound, without any of these findings.[82]

Management

Patients with ectopic pregnancy can be treated medically with methotrexate, or surgically via laparoscopy. Treatment decisions should be made in consultation with a gynecologist. The indications, relative contraindications, and absolute contraindications to methotrexate therapy are summarized in **Table 4**.[32,33,35,36] After receiving methotrexate, women should have β-hCG levels checked weekly. The level may increase in the first few days, but should decline by 15% to 25% by day 7; if it has not, consideration should be given to a second dose, which is needed in 15% to 20% of patients.[35,76] There is no consensus on predictors of success for medical therapy, and most patients who receive methotrexate therapy develop abdominal cramping and pain by day 3 to 7 after treatment. When such patients present to the ED, pelvic ultrasonography should be performed to assess for free fluid. Hemoperitoneum could indicate failure of therapy and rupture of the ectopic pregnancy, which occurs in 7% to 14% of patients treated with methotrexate.[32,33,36,83] These patients may require either a second dose of methotrexate, or surgical intervention, and should be managed in consultation with the patient's gynecologist.[32,33,36] Unless the affected tube is completely removed, it is possible for trophoblastic tissue to regrow. Thus, whether the patient is managed medically or surgically, the β-hCG level should be trended until it is undetectable to ensure complete resolution.[32,33]

Many studies have evaluated expectant management of ectopic pregnancy with conflicting results. A few recent trials have found that women with an ultrasound-confirmed ectopic pregnancy, without fetal heart beat or hemoperitoneum, and an initial β-hCG less than 1500 to 2000 mIU/mL, could be safely managed expectantly, without methotrexate or laparoscopy.[84,85] However, these studies included very few patients, and further study is needed before this becomes a widely accepted recommendation.

PREGNANCY OF UNKNOWN LOCATION

When there is neither a clear IUP nor ectopic pregnancy, and there is no specimen provided for pathology, a PUL is diagnosed. Patients initially diagnosed with PUL

Table 4
Indications and contraindications for the use of methotrexate

Indications	Relative Contraindications	Absolute Contraindications
Hemodynamic stability	Hemodynamic instability	Breastfeeding
Adnexal mass <3.5 cm	Adnexal mass >3.5–4 cm	Immunodeficiency
No fetal cardiac activity	Fetal cardiac activity	Renal insufficiency
β-hCG <5000–15,000	β-hCG >5000–15,000	Liver dysfunction
No signs of rupture	Signs of rupture	Blood dyscrasias
Desire for future fertility	Unreliable follow-up	Peptic ulcer disease
		Pulmonary disease
		Known sensitivity

β-hCG, β human chorionic gonadotropin, measured in mIU/mL.

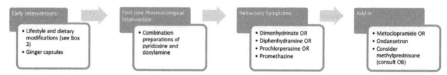

Fig. 1. Flowchart for Nausea and vomiting of pregnancy (NVP). (*Data from* Committee on Practice Bulletins-Obstetrics. ACOG Practice Bulletin No. 189: Nausea and Vomiting Of Pregnancy. Obstet Gynecol 2018;131(1):e15–30.)

can go on to have the diagnosis of nonviable pregnancy (including miscarriage), ectopic pregnancy, or normal IUP.[32,33] The challenge with this diagnosis is that failing to diagnose an ectopic pregnancy may lead to rupture, with subsequent hemorrhage and possible maternal death, whereas prematurely ruling out a normal IUP can result in termination of, or severe damage to, a desired normal pregnancy.[55] Between 8% and 42% of early pregnancies are initially classified as PUL.[33,86,87] The evaluation of these patients is based on both β-hCG testing and ultrasonography. Between 7% and 16% of patients initially diagnosed with PUL will ultimately receive the diagnosis of ectopic pregnancy, whereas between 10% and 40% will have normal IUPs. The remainder will have nonviable pregnancies. Ultrasound findings can include an empty uterus, nonspecific intrauterine fluid, an abnormal gestational sac, or echogenic debris within the uterus.[32,33,86–88]

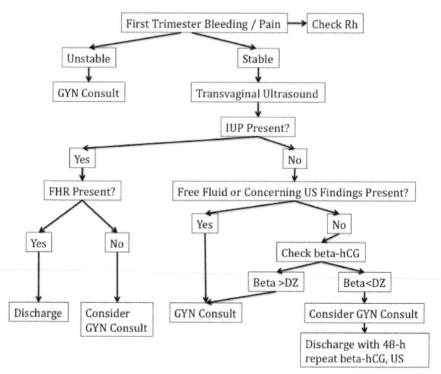

Fig. 2. Management of the patient with first-trimester bleeding or pain. DZ, discriminatory zone; GYN, gynecology; US, ultrasound.

Laboratory Testing

Serial β-hCG testing is frequently used to follow patients with PUL. Stable patients without a definite IUP should return in 48 hours for repeat β-hCG assessment. The β-hCG should be expected to rise by at least 53% in this time frame and this is seen in 99% of patients with normal IUP, but also seen in 15% to 30% of patients with ectopic pregnancy. A rise of less than 53% suggests ectopic pregnancy, occurring in 85% of ectopic pregnancies, but also occurs in 15% of normal pregnancies.[32,33,76,89] A declining β-hCG value indicates a nonviable pregnancy, either intrauterine or ectopic.[32,55] The β-hCG value should be used in conjunction with ultrasonography to follow patients with PUL.

SUMMARY

Complications in early pregnancy include nausea, vomiting, and vaginal bleeding. Nausea and vomiting can range from mild symptoms, which are controlled by dietary modifications and oral medications, to HG, requiring intravenous fluids and medication. Any patient presenting with vaginal bleeding or abdominal pain in early pregnancy should first undergo ultrasonography (**Figs. 1** and **2**). If an ectopic pregnancy is seen, immediate gynecologic consultation is warranted. If an IUP is seen, patients should be counseled for threatened miscarriage. If neither ectopic pregnancy nor IUP is established, PUL is diagnosed and patients should be followed with serial ultrasound and β-hCG measurements.

REFERENCES

1. Jarvis S, Nelson-Piercy C. Management of nausea and vomiting in pregnancy. BMJ 2011;342:d3606.
2. Niemeijer MN, Grooten IJ, Vos N, et al. Diagnostic markers for hyperemesis gravidarum: a systematic review and metaanalysis. Am J Obstet Gynecol 2014; 211(2):150 e1–15.
3. Bustos M, Venkataramanan R, Caritis S. Nausea and vomiting of pregnancy - what's new? Auton Neurosci 2017;202:62–72.
4. Piwko C, Koren G, Babashov V, et al. Economic burden of nausea and vomiting of pregnancy in the USA. J Popul Ther Clin Pharmacol 2013;20(2):e149–60.
5. Boelig RC, Barton SJ, Saccone G, et al. Interventions for treating hyperemesis gravidarum: a Cochrane systematic review and meta-analysis. J Matern Fetal Neonatal Med 2018;31(18):2492–505.
6. Nuangchamnong N, Niebyl J. Doxylamine succinate-pyridoxine hydrochloride (Diclegis) for the management of nausea and vomiting in pregnancy: an overview. Int J Womens Health 2014;6:401–9.
7. Erick M, Cox JT, Mogensen KM. ACOG practice bulletin 189: nausea and vomiting of pregnancy. Obstet Gynecol 2018;131(5):935.
8. Matthews A, Haas DM, O'Mathuna DP, et al. Interventions for nausea and vomiting in early pregnancy. Cochrane Database Syst Rev 2015;(9):CD007575.
9. Niebyl JR. Clinical practice. Nausea and vomiting in pregnancy. N Engl J Med 2010;363(16):1544–50.
10. Mitchell-Jones N, Farren JA, Tobias A, et al. Ambulatory versus inpatient management of severe nausea and vomiting of pregnancy: a randomised control trial with patient preference arm. BMJ Open 2017;7(12):e017566.
11. Tan PC, Omar SZ. Contemporary approaches to hyperemesis during pregnancy. Curr Opin Obstet Gynecol 2011;23(2):87–93.

12. Quinla JD, Hill DA. Nausea and vomiting of pregnancy. Am Fam Physician 2003; 68(1):121–8.
13. Tian R, MacGibbon K, Martin B, et al. Analysis of pre- and post-pregnancy issues in women with hyperemesis gravidarum. Auton Neurosci 2017;202:73–8.
14. Morgan SR, Long L, Johns J, et al. Are early pregnancy complications more common in women with hyperemesis gravidarum? J Obstet Gynaecol 2017;37(3): 355–7.
15. Siminerio LL, Bodnar LM, Venkataramanan R, et al. Ondansetron use in pregnancy. Obstet Gynecol 2016;127(5):873–7.
16. Tan PC, Norazilah MJ, Omar SZ. Dextrose saline compared with normal saline rehydration of hyperemesis gravidarum: a randomized controlled trial. Obstet Gynecol 2013;121(2 Pt 1):291–8.
17. Slaughter SR, Hearns-Stokes R, van der Vlugt T, et al. FDA approval of doxylamine-pyridoxine therapy for use in pregnancy. N Engl J Med 2014;370(12):1081–3.
18. Koren G, Clark S, Hankins GD, et al. Maternal safety of the delayed-release doxylamine and pyridoxine combination for nausea and vomiting of pregnancy; a randomized placebo controlled trial. BMC Pregnancy Childbirth 2015;15:59.
19. Koren G, Clark S, Hankins GD, et al. Effectiveness of delayed-release doxylamine and pyridoxine for nausea and vomiting of pregnancy: a randomized placebo controlled trial. Am J Obstet Gynecol 2010;203(6):571.e1-7.
20. Thomas BR, Rouf PVA, Al-Hail M, et al. Medication used in nausea and vomiting of pregnancy - a review of safety and efficacy. Gynecol Obstet 2015;5(2):270.
21. Ebrahimi N, Maltepe C, Einarson A. Optimal management of nausea and vomiting of pregnancy. Int J Womens Health 2010;2:241–8.
22. McParlin C, O'Donnell A, Robson SC, et al. Treatments for hyperemesis gravidarum and nausea and vomiting in pregnancy: a systematic review. JAMA 2016; 316(13):1392–401.
23. Parker SE, Van Bennekom C, Anderka M, et al. Ondansetron for treatment of nausea and vomiting of pregnancy and the risk of specific birth defects. Obstet Gynecol 2018;132(2):385–94.
24. Oliveira LG, Capp SM, You WB, et al. Ondansetron compared with doxylamine and pyridoxine for treatment of nausea in pregnancy: a randomized controlled trial. Obstet Gynecol 2014;124(4):735–42.
25. Anderka M, Mitchell AA, Louik C, et al. Medications used to treat nausea and vomiting of pregnancy and the risk of selected birth defects. Birth Defects Res A Clin Mol Teratol 2012;94(1):22–30.
26. Pasternak B, Svanstrom H, Hviid A. Ondansetron in pregnancy and risk of adverse fetal outcomes. N Engl J Med 2013;368(9):814–23.
27. Andersen JRJ-SE, Andersen NL, Poulsen HE. Ondansetron use in early pregnancy and the risk of congenital malformations—a registry based nationwide cohort study. Pharmacoepidemiol Drug Saf 2013;22:13–4.
28. Danielsson B, Wikner BN, Kallen B. Use of ondansetron during pregnancy and congenital malformations in the infant. Reprod Toxicol 2014;50:134–7.
29. Fejzo MS, MacGibbon KW, Mullin PM. Ondansetron in pregnancy and risk of adverse fetal outcomes in the United States. Reprod Toxicol 2016;62:87–91.
30. Tiran D. Ginger to reduce nausea and vomiting during pregnancy: evidence of effectiveness is not the same as proof of safety. Complement Ther Clin Pract 2012;18(1):22–5.
31. Viljoen E, Visser J, Koen N, et al. A systematic review and meta-analysis of the effect and safety of ginger in the treatment of pregnancy-associated nausea and vomiting. Nutr J 2014;13:20.

32. Della-Giustina D, Denny M. Ectopic pregnancy. Emerg Med Clin North Am 2003; 21(3):565–84.

33. Barnhart KT. Clinical practice. Ectopic pregnancy. N Engl J Med 2009;361(4): 379–87.

34. Mausner Geffen E, Slywotzky C, Bennett G. Pitfalls and tips in the diagnosis of ectopic pregnancy. Abdom Radiol (NY) 2017;42(5):1524–42.

35. Murray H, Baakdah H, Bardell T, et al. Diagnosis and treatment of ectopic pregnancy. CMAJ 2005;173(8):905–12.

36. Huancahuari N. Emergencies in early pregnancy. Emerg Med Clin North Am 2012;30(4):837–47.

37. Promes SB, Nobay F. Pitfalls in first-trimester bleeding. Emerg Med Clin North Am 2010;28(1):219–34, x.

38. Committee on Practice Bulletins-Obstetrics. Practice bulletin no. 181: prevention of Rh D alloimmunization. Obstet Gynecol 2017;130(2):e57–70.

39. Hannafin B, Lovecchio F, Blackburn P. Do Rh-negative women with first trimester spontaneous abortions need Rh immune globulin? Am J Emerg Med 2006;24(4): 487–9.

40. Jabara S, Barnhart KT. Is Rh immune globulin needed in early first-trimester abortion? A review. Am J Obstet Gynecol 2003;188(3):623–7.

41. Committee on Practice Bulletins—Gynecology. The American College of Obstetricians and Gynecologists Practice Bulletin no. 150. Early pregnancy loss. Obstet Gynecol 2015;125(5):1258–67.

42. Nanda K, Lopez LM, Grimes DA, et al. Expectant care versus surgical treatment for miscarriage. Cochrane Database Syst Rev 2012;(3):CD003518.

43. Bourne T, Bottomley C. When is a pregnancy nonviable and what criteria should be used to define miscarriage? Fertil Steril 2012;98(5):1091–6.

44. Jurkovic D, Overton C, Bender-Atik R. Diagnosis and management of first trimester miscarriage. BMJ 2013;346:f3676.

45. Bardos J, Hercz D, Friedenthal J, et al. A national survey on public perceptions of miscarriage. Obstet Gynecol 2015;125(6):1313–20.

46. Jeve Y, Rana R, Bhide A, et al. Accuracy of first-trimester ultrasound in the diagnosis of early embryonic demise: a systematic review. Ultrasound Obstet Gynecol 2011;38(5):489–96.

47. Makhlouf MA, Clifton RG, Roberts JM, et al. Adverse pregnancy outcomes among women with prior spontaneous or induced abortions. Am J Perinatol 2014;31(9):765–72.

48. Gracia CR, Sammel MD, Chittams J, et al. Risk factors for spontaneous abortion in early symptomatic first-trimester pregnancies. Obstet Gynecol 2005;106(5 Pt 1):993–9.

49. Nybo AA, Wohlfahrt J, Christens P, et al. Is maternal age an independent risk factor for fetal loss? West J Med 2000;173(5):331.

50. Poorolajal J, Cheraghi P, Cheraghi Z, et al. Predictors of miscarriage: a matched case-control study. Epidemiol Health 2014;36:e2014031.

51. Maconochie NDP, Prior S, Simmons R. Risk factors for first trimester miscarriage: results from a UK-population-based case-control study. BJOG 2006;114:170–86.

52. Feodor Nilsson S, Andersen PK, Strandberg-Larsen K, et al. Risk factors for miscarriage from a prevention perspective: a nationwide follow-up study. BJOG 2014;121(11):1375–84.

53. Prine LW, MacNaughton H. Office management of early pregnancy loss. Am Fam Physician 2011;84(1):75–82.

54. Wilcox AJ, Weinberg CR, O'Connor JF, et al. Incidence of early loss of pregnancy. N Engl J Med 1988;319(4):189–94.

55. Doubilet PM, Benson CB, Bourne T, et al. Diagnostic criteria for nonviable pregnancy early in the first trimester. N Engl J Med 2013;369(15):1443–51.

56. Hasan R, Baird DD, Herring AH, et al. Association between first-trimester vaginal bleeding and miscarriage. Obstet Gynecol 2009;114(4):860–7.

57. Hasan R, Baird DD, Herring AH, et al. Patterns and predictors of vaginal bleeding in the first trimester of pregnancy. Ann Epidemiol 2010;20(7):524–31.

58. Lykke JA, Dideriksen KL, Lidegaard O, et al. First-trimester vaginal bleeding and complications later in pregnancy. Obstet Gynecol 2010;115(5):935–44.

59. Weiss JL, Malone FD, Vidaver J, et al. Threatened abortion: a risk factor for poor pregnancy outcome, a population-based screening study. Am J Obstet Gynecol 2004;190(3):745–50.

60. Isoardi K. Review article: the use of pelvic examination within the emergency department in the assessment of early pregnancy bleeding. Emerg Med Australas 2009;21(6):440–8.

61. Seymour A, Abebe H, Pavlik D, et al. Pelvic examination is unnecessary in pregnant patients with a normal bedside ultrasound. Am J Emerg Med 2010;28(2):213–6.

62. Johnstone C. Vaginal examination does not improve diagnostic accuracy in early pregnancy bleeding. Emerg Med Australas 2013;25(3):219–21.

63. Linden JA, Grimmnitz B, Hagopian L, et al. Is the pelvic examination still crucial in patients presenting to the emergency department with vaginal bleeding or abdominal pain when an intrauterine pregnancy is identified on ultrasonography? A randomized controlled trial. Ann Emerg Med 2017;70(6):825–34.

64. Datta MR, Raut A. Efficacy of first-trimester ultrasound parameters for prediction of early spontaneous abortion. Int J Gynaecol Obstet 2017;138(3):325–30.

65. Tuuli MG, Norman SM, Odibo AO, et al. Perinatal outcomes in women with subchorionic hematoma: a systematic review and meta-analysis. Obstet Gynecol 2011;117(5):1205–12.

66. Aleman A, Althabe F, Belizan J, et al. Bed rest during pregnancy for preventing miscarriage. Cochrane Database Syst Rev 2005;(2):CD003576.

67. Kim C, Barnard S, Neilson JP, et al. Medical treatments for incomplete miscarriage. Cochrane Database Syst Rev 2017;(1):CD007223.

68. Lemmers M, Verschoor MAC, Overwater K, et al. Fertility and obstetric outcomes after curettage versus expectant management in randomised and non-randomised women with an incomplete evacuation of the uterus after misoprostol treatment for miscarriage. Eur J Obstet Gynecol Reprod Biol 2017;211:78–82.

69. Trinder J, Brocklehurst P, Porter R, et al. Management of miscarriage: expectant, medical, or surgical? Results of randomised controlled trial (miscarriage treatment (MIST) trial). BMJ 2006;332(7552):1235–40.

70. Torre A, Huchon C, Bussieres L, et al. Immediate versus delayed medical treatment for first-trimester miscarriage: a randomized trial. Am J Obstet Gynecol 2012;206(3):215.e1-6.

71. Schreiber CA, Creinin MD, Atrio J, et al. Mifepristone pretreatment for the medical management of early pregnancy loss. N Engl J Med 2018;378(23):2161–70.

72. Mehta MPR. Follow-up for improving psychological well-being for women after a miscarriage: RHL commentary. The WHO Reproductive Health Library. Geneva (Switzerland): World Health Organization; 2013.

73. Haas DM, Ramsey PS. Progestogen for preventing miscarriage. Cochrane Database Syst Rev 2013;(10):CD003511.

74. Seeber BE, Sammel MD, Guo W, et al. Application of redefined human chorionic gonadotropin curves for the diagnosis of women at risk for ectopic pregnancy. Fertil Steril 2006;86(2):454–9.
75. Robertson JJ, Long B, Koyfman A. Emergency medicine myths: ectopic pregnancy evaluation, risk factors, and presentation. J Emerg Med 2017;53(6): 819–28.
76. Alkatout I, Honemeyer U, Strauss A, et al. Clinical diagnosis and treatment of ectopic pregnancy. Obstet Gynecol Surv 2013;68(8):571–81.
77. Hoover RN, Hyer M, Pfeiffer RM, et al. Adverse health outcomes in women exposed in utero to diethylstilbestrol. N Engl J Med 2011;365(14):1304–14.
78. American College of Emergency Physicians Clinical Policies Subcommittee on Early Pregnancy, Hahn SA, Promes SB, Brown MD. Clinical policy: critical issues in the initial evaluation and management of patients presenting to the emergency department in early pregnancy. Ann Emerg Med 2017;69(2):241–50.e20.
79. Hsu S, Euerle BD. Ultrasound in pregnancy. Emerg Med Clin North Am 2012; 30(4):849–67.
80. Lane BF, Wong-You-Cheong JJ, Javitt MC, et al. ACR appropriateness Criteria(R) first trimester bleeding. Ultrasound Q 2013;29(2):91–6.
81. Nadim B, Infante F, Lu C, et al. Morphological ultrasound types known as 'blob' and 'bagel' signs should be reclassified from suggesting probable to indicating definite tubal ectopic pregnancy. Ultrasound Obstet Gynecol 2018;51(4):543–9.
82. Bhatt S, Ghazale H, Dogra VS. Sonographic evaluation of ectopic pregnancy. Radiol Clin North Am 2007;45(3):549–60, ix.
83. Dudley PS, Heard MJ, Sangi-Haghpeykar H, et al. Characterizing ectopic pregnancies that rupture despite treatment with methotrexate. Fertil Steril 2004;82(5): 1374–8.
84. Jurkovic D, Memtsa M, Sawyer E, et al. Single-dose systemic methotrexate vs expectant management for treatment of tubal ectopic pregnancy: a placebo-controlled randomized trial. Ultrasound Obstet Gynecol 2017;49(2):171–6.
85. Silva PM, Araujo Junior E, Cecchino GN, et al. Effectiveness of expectant management versus methotrexate in tubal ectopic pregnancy: a double-blind randomized trial. Arch Gynecol Obstet 2015;291(4):939–43.
86. Fields L, Hathaway A. Key concepts in pregnancy of unknown location: identifying ectopic pregnancy and providing patient-centered care. J Midwifery Womens Health 2017;62(2):172–9.
87. Bobdiwala S, Al-Memar M, Farren J, et al. Factors to consider in pregnancy of unknown location. Womens Health (Lond) 2017;13(2):27–33.
88. Dart R, Howard K. Subclassification of indeterminate pelvic ultrasonograms: stratifying the risk of ectopic pregnancy. Acad Emerg Med 1998;5(4):313–9.
89. Barnhart KT, Sammel MD, Rinaudo PF, et al. Symptomatic patients with an early viable intrauterine pregnancy: HCG curves redefined. Obstet Gynecol 2004; 104(1):50–5.

Complications of Assisted Reproductive Technology

SueLin M. Hilbert, MD, MPH[a],*, Stephanie Gunderson, MD[b]

KEYWORDS

- Assisted reproductive technology • Complications
- Ovarian hyperstimulation syndrome

KEY POINTS

- Assisted reproductive technology (ART) accounts for 1.7% of all infants in the United States.
- ART is a careful manipulation of the menstrual cycle that involves combinations of multiple medications, intricate timing, and a close patient-physician relationship.
- Although much of the literature focuses on perinatal and pregnancy-related complications, ovarian hyperstimulation syndrome (OHSS), ectopic pregnancy, and ovarian torsion are potentially life-threatening diagnoses that are particularly relevant to emergency medicine.
- All patients undergoing an ART procedure who present to the emergency department with abdominal pain or distension should have a pelvic ultrasound to evaluate for ovarian enlargement and/or free fluid.
- The primary focus of treatment of OHSS is initial resuscitation and stabilization, followed by supportive care and close consultation with obstetrics and gynecology.

INTRODUCTION

In Oldham, England on July 25, 1978, Louise Joy Brown was the first human born as the result of in vitro fertilization (IVF). Four years later, Elizabeth Jordan Carr was the first IVF baby born in the United States. In 2015, 464 fertility clinics in the United States performed 182,111 assisted reproductive technology (ART) procedures, which resulted in 59,334 live-birth deliveries and accounted for 1.7% of all infants in the United States.[1] Use of ART is becoming more common, and emergency physicians should be familiar with the process and complications that can arise.

The Centers for Disease Control and Prevention (CDC) defines ART as "any treatment where oocytes and sperm are handled outside the body for the purpose of

a Division of Emergency Medicine, Washington University in St. Louis, 660 South Euclid, Campus Box 8072, Saint Louis, MO 63110, USA; b Department of Obstetrics and Gynecology, Washington University in St. Louis, 660 South Euclid, Mailbox 8064-37-905, Saint Louis, MO 63110, USA
* Corresponding author.
E-mail address: hilberts@wustl.edu

Emerg Med Clin N Am 37 (2019) 239–249
https://doi.org/10.1016/j.emc.2019.01.005
0733-8627/19/© 2019 Elsevier Inc. All rights reserved.
emed.theclinics.com

establishing a pregnancy."[2] Generally, this process consists of controlled ovarian stimulation (COS), oocyte retrieval, IVF, and transfer of the embryo or embryos into the uterus. Many women, however, conceive with the assistance of ovarian stimulation alone, and although this does not strictly fall within the CDC definition of ART, emergency physicians should evaluate these patients similarly.

THE ASSISTED REPRODUCTIVE TECHNOLOGY PROCESS

Infertility is defined as unprotected intercourse without conception for 1 year, the time during which 85% of couples will conceive.[3] When couples struggling with infertility present to a reproductive endocrinologist's office, they will often undergo a specialized workup beyond the basic history and physical examination (**Fig. 1**). Once this workup is complete, and depending on the diagnosis made, a couple will typically undergo a trial of oral ovulation induction using either letrozole or clomiphene citrate and intrauterine insemination. Some patients, such as women with functional hypothalamic amenorrhea, do not produce sufficient endogenous gonadotropins and therefore do not respond to oral ovulation induction. They will require gonadotropin stimulation in conjunction with intrauterine insemination. If a couple fails to conceive with this initial treatment approach, typically the next step in management is IVF.

At this point, a consultation often occurs to discuss logistics, procedures, and follow-up associated with the IVF process (**Fig. 2**). Typically, the first step is to place the patient on combined oral contraceptives to allow more predictable timing of gonadotropin use and the egg retrieval procedure. Once she begins her menses, on cycle day 2 or 3, the patient undergoes a baseline pelvic ultrasound and has serum follicle stimulating hormone (FSH) and estradiol levels drawn. If the estradiol is not elevated as a result of a dominant follicle being recruited, the patient is considered "suppressed" and she will begin COS with exogenous gonadotropin.

During COS, there are multiple office visits for monitoring serum estradiol levels as well as follicular development on ultrasound. Depending on the stimulation protocol, gonadotropin releasing hormone (GnRH) agonists or antagonists are used to prevent premature ovulation. Once follicular development reaches a certain threshold (usually defined at 2–3 follicles measuring ≥ 18 mm^3)[7], final maturation of the oocytes is

- Semen analysis

- Uterine Cavity
  - Saline sonohysterography
  - Hysterosalpingogram
- Tubal Patency
  - Hysterosalpingogram
- Ovarian Reserve
  - Serum antimullerian hormone level
  - Cycle day 3 follicle stimulation hormone and estradiol levels
  - Antral follicle count (transvaginal ultrasound)

Fig. 1. Initial evaluation of couples struggling with infertility.[4–6]

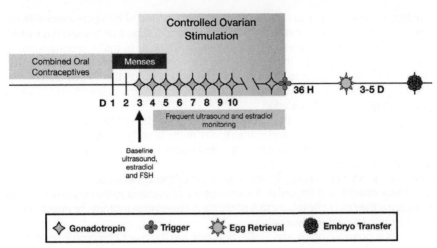

Fig. 2. The process of IVF.

triggered with either recombinant hCG or leuprolide. Egg retrieval, or "ultrasound-guided follicle aspiration," is scheduled approximately 36 hours later to avoid spontaneous ovulation, which typically occurs 40 hours after the trigger injection. The procedure is done under local anesthesia or monitored anesthetic care, often in an outpatient center. Using a vaginal ultrasound probe, a small-gauge needle attached to suction is guided through the vaginal wall and into the follicles allowing for oocyte aspiration. The whole procedure is typically well tolerated with minimal pain medication requirements. As with any procedure, however, there is a risk of bleeding, injury to surrounding structures (which include bladder, bowel, and iliac vessels), as well as infection.

Once retrieved, mature oocytes are fertilized using either a standard method in which 100,000 sperm are sprinkled around the oocyte or an intracytoplasmic sperm injection, whereby a single sperm is injected into one oocyte. Frequent monitoring of fertilization and early embryologic development then ensue. Although embryos are incubating, patients undergoing a fresh embryo transfer will start progesterone supplementation as the process of IVF negatively impacts the body's natural production of progesterone. Embryo transfer occurs on postfertilization days 3 to 6 depending on the number of embryos created and other patient factors. Embryo transfers occur under ultrasound guidance typically with minimal or no sedation and include a sterile speculum examination allowing careful and controlled placement of a small catheter containing the embryo or embryos into the uterine cavity. After embryo transfer, patients will continue progesterone supplementation until either 8 to 10 weeks' gestation or a negative pregnancy test.

ASSISTED REPRODUCTIVE TECHNOLOGY MEDICATIONS

A familiarity of the physiology of the menstrual cycle aids in the understanding of the ART process and the frequently used medications. To review briefly, the typical menstrual cycle begins with an increase in endogenous FSH to recruit a Graafian or dominant follicle. The dominant follicle begins producing estradiol that feeds back to the hypothalamus and pituitary, decreasing FSH production. When estradiol reaches a peak level, stimulation of luteinizing hormone (LH) secretion from the pituitary is promoted, resulting in the LH surge. LH, through a series of complex mechanisms, triggers ovulation to occur and the resultant collapsed follicle that housed the mature egg becomes the corpus luteum, the purpose of which is to make progesterone. If pregnancy does not occur, the corpus luteum regresses, progesterone levels fall, and the menstrual cycle starts again. If pregnancy does occur, the corpus luteum production of progesterone supports the early pregnancy until the placenta takes over at approximately 10 weeks' gestation.

ART elegantly manipulates the menstrual cycle in an attempt to hyperstimulate the ovaries to promote the growth and maturation of multiple oocytes, control the timing of oocyte final maturation, and support any subsequent pregnancy. This complex and delicately timed process requires a carefully crafted combination of exogenous hormones and medications (**Table 1**). Although most of these medications have relatively minimal side effects, it is important for emergency physicians to be cognizant of their use because they may contribute to a patient's presenting symptoms or affect the results of certain laboratory evaluations.

Exogenous gonadotropins and GnRH agonists are the most commonly used medications to promote the growth and maturation of multiple oocytes during the process of COS. These medications are self-administered subcutaneous injections and are generally well tolerated. Common side effects include bloating, nausea, mood changes, and injection site reactions. Patients will typically be on exogenous gonadotropins for 7 to 12 days and GnRH agonists for 21 to 28 days. In order to prevent premature ovulation during COS, patients may also receive a GnRH antagonist, which is also a subcutaneous injection and equally well tolerated. None of these medications should affect laboratory values obtained in the emergency department (ED).

Once the ovaries have been adequately stimulated, final maturation of oocytes must be "triggered," much like an endogenous LH surge triggers ovulation. Medications used to trigger final oocyte maturation include recombinant human chorionic gonadotropin (hCG) and/or a GnRH agonist. These medications are administered intramuscularly or subcutaneously one time during the process of COS. Side effects are minimal. When hCG is used to trigger final maturation, typical doses range from 2500 to 10,000 IU. The half-life is approximately 28 hours; therefore, a one-time dose of 10,000 IU of hCG will result in an elevated serum hCG for 14 days.

Last, intramuscular injections of progesterone in oil, or some form of vaginal progesterone, is administered for luteal support of a pregnancy and can be continued until 8 to 10 weeks' gestation. Progesterone in oil can be very irritating to surrounding tissues, causing injection site reactions and sometimes even systemic allergic reactions. Treatment is often as simple as switching the suspension oil, which is typically sesame, in addition to standard allergic reaction therapies, such as antihistamines.

ASSISTED REPRODUCTIVE TECHNOLOGY COMPLICATIONS

In terms of significant complications of ART beyond medication side effects, much of the literature focuses primarily on pregnancy-related and perinatal outcomes, such as gestational diabetes, pregnancy-induced hypertension, low birth weight, and preterm delivery.[8] There are several complications, however, that are more germane to emergency medicine, particularly OHSS, ectopic and heterotopic pregnancy, and ovarian torsion.

Of note, the use of ART for the purpose of fertility preservation is increasing, and special consideration should be given to these patients and the potential for unusual complications in light of their comorbidities. For example, a patient with aplastic anemia undergoing ART for the purposes of fertility preservation will have a higher risk of

Table 1
Common assisted reproductive technology medications

	Purpose	Examples	Administration Route	Average Duration	Common Side Effects	Notes
Exogenous gonadotropins, recombinant FSH	Promote growth and maturation of multiple oocytes	Follitropin beta	Subcutaneous injection	7–12 d	Bloating, nausea, mood changes, and injection site reactions	
Exogenous gonadotropins, urinary combined FSH and LH	Promote growth and maturation of multiple oocytes	Menotropin	Subcutaneous injection	7–12 d	Bloating, nausea, mood changes, and injection site reactions	
GnRH agonist	Promote growth and maturation of multiple oocytes and prevent premature ovulation during gonadotropin stimulation	Leuprolide	Subcutaneous injection	21–28 d	Typically well tolerated	Can also be used in conjunction with, or in place of, recombinant hCG for "triggering" oocyte final maturation
GnRH antagonist	Prevent premature ovulation during gonadotropin stimulation	Cetrorelix, ganirelix acetate	Subcutaneous injection	4–7 d	Typically well tolerated	
Recombinant hCG	"Trigger" oocyte final maturation	hCG	Intramuscular or subcutaneous injection	1 time	Typically well tolerated	Will result in an elevated serum hCG for 14 d
Progesterone	Luteal support of a pregnancy	Progesterone	Vaginal suppository	8–10 wk gestation	Abnormal vaginal discharge, occasional spotting	
		Progesterone in oil	Intramuscular injection	8–10 wk gestation	Injection site reactions, occasional systemic allergic reactions	Allergic reactions often treated by changing the suspending oil

internal bleeding after oocyte retrieval. All patients undergoing ART are considered to have "high-risk pregnancies" and are often followed very closely by their obstetricians. Close communication with these providers will likely facilitate ED evaluation and management, and obstetric colleagues should be consulted early in the ED course.

OVARIAN HYPERSTIMULATION SYNDROME
Background

If there is one complication of ART that emergency physicians should be aware of, it is OHSS. Although up to one-third of cases are mild and amenable to outpatient treatment,[9] this iatrogenic condition can rapidly progress to a much more critical and potentially life-threatening diagnosis. The overall incidence of OHSS across all COS cycles is estimated to be 3% to 8% and has a higher association with injected infertility medications compared with oral infertility medications.[9,10]

Several risk factors for the development of OHSS have been identified. Those most relevant to emergency medicine include young age, low body mass index, history of polycystic ovarian syndrome, and prior history of OHSS.[11,12] Rapidly rising or peak estradiol levels greater than 3500 pg/mL and the presence of multiple follicles (>20) also increase the risk of OHSS, but this information is not often readily available in the ED.

The pathophysiology of OHSS is based on increased vascular permeability likely related to high levels of vascular endothelial growth factors secreted by the ovaries in response to rapid increases in hCG.[9,10] The bimodal distribution of peak incidence therefore correlates with spikes in hCG during the ART process: first 3 to 7 days after hCG administration for final oocyte maturation and again at 10 to 17 days with implantation.[9] There have been cases of spontaneous OHSS unrelated to ART, but they are extremely rare. The increase in vascular permeability leads to a "third-spacing" of fluid and subsequent ascites, lower extremity edema, intravascular hypovolemia, and decreased renal perfusion. Secondary effects include hemoconcentration, hypercoagulability, and electrolyte abnormalities.[11,12]

Diagnosis

OHSS is generally classified as "mild," "moderate," or "severe" depending on the patient's clinical presentation, diagnostics, and imaging results (**Table 2**). Although most cases are mild or moderate, progression to severe can occur rapidly, and therefore, emergency physicians should consider the diagnosis in any woman undergoing ovarian stimulation who presents with abdominal pain or distension. Additional signs and symptoms may include nausea, vomiting, diarrhea, shortness of breath, and lower-extremity edema. In its most severe or critical form, patients will also display secondary characteristics related to intravascular volume depletion, such as hypotension and tachycardia. Physical examination findings are also consistent with third-spacing of fluid and depend on severity of illness, ranging from mild abdominal tenderness and lower-extremity edema to tense ascites with respiratory compromise. A pelvic examination is not routinely recommended for these patients because they often have multiple, large ovarian cysts that can hemorrhage and/or rupture.

Laboratory diagnostics are helpful in characterizing the severity of OHSS. As more fluid accumulates extravascularly, patients will become more hemoconcentrated as demonstrated by elevations of hematocrit, hemoglobin, and white blood cells. Renal hypoperfusion and fluid shifts contribute to electrolyte abnormalities and elevations in creatinine. In severe cases, hepatic function may also become compromised.

Transabdominal pelvic ultrasound is the imaging modality of choice to diagnose OHSS, and all patients undergoing ART who present to the ED with abdominal pain

Table 2
Modified Golan classification and treatment of ovarian hyperstimulation syndrome

	Signs and Symptoms	Diagnostic Testing	Imaging	Treatment
Mild	Abdominal discomfort Mild distention	No laboratory abnormalities	Ovaries <5 cm Trace ascites	Analgesia Close OB/GYN follow-up
Moderate	Abdominal tenderness Moderate distention Nausea/vomiting/diarrhea Peripheral edema	Hematocrit (Hct) >41% White blood cell count (WBC) >15,000/μL Hypoproteinemia	Ovaries 5–12 cm Mild to moderate ascites	Analgesia Antiemetics Ensure adequate fluid intake Close OB/GYN follow-up
Severe	Severe abdominal pain, severe distention, palpable ovaries, anasarca Oliguria Dyspnea, acute respiratory distress Shock (eg, hypotension, tachycardia)	Hct >45% WBC >25,000/μL Renal insufficiency Electrolyte abnormalities Elevated liver enzymes	Ovaries >12 cm, large ascites, pleural effusion, thromboembolism	IV fluid bolus, electrolyte repletion, monitor urine output, paracentesis, supplemental oxygen Thromboembolism prophylaxis Adequate analgesia and antiemetics

Data from Refs.[9–15]

or distension should have a pelvic ultrasound.[14–16] Findings include enlarged ovaries, multiple ovarian cysts, and pelvic ascites (**Fig. 3**).[14–16] In the ED, bedside ultrasound can also be useful for detecting free fluid in other extravascular compartments, including the abdomen, thorax, and pericardium. Chest radiographs are also helpful for identifying pleural effusions. Because many patients with OHSS may present to the ED with undifferentiated abdominal pain, abdominal/pelvic CT with intravenous (IV) contrast may also be considered to evaluate for other pathologic conditions.

Treatment and Disposition

Treatment of OHSS is largely supportive. Early consultation with the patient's obstetrician is essential for any patient with OHSS, regardless of severity. Mild and moderate cases may require analgesics, antiemetics, or thromboprophylaxis for hematocrit greater than 45 and can be discharged home with clear return precautions and close follow-up after discussion with the patient's obstetrician. Some patients may also benefit from therapeutic paracentesis before discharge.[17] Patients with any signs of hemodynamic instability, respiratory compromise, or significant laboratory abnormalities, however, should receive focused resuscitation and close inpatient or intensive care monitoring,[15] including:

- IV fluid boluses for intravascular and electrolyte repletion
- Adequate analgesia and antiemetics
- Close monitoring of urine output
- Therapeutic paracentesis for significant ascites, especially if there is concern for abdominal compartment syndrome or respiratory compromise[18]
- Supplemental oxygen, including the use of noninvasive positive pressure ventilation if necessary to maintain adequate oxygen saturations
- Low-molecular-weight heparin for thromboembolic prophylaxis[19]

ECTOPIC AND HETEROTOPIC PREGNANCY

Ectopic pregnancy is defined as any pregnancy outside the uterus. Traditionally, ART has been associated with an increased risk of ectopic pregnancies with rates reported in the 1990s as high as 8.6%, compared with 2% in the general population during that same time period.[2,14] Over the years, however, the rate has steadily decreased, and recent analysis of data from 2011 suggests a rate of 1.6%.[20] Factors contributing to this decline include advances in ART procedures, fewer multiple embryo transfers,

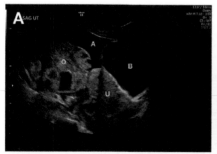
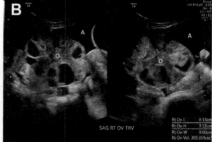

Fig. 3. (*A*) Pelvic ultrasound findings in OHSS. Transabdominal pelvic ultrasound of a patient with OHSS demonstrating a hyperstimulated ovary (O), surrounding ascites (A), uterus (U), and bladder (B). (*B*) Two transabdominal views of a large volume (309.4 cm³) right ovary with multiple cystic lesions (O) that create a "wheel spoke" appearance, and surrounding ascites (A), both of which are characteristic of OHSS.

and lower rates of tubal factor infertility among women undergoing ART procedures. Heterotopic pregnancy is the occurrence of simultaneous intrauterine and ectopic pregnancies. Overall, the incidence of heterotopic pregnancies is estimated to be between 1 in 4000 and 8000 in the general population, but the incidence of heterotopic pregnancies occurring in patients undergoing ART has been reported to be as high as 1/100.[21]

The presentation, diagnosis, and management of ectopic and heterotopic pregnancies are covered in a separate section (see Elizabeth Pontius and Julie T. Vieth's article, "Complications in Early Pregnancy", in this issue), but it is worth noting that the diagnosis may be especially challenging in the setting of ART use and particularly for women with OHSS. Pelvic pain and free fluid, two hallmarks of ectopic pregnancies, are common findings during COS. As use of ART is a risk factor for heterotopic pregnancy, close attention must be paid to the entire pelvis on ultrasound, even if an intrauterine pregnancy is seen. In addition, visualizing an extrauterine pregnancy on ultrasound may be complicated by enlarged ovaries or abnormal anatomy. Lastly, unusual ectopic pregnancies can arise of ART, including cervical and cesarean scar ectopic pregnancies requiring specialized evaluation and treatment. Therefore, although the rate of ectopic pregnancy may not be higher among women undergoing ART procedures, these patients may present a unique diagnostic challenge in the ED, and early consultation with gynecology is often warranted.

OVARIAN TORSION

There are few pieces of data on the specific incidence of ovarian torsion in patients undergoing ART procedures.[14] However, ovarian enlargement is a significant risk factor, and torsion should be considered when patients undergoing ART present with sudden onset, unilateral pelvic pain.[12] Like ectopic pregnancy, ovarian torsion in the setting of ART may present a diagnostic challenge in that ovarian enlargement and free pelvic fluid can occur following ovarian stimulation and may be a normal result of ART. A complete discussion of ovarian torsion can be found in Kayla Dewey and Cory Wittrock's article, "Acute Pelvic Pain", in this issue.

SUMMARY

Use of ART is becoming more common, and it is important for emergency physicians to have an understanding of the process, common medications used, and potential complications.

Patients undergoing ART procedures are most likely to present to the ED for complications related to the process of COS. Emergency physicians should be vigilant to assess all patients using ART for the potentially life-threatening complications of OHSS, ectopic pregnancy, and ovarian torsion. In addition to standard examination and basic laboratory tests, the ED evaluation should also include a pelvic ultrasound to assess ovarian size and presence of free fluid. Treatment is generally focused on initial resuscitation and stabilization, followed by symptomatic management and close consultation with gynecology.

REFERENCES

1. Sunderam S, Kissin DM, Crawford SB, et al. Assisted reproductive technology surveillance - United States, 2015. MMWR Surveill Summ 2018;67(3):1–28.

2. Clayton HB, Schieve LA, Peterson HB, et al. Ectopic pregnancy risk with assisted reproductive technology procedures. Obstet Gynecol 2006;107(3): 595–604.
3. The Practice Committee of the American Society of Reproductive Medicine. Optimizing natural fertility a committee opinion. Fertil Steril 2017;107:52–8.
4. The Practice Committee of the American Society of Reproductive Medicine. Diagnostic evaluation of the infertility male a committee opinion. Fertil Steril 2012;98: 294–301.
5. The Practice Committee of the American Society of Reproductive Medicine. Diagnostic evaluation of the infertility female a committee opinion. Fertil Steril 2012;98: 302–7.
6. The Practice Committee of the American Society of Reproductive Medicine. Testing and interpreting measures of ovarian reserve a committee opinion. Fertil Steril 2012;98:1407–15.
7. The Practice Committee of the American Society of Reproductive Medicine. Use of exogenous gonadotropins in anovulatory women: a technical bulletin. Fertil Steril 2008;90:S7–12.
8. Qin J, Liu X, Sheng X, et al. Assisted reproductive technology and the risk of pregnancy-related complications and adverse pregnancy outcomes in singleton pregnancies: a meta-analysis of cohort studies. Fertil Steril 2016;105(1): 73–85.e1-6.
9. Zivi E, Simon A, Laufer N. Ovarian hyperstimulation syndrome: definition, incidence, and classification. Semin Reprod Med 2010;28(6):441–7.
10. Nastri CO, Teixeira DM, Moroni RM, et al. Ovarian hyperstimulation syndrome: pathophysiology, staging, prediction and prevention. Ultrasound Obstet Gynecol 2015;45(4):377–93.
11. The Practice Committee of the American Society for Reproductive Medicine. Ovarian hyperstimulation syndrome. Fertil Steril 2008;90(5 Suppl):S188–93.
12. Yang-Kauh C. Complications of gynecologic procedures, abortion, and assisted reproductive techonology. In: Adams J, editor. Emergency medicine, clinical essentials. Volume 125. Philadelphia: Saunders; 2013. p. 1079–96.e1.
13. Chen CD, Chen SU, Yang YS. Prevention and management of ovarian hyperstimulation syndrome. Best Pract Res Clin Obstet Gynaecol 2012;26(6):817–27.
14. Baron KT, Babagbemi KT, Arleo EK, et al. Emergent complications of assisted reproduction: expecting the unexpected. Radiographics 2013;33(1):229–44.
15. Sansone P, Aurilio C, Pace MC, et al. Intensive care treatment of ovarian hyperstimulation syndrome (OHSS). Ann N Y Acad Sci 2011;1221:109–18.
16. Frasure SE, Rempell JS, Noble VE, et al. Emergency ultrasound diagnosis of ovarian hyperstimulation syndrome: case report. J Emerg Med 2012;43(2): e129–32.
17. Csokmay JM, Yauger BJ, Henne MB, et al. Cost analysis model of outpatient management of ovarian hyperstimulation syndrome with paracentesis: "tap early and often" versus hospitalization. Fertil Steril 2010;93(1):167–73.
18. Grossman LC, Michalakis KG, Browne H, et al. The pathophysiology of ovarian hyperstimulation syndrome: an unrecognized compartment syndrome. Fertil Steril 2010;94(4):1392–8.
19. Chan WS, Dixon ME. The "ART" of thromboembolism: a review of assisted reproductive technology and thromboembolic complications. Thromb Res 2008; 121(6):713–26.

20. Perkins KM, Boulet SL, Kissin DM, et al. Risk of ectopic pregnancy associated with assisted reproductive technology in the United States, 2001-2011. Obstet Gynecol 2015;125(1):70–8.
21. Felekis T, Akrivis C, Tsirkas P, et al. Heterotopic triplet pregnancy after in vitro fertilization with favorable outcome of the intrauterine twin pregnancy subsequent to surgical treatment of the tubal pregnancy. Case Rep Obstet Gynecol 2014; 2014:356131.

Vaginal Bleeding in Late Pregnancy

Janet S. Young, MD[a],*, Lindsey M. White, MD[b]

KEYWORDS

- Placenta previa • Abruption • Bleeding • Antepartum • Hemorrhage • Pregnancy
- Disseminated intravascular coagulopathy • Thromboelastography

KEY POINTS

- The clinical presentation of vaginal bleeding in the late-term pregnancy (>26 weeks) is associated with increased maternal and fetal mortality.
- Causes of life-threatening vaginal bleeding in late-term pregnancy are placenta previa, vasa previa, placental abruption, uterine rupture, invasive placentation, and coagulopathy.
- Resuscitation of the bleeding pregnant patient should be modified for the physiologic changes associated with advanced pregnancy.
- During resuscitation for serious antepartum hemorrhage, blood product replacement can be given in a balanced approach versus a targeted approach.

INTRODUCTION

The clinical presentation of vaginal bleeding in the late-term pregnancy (>26 weeks estimated gestational age [EGA]) is associated with increased maternal and fetal mortality. The need for emergency delivery is more common in women with a first episode of bleeding before 29 weeks EGA and greater than or equal to 3 episodes of antepartum bleeding.[1] The emergency department (ED) management of late-term bleeding can be challenging, especially when providing stabilizing care in a limited-resource environment. Early recognition of life-threatening bleeding, potential causes, maternal-fetal distress, and prompt obstetric consultation or transfer are essential to the effective management of late-term vaginal bleeding.

Disclosure Statement: The authors have no relevant financial disclosures for any direct financial interest in the subject matter presented in this article or with any competing company or product.
 a Department of Emergency Medicine, Virginia Tech Carilion School of Medicine, Carilion Medical Center, 1 Riverside Circle, 4th Floor Admin, Roanoke, VA 24016, USA; b Department of Emergency Medicine, Virginia Tech Carilion School of Medicine, 1 Riverside Circle, 4th Floor Admin, Roanoke, VA 24016, USA
* Corresponding author.
E-mail address: jsyoung@carilionclinic.org

Emerg Med Clin N Am 37 (2019) 251–264
https://doi.org/10.1016/j.emc.2019.01.006
0733-8627/19/© 2019 Elsevier Inc. All rights reserved.

RECOGNITION AND ASSESSMENT OF LATE-TERM BLEEDING

Cervical ripening occurs in late pregnancy, resulting in increased tissue elasticity and friability. Minor trauma, such as sexual intercourse or a vaginal examination, can result in spotting or minor vaginal bleeding. Other causes of minor bleeding include cervical cancer, cervicitis, cervical ectropion, or cervical polyps.[2] Cervical dilatation during the early phase of labor can be accompanied by a small amount of blood or blood-tinged mucus, termed a bloody show, which may cause the patient to seek medical care. Benign causes of late-term vaginal bleeding often present with small amounts of self-limited bleeding or blood-streaked mucus. A detailed history, ultrasound for excluding placenta previa, and careful pelvic examination are usually sufficient to distinguish minor from more serious causes of vaginal bleeding. Short-term observation in a monitored antepartum unit may be advisable after consultation with an obstetrician.

Signs and symptoms for serious late-term vaginal bleeding include a sudden gush of bright red blood, presence of clotted vaginal bleeding, or bleeding accompanied by severe pain and cramping. These red flags, which may or may not be accompanied by a history of minor trauma, require an immediate assessment of maternal and fetal well-being. Although mild tachycardia can be physiologic in pregnancy, significant orthostatic changes in vital signs can indicate hypovolemia. Overt signs of shock, such as tachycardia and hypotension, may be may be late findings in a pregnant woman and indicate the need for immediate resuscitation with fluids and/or blood products. See later discussion of resuscitation of the late-term, bleeding pregnant patient.

ETIOLOGIC FACTORS

The most common causes of serious vaginal bleeding in late-term pregnancy are placenta previa, placental abruption, uterine rupture, and vasa previa. Less common, although historically increasing in frequency, are placenta accreta (adherence of the placenta directly on the superficial myometrium), placenta increta (placental invasion into the uterine myometrium), and placenta percreta (placental invasion through the uterine myometrium into the uterine serosa or beyond the uterus). **Box 1** lists the risk factors associated with common causes of vaginal bleeding in late pregnancy.

ABNORMAL PLACENTATION
Placenta Previa

Placenta previa occurs when the placenta covers any portion of the endocervical os. The incidence is estimated at 1 per 200 term pregnancies and has been increasing with the increasing utilization of cesarean sections.[3] Other risk factors include prior previa, increased parity, increased maternal age, maternal smoking, cocaine use, and previous uterine surgeries, as well as elective and spontaneous abortions. Placenta previa can present as painless, bright red vaginal bleeding in the second or third trimester but may be accompanied by cramping. Many previas are diagnosed on routine prenatal screening with ultrasonography (**Fig. 1**). Because previa or low-lying placentas detected after 20 weeks EGA are associated with vasa previa and, consequently, elevated perinatal mortality rates, transvaginal ultrasonography with Doppler is recommended to rule out vasa previa.[4] If placenta previa is suspected in the ED, placental location should be confirmed with point-of-care transabdominal ultrasound. Although there is evidence to suggest a careful transvaginal ultrasound or

---

Box 1
Risk factors for major causes of vaginal bleeding in late pregnancy

Abnormal placentation
Placenta previa
  Advanced maternal age (>40 years)
  Chronic hypertension
  Multiparity
  Multiple gestations
  Previous cesarean delivery
  Tobacco use
  Uterine curettage
  Previous uterine surgery, including uterine curettage
  Cocaine use
  History of placenta previa
  Chronic hypertension
  In vitro fertilization
Vasa previa
  In vitro fertilization
  Low-lying and second trimester placenta previa
  Multiple gestation
  Succenturiate-lobed and bilobed placenta
  Velamentous cord insertion
Invasive placenta (accreta, increta, percreta)
  Prior gynecologic procedure
  Advanced maternal age
  Placenta previa
  Hypertension
  Female fetal sex

Uteroplacental trauma
Placental abruption
  Chronic hypertension
  History of domestic violence
  Multiparity
  Preeclampsia
  Previous abruption
  Short umbilical cord
  Sudden decompression of an overdistended uterus
  Thrombophilias
  Tobacco, cocaine, or methamphetamine use
  Trauma: blunt abdominal or sudden deceleration
  Unexplained elevated maternal alpha fetoprotein level
  Uterine fibroids
Uterine rupture
  Abnormal placentation
  History of uterine surgery
  Labor induction (especially prostaglandins)
  Maternal connective tissue disease
  Non-European ethnicity
  Trauma
  Trial of labor after cesarean delivery
  Uterine anomalies

Data from Refs.[34,35]

---

speculum examination may be safe, a digital cervical examination is contraindicated.[5] Early consultation with obstetrics is warranted, even in cases of minor bleeding from a known placenta previa. The patient may require extended antepartum monitoring in a tertiary care institution.

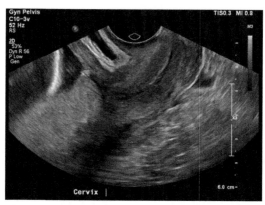

Fig. 1. Ultrasound of placenta previa. (*Courtesy of* Allison R. Durica, MD, Roanoke, VA.)

Vasa Previa

Vasa previa occurs when fetal blood vessels that are unprotected by the placenta or umbilical cord run through the amniotic membranes and across or within 2 cm of the cervix, leaving the vessels at risk of rupture following membrane rupture. It is thought vasa previa arises from early placenta previa, in which the segment of placental tissue overlying the cervix undergoes atrophy, leaving blood vessels exposed and unprotected. Vasa previa is rare, occurring in only 1 per 2500 deliveries and risk factors include velamentous insertion, bilobed or succenturiate-lobed placenta, in vitro fertilization, multiple gestation, and placenta previa.[6] Ideally, vasa previa should be detected in antenatal screening but some patients present to the ED without any prenatal care. Even with diagnosis and surveillance in the antenatal setting, nearly one-third of vasa previa patients undergo emergency preterm delivery.[7] Classic presentation of vasa previa hemorrhage includes rupture of membranes, painless vaginal bleeding, and signs of fetal distress; for example, fetal bradycardia, or death. With fetal blood volume averaging only 275 mL, bleeding from a vasa previa drains the fetoplacental circulation and rapidly results in devastating consequences for the fetus.[6] Approximately 50% of neonates die when the diagnosis of vasa previa is not made antenatally.[8] Although options exist to test if vaginal blood is fetal or maternal in origin, they often take too long to be clinically useful in an emergency setting. Emergency management of hemorrhage from vasa previa is limited to emergency cesarean section delivery of the fetus, followed by fetal resuscitation and maternal stabilization. Management for vasa previa in a low-resource environment is immediate maternal stabilization and transfer to a tertiary care obstetrics unit.

INVASIVE PLACENTATION: PLACENTA ACCRETA, INCRETA, AND PERCRETA

Invasive placentation, which includes placenta accreta, increta, and percreta, is an uncommon cause of late-term vaginal bleeding but is a significant cause of maternal morbidity and postpartum hemorrhage. Placenta accreta, the invasion of placental villi into the surface of the myometrium, has steadily increased in frequency as a result of increased cesarean delivery utilization. It now occurs in approximately 1 in 300 to 500 pregnancies.[9,10] In a patient having 3 or more prior cesarean deliveries, the risk of placenta accreta is 40% if the placenta is a previa.[11] Other risk factors for invasive placentation include concomitant placenta previa, history of placenta accreta, uterine surgery (eg, myomectomy), and assisted reproductive therapies.[12,13] The emergency presentation resulting from invasive placentation is one of marked intrapartum or postpartum hemorrhage after preterm or precipitous delivery. Placenta accreta is usually associated with a prolonged third stage of labor (delivery of placenta >30 minutes) even when uterotonics are administered. Estimates of typical blood loss from unrecognized placenta accreta range from 3000 mL to 5000 mL.[14] Overaggressive traction on the umbilical cord can result in uterine inversion due to a morbidly adherent placenta. It is critical, therefore, to maintain an elevated clinical suspicion for invasive placentation because there is a high rate of maternal morbidity (blood loss, postpartum hysterectomy). Emergency management consists of early recognition of abnormal bleeding (>500 mL), active management of the third stage of labor, early transfusion or initiation of massive transfusion protocol (MTP), and consultation with obstetrics and interventional radiology, if available. Fertility-sparing maneuvers, such as uterine artery embolization, may not be possible, and emergency hysterectomy may be necessary to prevent maternal exsanguination. Management in a low-resource ED depends on the availability of blood products and surgical services. Maternal stabilization and resuscitation, to the best ability of the transferring physician, must be initiated before emergency transfer.

UTEROPLACENTAL TRAUMA
Abruption

Placental abruption is generally defined as any premature antenatal separation of the placenta from the endometrium, potentially resulting in the catastrophic loss of fetal perfusion. A recent cohort analysis of more than 27 million singleton births revealed a prevalence of 9.6 cases of abruption per 1000 births in the United States, with a notable increase in serious maternal complications (acute heart failure and respiratory failure) since 2010.[15] An increased risk of abruption is associated with advanced maternal age, multiparity, black race, cigarette smoking, chronic hypertension, intrauterine infection, recent traumatic injury, and the use of illicit drugs or alcohol during pregnancy. Presentation of abruption is widely variable but the most common presenting clinical signs and symptoms are vaginal bleeding associated with severe abdominal or back pain, uterine fundal tenderness, and abnormal (tetanic) uterine contractions. The amount of vaginal bleeding correlates poorly with the degree of placental separation; a large abruption can be concealed behind the placenta with no evidence of vaginal bleeding. The risk of intrauterine fetal demise is significantly increased in patients with concealed abruptions.[16] Clinical suspicion for abruption should remain high in women who present with a history of proximate trauma, even a relatively low-energy mechanism that would not normally be expected to cause maternal injury. Inquiry for possible intimate partner violence should be included in the history. Placental abruption is primarily a clinical diagnosis. Ultrasound may be useful but has poor sensitivity for abruption.[17] Placental abruption is usually diagnosed at the time of placental delivery; however, management of potential abruption is determined by any evidence of fetal distress and EGA greater than or equal to 23 weeks at time of presentation. Current practice guidelines recommend immediate obstetric consultation and expedited delivery for evidence of fetal distress if institutional resources are available or immediate transfer to a tertiary care facility.[17] Abruption can result in a consumptive coagulopathy, and maternal resuscitation with repletion of fibrinogen, if available, must be considered.

UTERINE RUPTURE

Uterine rupture is the breach of the myometrial wall of the uterus. It can range from a dehiscence of a previous cesarean section scar with peritoneum intact, or complete rupture when uterine contents spill into the broad ligament or the peritoneal cavity. Rupture occurs in 0.8% of women with prior uterine surgery but only 0.03% to 0.08% of all delivering women.[18] Trauma can cause uterine rupture and should be high on the differential diagnosis of a gravid trauma patient. Classic signs of uterine rupture include severe abdominal pain and vaginal bleeding; however, most cases of rupture initially present with abnormal fetal heart tones. Loss of fetal station, absence of fetal heart tones, and easily palpable fetal body parts through the abdomen are also suggestive of a ruptured uterus. Uterine rupture can lead to maternal hemorrhage and anemia, as well as profound hypotension and tachycardia. If uterine rupture is suspected, initiate maternal and fetal resuscitation immediately with uterine displacement, intravenous (IV) fluids, and oxygen administration. Consider subcutaneous administration of a beta agonist (eg, terbutaline) to slow contractions. The definitive management of uterine rupture is emergent operative delivery, and consultation of an obstetrician or immediate transfer to an obstetric service is essential.

OTHER CAUSES
Disseminated Intravascular Coagulation

As pregnancy advances, physiologic changes occur systemically (elevation of factors VII, X, VIII, von Willebrand factor, and fibrinogen) and at the uteroplacental junction that serves to preserve maternal hemostasis at term. The placenta develops a prothrombogenic state, which increases the risk of maternal thrombosis if localized coagulation activation is transmitted into maternal circulation at the time of placental separation.[19] Disseminated intravascular coagulation (DIC) is a pathologic activation of blood coagulation that leads to intravascular fibrin deposition. A consumptive coagulopathy occurs, resulting in bleeding due to insufficient platelets and clotting factors with concomitant increase in fibrinolysis. In late pregnancy, DIC can occur in many conditions, including sepsis; intrauterine infection; placental abruption; acute peripartum hemorrhage; cervical or vaginal lacerations; amniotic fluid embolism; preeclampsia; the syndrome of hemolysis, elevated liver enzymes, and low platelets (HELLP); intrauterine fetal demise; pancreatitis; and acute fatty liver of pregnancy.[20,21] The clinical symptoms of DIC can present as vaginal bleeding with other sites of bleeding (rectal, gingival, epidermal) and signs of maternal shock. The laboratory findings of DIC demonstrate elevated prothrombin time (PT) and partial thromboplastin time (PTT), low platelets, low fibrinogen, elevated fibrin split products (fibrin degradation products or FDP), and elevated D-dimer. Management of maternal DIC should focus on maternal resuscitation with attention to restoration of circulating blood volume, taking care to avoid hypothermia and worsening acidosis. Platelets can be administered for platelets less than 50 K/μL with active bleeding or less than 30 K/μL with no bleeding. With prolonged PTT and PT, 10 to 20 mg/kg of fresh frozen plasma (FFP) is or cryoprecipitate may be administered. Alternatively, 25 to 30 U/kg of nonactivated prothrombin complex concentrate (PCC) can be given if there are signs of volume overload.[21] The crucial step in managing DIC in pregnancy is simultaneously identifying and treating the inciting event. Placental abruption has historically been the most common precipitant of maternal DIC. However, when faced with diagnostic uncertainty, using point-of-care ultrasound screening examination to evaluate the heart, inferior vena cava, Morison's pouch, aorta, and lungs (eg, rapid ultrasound for shock and hypotension [RUSH] examination) may facilitate rapid evaluation of other causes for hypotension.[22-24] In a study of pregnant patients admitted to an intensive care unit for sepsis, pyelonephritis was found to be the most common source of sepsis with patients in septic shock and DIC.[25] Despite advanced medical and obstetric management, perinatal mortality secondary to DIC has been reported in from 30% to 44% of affected pregnancies in large cohort studies.[26,27]

MATERNAL RESUSCITATION AND STABILIZATION
Low-Resource Facility

Each emergency physician or practitioner must be prepared to stabilize and transfer a pregnant patient presenting with vaginal hemorrhage, regardless of institutional capabilities. Typical resuscitation measures for maternal-fetal distress in a low-resource or critical access hospital (no available obstetrician or labor and delivery unit) should include the following:

1. Obtaining IV access: preferably 2 large-bore IVs (16 gauge or higher)
2. Maternal monitoring–continuous telemetry, blood pressure, and pulse oximetry
3. Continuous electronic fetal monitoring if available, or periodic fetal heart tones by Doppler
4. Focused history and physical examination to evaluate for signs of trauma, coagulopathy, or shock
5. Ultrasound for placental location, fetal heart activity if readily available
6. Pelvic examination to assess vaginal bleeding, estimate blood loss, or impending fetal delivery
7. Laboratory tests, including complete blood count, blood type, and cross-match, fibrinogen, PT or PTT, type and screen, basic metabolic profile and liver function testing
8. Consider transfusing O negative packed red blood cells, FFP, and platelets in a 1:1:1 ratio
9. Rho (D) immune globulin for known maternal Rh negative blood type
10. Arrange for immediate transfer to higher level of care with obstetric capabilities (will occur simultaneously with these steps).

For the pregnant patient presenting in significant cardiovascular distress, emergency resuscitation should be modified for the physiologic changes associated with advanced pregnancy. **Table 1** summarizes these modifications. The upper airways are functionally narrowed by the third trimester; consider choosing an endotracheal tube 1 size smaller for intubation. There is an increased risk of aspiration in

Table 1	
Modifications for pregnancy resuscitations	
Airway	Endotracheal tube 1 size smaller
	Same rapid sequence intubation (RSI) medications
	Use RSI to avoid aspiration
Breathing	Supplemental O$_2$ on all gravid patients
	10% reduction in estimated tidal volumes
	Small increase in ventilation rate
Circulation	Uterine displacement immediately-left lateral decubitus position
	Aggressive volume resuscitation despite reassuring blood pressure (packed red blood cells/ ffp/platelets in 1:1:1 ratio if needed)

pregnancy; rapid sequence intubation (RSI) is preferred over delayed sequence intubation. Induction agents and paralytic medications are the same dose and route as for a nongravid patient. Supplemental oxygen and passive oxygenation should be provided because pregnant patients have a rapid decline in Pao_2 with apnea. A growing uterus can cause elevation of the diaphragm and decrease functional residual capacity by 20%. Use reduced tidal volumes and end-tidal CO-oximetry to guide appropriate mechanical ventilation. Finally, blood volume and cardiac output have increased by 35% to 40% at 28 weeks gestation, which results in blunted clinical signs of shock. Blood loss may not be evident before significant volume loss. Tachycardia and tachypnea should be red flags in the pregnant patient. Suspect hypovolemia before clinical signs of hypotension and initiate aggressive fluid resuscitation with warmed crystalloid and/or blood products. In the second half of pregnancy, compression of the inferior vena cava by the gravid uterus can cause significant hypotension by decreasing venous return when the patient lies supine. Perform immediate uterine displacement regardless of gestational age by tilting the patient to the left (wedge under left flank) or manually displacing the patient's uterus to the left side of the body (manual decompression).

MATERNAL RESUSCITATION IN THE TERTIARY CARE EMERGENCY DEPARTMENT

In addition to obtaining IV access, continuous maternal cardiopulmonary monitoring, and providing supplemental oxygen, the emergency team should initiate immediate continuous external fetal monitoring to determine the presence of fetal distress and contractions. Obstetric consultation must be obtained simultaneously to determine the need for urgent operative delivery. Operative delivery is indicated with persistent fetal heart rate abnormalities or other signs of fetal distress. Aggressive maternal resuscitation may be successful at resolving fetal heart rate decelerations, tachycardia, or loss of heart rate variability.

Replacement of Blood Products

During resuscitation of a large antepartum hemorrhage, care must be taken to avoid hypothermia, acidosis, and hypocalcemia, all of which can contribute to coagulopathy (**Table 2**). Based on large trauma center registries, a balanced approach to hemorrhagic resuscitation is recommended, thereby avoiding excess crystalloid therapy. O negative, uncrossmatched blood is indicated for initial therapy. A single unit of 300 mL will increase maternal hemoglobin by 1 mg/dL if ongoing bleeding is not present. FFP, which contains multiple coagulation factors, is indicated to treat DIC or when initiating MTP). The general approach to dosing FFP is to transfuse 1 unit (250 mL) for each unit of packed red cells or 1 unit per 20 kg of body weight to obtain PT less than or equal to 15 seconds and a PTT less than or equal to 35 seconds. Platelets are also indicated in MTP protocols or when coagulopathy is suspected (eg, abruption, DIC). A single unit of platelets increases platelet count by 5000 to 10,000 mm^3, and should be considered after each dose of FFP. Finally, replacement of fibrinogen by means of cryoprecipitate, fibrinogen concentrate, or PCC should be considered in any bleeding pregnant patient because uteroplacental coagulation may precipitate a consumptive coagulopathy.

Viscoelastic Testing

If there is concern for massive hemorrhage or DIC, viscoelastic testing, such as thromboelastography (TEG) or rotational thromboelastometry (ROTEM) can be of clinical use, if available. Both testing modalities measure the clot formation,

Table 2
Blood product utilization for maternal hemorrhage

Red cells	1 unit: 300 mL, hematocrit of 70%, increased hemoglobin concentration by 1 mg/dL without ongoing bleeding Use O negative red cells first Type and crossmatch additional blood Replace red cells to maintain volume
FFP	1 unit: 250 mL, contains coagulation factors Indicated in massive transfusion and DIC: PT 1.5 × normal, international normalized ratio >2.0, PTT 2 × normal Give 1 unit plasma per unit of red cells or 1 unit FFP per 20 kg body weight Aim for PT of 15 s and a PTT of 35 s
Platelets	I unit increases platelet count 5000–10,000 mm^3 Indicated in active bleeding with platelets <50,000 1 to 2 adult doses every 1.5–2 × blood volume replacement Aim for platelets count >50 × 10^9/l
Fibrinogen	Contains fibrinogen, factor VIII, vW, fibronectin and factor XIII Used to replace fibrinogen 2 donation pools cryoprecipitate 4 g fibrinogen concentrates Aim for fibrinogen level >1 g/L

Data from Erez O, Mastrolia SA, Thachil J. Disseminated intravascular coagulation in pregnancy: insights in pathophysiology, diagnosis and management. Am J Obstet Gynecol 2015;213(4):452–63.

initiation, strength, and lysis in whole blood and can help guide which blood products are needed. TEG and ROTEM allow for rapid identification of excessive fibrinolysis.

In TEG-guided resuscitations, the repletion of blood products can be directed by the graphical and numerical results of the viscoelastic testing. The typical parameters are noted in **Fig. 2**A. The variables for TEG include the following:

- R time: measures the initiation of clot formation or the time from start of the test to the start of fibrin formation.
- K time: measures the amplification of clotting with the time taken to achieve a 20 mm amplitude of clot strength
- Alpha angle: measures rate clot formation with the speed of fibrin buildup
- Maximum amplitude (MA) represents strength and overall stability of clot
- Time to MA measures the time it takes to get to this point
- A30 measures the percentage of decrease in amplitude at 30 minutes post-MA and demonstrates the degree of fibrinolysis

Similar variables exist for ROTEM (**Fig. 2**):

- Clotting time: start of test to clot formation start
- Clot formation time: time from clot start to 20 mm amplitude
- Clot lysis (LY30): clot lysis at 30 minutes
- Alpha angle: measures the rate of clot formation
- Maximum clot firmness.

ROTEM can detect hypofibrinogenemia, which has been shown to predict the severity of hemorrhage.[28] In a prospective, observational study, women experiencing postpartum hemorrhage (PPH) of greater than 1000 mL, standard fibrinogen

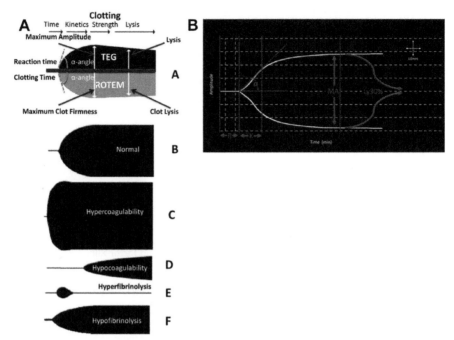

Fig. 2. (*A*) Normal TEG, and common pathologic conditions resulting in aberrantly shaped TEG or ROTEM results. A: TEG compared with ROTEM, showing clotting or reaction parameters, including time, kinetics, strength, and lysis of the clot. B to F: various viscoelastic hemostatic assay tracings. B, normal (healthy); C, hypercoagulability; D, hypocoagulability; E, hyperfibrinolysis; F, hypofibrinolysis. (*B*) Normal TEG demonstrates clot development and fibrinolysis as a function of time. Factor-dependent development of the initial fibrin clot is measured by R. The kinetics of clot formation are reflected by K and α. The maximal clot strength is measured by maximum amplitude (MA). Percent clot lysis at 30 minutes after MA (Ly30%) reflects the rate of fibrinolysis. (*From [A]* Kell, DB, Pretorius, E. The simultaneous occurrence of both hypercoagulability and hypofibrinolysis in blood and serum during systemic inflammation, and the roles of iron and fibrin (ogen). Integr Biol (Camb) 2015;7(1):24–52; and [*B*] Hurwich M, Zimmer D, Guerra E, et al. A case of successful thromboelastographic guided resuscitation after postpartum hemorrhage and cardiac arrest. J Extra Corpor Technol 2016;48(4):194.

levels, and early assessment of fibrinogen by ROTEM were measured using the Fibtem A5 value, which reflects fibrinogen contribution to clot strength 5 minutes after onset of clot formation. The Fibtem A5 value was found to be predictive of PPH progression to 2500 mL blood loss.[29] **Table 3** illustrates the appropriate blood product replacement based on TEG or ROTEM abnormalities. Using a targeted approach may prevent volume overload, hypothermia, and lung injury, and potentially increase maternal survival, but has not been prospectively validated on any pregnancy-specific cohort.[30]

INSTITUTIONAL PREPAREDNESS FOR OBSTETRIC HEMORRHAGE

Despite significant medical advances in obstetrics, maternal hemorrhage continues to be a leading cause of maternal mortality in the United States and worldwide. As a result, standardized approaches for the institutional response for maternal

Table 3
Thromboelastographic-guided blood component therapy

TEG Result	Process Impaired	Problem	Treat with
R time prolonged	Start of clot formation slowed	Coagulation factors	FFP
K time prolonged	Time clot reaches fixed strength prolonged	Fibrinogen	Cryoprecipitate or fibrinogen
Reduced α angle	Speed of fibrin accumulation reduced	Fibrinogen	Cryoprecipitate or fibrinogen
MA reduced	Reduced vertical amplitude of TEG	Platelets, fibrinogen	Platelets, DDAVP, cryoprecipitate
LY30 elevated	Increased % of amplitude reduction 30 min after MA	Increased fibrinolysis	Antifibrinolytics: Tranexamic acid Aminocaproic acid

Adapted from Walsh M, Thomas SG, Howard JC, et al. Blood component therapy in trauma guided with the utilization of the perfusionist and thromboelastography. J Extra Corpor Technol 2011;43(3):162; and Rezaie S. Rebel review #54. Thromboelastogram (TEG). Available at: http://rebelem.com/rebel-reviews.com. Accessed July 17, 2018.

hemorrhage have been developed to aid in early recognition and management of hemorrhagic emergencies in antenatal, intrapartum, and postpartum patients.[31–33] **Box 2** outlines one such approach to guide institutional and ED preparedness for the management of the bleeding, pregnant patient.

Box 2
Institutional obstetric hemorrhage preparation

Readiness (every unit)
1. Hemorrhage cart with supplies, checklist, and instruction cards for intrauterine balloons and compression stitches
2. Immediate access to hemorrhage medications (kits or equivalent)
3. Establish a response team: who to call when help is needed (blood bank, advanced gynecologic surgery, other support, and tertiary services)
4. Establish massive and emergency release transfusion protocols (O negative uncrossmatched blood products)
5. Unit education on protocols: unit-based drills with after-drill debriefs; recognition and prevention (every patient)
6. Assessment of hemorrhage risk (prenatal, on admission, and at other appropriate times)
7. Measurement of cumulative blood loss (formal and as quantitative as possible)
8. Active management of the third stage of labor (department-wide protocol)

Response (every hemorrhage)
9. Unit-standard, stage-based obstetric hemorrhage emergency management plan with checklists
10. Support programs for patients, families, and staff for all significant hemorrhages

Reporting or systems learning (every unit)
11. Establish a culture of huddles for high-risk patients and after-event debriefs to identify successes and opportunities
12. Multidisciplinary review of serious hemorrhage for systems issues
13. Monitor outcomes and processes metrics in perinatal quality improvement committee

From Main EK, Goffman D, Scavone BM, et al. National partnership for maternal safety: consensus bundle on obstetric hemorrhage. Obstet Gynecol 2015;126(1):155–62.

SUMMARY

Bleeding in the second and third trimester of pregnancy can present as an innocuous start to parturition or a catastrophic maternal-fetal hemorrhage potentially masked by the physiologic adaptations of pregnancy. A careful assessment for the presence of compensated maternal shock, abnormal placentation, fetal distress, and immediate resuscitative efforts may reduce the risk of perinatal death. Early recognition and appropriate resuscitation of concealed hemorrhage (abruption, uterine rupture) or abnormal peripartum bleeding will reduce maternal morbidity and mortality. Maternal resuscitation with balanced (1:1:1) versus targeted blood products replacement will be guided by institutional capabilities and blood bank resources. ED readiness for such a patient encompasses not only the physician's preparation and knowledge but also an institutional response for resuscitating and stabilizing any pregnant patient before emergency transfer.

REFERENCES

1. Pivano A, Alessandrini M, Desbriere R, et al. A score to predict the risk of emergency caesarean delivery in women with antepartum bleeding and placenta praevia. Eur J Obstet Gynecol Reprod Biol 2015;195:173–6.
2. Royal College of Obstetricians and Gynaecologists. Green-top guideline No. 63. Antepartum haemorrhage. London: Royal College of Obstetricians and Gynaecologists; 2011.
3. Cresswell JA, Ronsmans C, Calvert C, et al. Prevalence of placenta praevia by world region: a systematic review and meta-analysis. Trop Med Int Health 2013;18:712–24.
4. Reddy UM, Abuhamad AZ, Levine D, et al. Fetal imaging. J Ultrasound Med 2014;33:745–57.
5. Young J. Maternal emergencies after 20 weeks of pregnancy and in the postpartum period. In: Tintinalli JE, Stapczynski J, editors. Tintinalli's emergency medicine. 8th edition. New York: McGraw-Hill; 2016. p. 644–51.
6. Silver RM. Abnormal placentation: placenta previa, vasa previa, and placenta accreta. Obstet Gynecol 2015;126(3):654–68.
7. Sinkey RG, Odibo AO, Dashe JS. # 37: diagnosis and management of vasa previa. Am J Obstet Gynecol 2015;213(5):615–9.
8. Oyelese Y. Re: Incidence of and risk factors for vasa praevia: a systematic review. BJOG 2017;124(1):162.
9. Silver RM, Fox KA, Barton JR, et al. Center of excellence for placenta accreta. Am J Obstet Gynecol 2015;212(5):561–8.
10. Belfort MA, Publications CommitteeSociety for Maternal-Fetal Medicine. Placenta accreta. Am J Obstet Gynecol 2010;203(5):430–9.
11. Reddy UM, Abuhamad AZ, Levine D, et al. Fetal imaging: executive summary of a Joint Eunice Kennedy Shriver National Institute of Child Health and Human Development, Society for Maternal-Fetal Medicine, American Institute of Ultrasound in Medicine, American College of Obstetricians and Gynecologists, American College of Radiology, Society for Pediatric Radiology, and Society of Radiologists in Ultrasound Fetal Imaging Workshop. J Ultrasound Med 2014;33(5):745–57.
12. Thurn L, Lindqvist PG, Jakobsson M, Colmorn LB, Klungsoyr K, Bjarnadóttir RI,, Krebs L. Abnormally invasive placenta—prevalence, risk factors and antenatal suspicion: results from a large population-based pregnancy cohort study in the Nordic countries. BJOG 2016;123(8):1348–55.

13. Kaser DJ, Melamed A, Bormann CL, et al. Cryopreserved embryo transfer is an independent risk factor for placenta accreta. Fertil Steril 2015;103(5):1176–84.

14. Shellhaas CS, Gilbert S, Landon MB, et al. The frequency and complication rates of hysterectomy accompanying cesarean delivery. Eunice Kennedy Shriver National Institutes of Health and Human Development Maternal-Fetal Medicine Units Network. Obstet Gynecol 2009;114:224–9.

15. Ananth CV, Lavery JA, Vintzileos AM, et al. Severe placental abruption: clinical definition and associations with maternal complications. Am J Obstet Gynecol 2016;214(2):272.e1-9.

16. Kasai M, Aoki S, Ogawa M, et al. Prediction of perinatal outcomes based on primary symptoms in women with placental abruption. J Obstet Gynaecol Res 2015; 41:850–6.

17. Jain V, Chari R, Maslovitz S, et al. Guidelines for the management of a pregnant trauma patient. J Obstet Gynaecol Can 2015;37(6):553–74.

18. American College of Obstetricians and Gynecologists. ACOG practice bulletin no. 115: vaginal birth after previous cesarean delivery. Obstet Gynecol 2010; 116(2 Pt 1):450–63.

19. Cromwell C, Paidas M. Hematologic changes in pregnancy. In: Hoffman R, Benz EJ Jr, Silberstein LE, et al, editors. Hematology: Basic Principles and Practice. Elsevier; 2018. p. 2203–14.

20. Tang SJ, Rodriguez–Frias E, Singh S, et al. Acute pancreatitis during pregnancy. Clin Gastroenterol Hepatol 2010;8(1):85–90.

21. Erez O, Mastrolia SA, Thachil J. Disseminated intravascular coagulation in pregnancy: insights in pathophysiology, diagnosis and management. Am J Obstet Gynecol 2015;213(4):452–63.

22. Perera P, Mailhot T, Riley D, et al. The RUSH exam 2012: rapid ultrasound in shock in the evaluation of the critically ill patient. Ultrasound Clin 2012;7(2): 255–78.

23. Richards JR, McGahan JP. Focused assessment with sonography in trauma (FAST) in 2017: what radiologists can learn. Radiology 2017;283(1):30–48.

24. Blanco P, Aguiar FM, Blaivas M. Rapid ultrasound in shock (RUSH) velocity-time integral: a proposal to expand the RUSH protocol. J Ultrasound Med 2015;34(9): 1691–700.

25. Snyder CC, Barton JR, Habli M, et al. Severe sepsis and septic shock in pregnancy: indications for delivery and maternal and perinatal outcomes. J Matern Fetal Neonatal Med 2013;26(5):503–6.

26. Rattray DD, O'Connell CM, Baskett TF. Acute disseminated intravascular coagulation in obstetrics: a tertiary centre population review (1980 to 2009). J Obstet Gynaecol Can 2012;34(4):341–7.

27. Erez O, Novack L, Beer-Weisel R, et al. DIC score in pregnant women–a population based modification of the International Society on Thrombosis and Hemostasis score. PLoS One 2014;9(4):e93240.

28. Lockhart E. Postpartum hemorrhage: a continuing challenge. Hematology Am Soc Hematol Educ Program 2015;2015:132–7.

29. Collins PW, Lilley G, Bruynseels D, et al. Fibrin-based clot formation as an early and rapid biomarker for progression of postpartum hemorrhage: a prospective study. Blood 2014;124(11):1727–36.

30. Walsh M, Thomas SG, Howard JC, et al. Blood component therapy in trauma guided with the utilization of the perfusionist and thromboelastography. J Extra Corpor Technol 2011;43(3):162.

31. Main EK, Goffman D, Scavone BM, et al. National partnership for maternal safety: consensus bundle on obstetric hemorrhage. J Obstet Gynecol Neonatal Nurs 2015;44(4):462–70.

32. American College of Obstetricians and Gynecologist. ACOG Practice Bulletin. Postpartum hemorrhage. Number 183. Obstet Gynecol 2017;130(4):e168–86.

33. Simpson KR. Update on evaluation, prevention, and management of postpartum hemorrhage. MCN Am J Matern Child Nurs 2018;43(2):120.

34. Frank J, Baeseman Z, Leeman L, Chapter C. Vaginal bleeding in late pregnancy. In: Leeman L, Quinlan JD, Dresang LT, et al, editors. ALSO: Advanced Life Support in Obstetrics Provider Manual. 8th edition. Leawood, Kansas: American Academy of Family Physicians; 2017. p. 1–14.

35. Baldwin HJ, Patterson JA, Nippita TA, et al. Antecedent of abnormally invasive placenta in primiparous women: risk associated with gynecologic procedures. Obstet Gynecol 2018;131(2):227–33.

Precipitous Labor and Emergency Department Delivery

Joelle Borhart, MD*, Kathryn Voss, MD

KEYWORDS

- Precipitous delivery • Nuchal cord • Shoulder dystocia • McRoberts maneuver
- Breech presentation

KEY POINTS

- A vast majority of ED deliveries are cephalic (head-first) fetal presentation and result in good outcomes for mother and baby, with adequate preparation.
- Nuchal cords are common, are usually loose, and often do not cause harm.
- The combination of McRoberts maneuver and suprapubic pressure alleviates a majority of cases of shoulder dystocia.
- For breech presentation, hands should be maintained off the breech as much as possible.

INTRODUCTION

A precipitous, emergency department (ED) delivery can be among the most stressful events an emergency physician encounters. Physicians must assess 2 patients (mother and fetus), be prepared to manage a variety of complications that may arise during delivery, and lead both maternal and neonatal resuscitations in the immediate postpartum period. A majority of precipitous deliveries result in good outcomes for both mother and baby, but emergency physicians must be prepared to manage feared complications, such as tight nuchal cords, shoulder dystocia, and breech presentation. An understanding of the labor process, as well as advanced planning, including development of delivery checklists, kits, and consultant paging lists, can help decrease the stress and chaos inherent to any precipitous delivery.

Precipitous delivery is defined as labor that lasts for 3 hours or less from the onset of regular contractions to birth.[1] Many factors contribute to a precipitous delivery and include abnormally strong contractions, abnormally low resistance in the birth canal,

The authors have no disclosures.
Department of Emergency Medicine, MedStar Georgetown University, MedStar Washington Hospital Center, 3800 Reservoir Road, Washington, DC 20007, USA
* Corresponding author.
E-mail address: joelle.borhart@gmail.com

Emerg Med Clin N Am 37 (2019) 265–276
https://doi.org/10.1016/j.emc.2019.01.007
0733-8627/19/© 2019 Elsevier Inc. All rights reserved.
emed.theclinics.com

and a lack of awareness of painful sensations.[2] Prehospital and ED deliveries are associated with a high rate of maternal and fetal complications, including cervical and high-degree perineal lacerations, retained placenta, and postpartum hemorrhage.[3–5] Any ED delivery should be approached as a precipitous delivery.

EVALUATION OF THE PATIENT PRESENTING IN LABOR

Evaluation should begin by obtaining as much history as time allows, including frequency of contractions, loss of fluid, bleeding, and presence of fetal movement. The physician should ask about any prior births and complications, prenatal care, and estimated due date. If the due date is unknown, the last menstrual period can be used as an estimate. Uterine fundal height also can provide a rapid assessment of gestational age. In general, the fundus can be palpated at the level of the umbilicus at 20 weeks and grows 1 cm for every week until 36 weeks, when the fetus drops in the pelvis.[6] If available, bedside ultrasound also can provide an estimate of gestational age.

Normal Labor

Symptoms of labor include contractions but also back pain, abdominal pain, pelvic cramping or pressure, vomiting, and urinary urgency.[6] False labor is defined as uterine contractions that do not lead to cervical change (Braxton Hicks contractions).[7] Normal labor proceeds through 3 stages, leading to the delivery of the fetus and the placenta. Stage 1, cervical stage, begins with the onset of regular contractions and ends with complete cervical effacement and dilatation. Stage 1 lasts an average of 8 hours in nulliparous women and 5 hours in multiparous women. Stage 2, expulsion stage, starts once the cervix is completely effaced and dilated and continues to the delivery of the fetus. This stage lasts a median of 50 minutes in nulliparous women and 20 minutes in multiparous women.[6] Stage 3, placental stage, includes separation and delivery of the placenta. Most women who present to the ED in labor are in stage 1 or early stage 2. The length of these stages usually allows enough time for a patient to be transferred to a labor and delivery (L&D) unit; however, emergency physicians must be prepared to act if delivery is imminent.

Emergency Department Evaluation

To establish if delivery is imminent, a sterile vaginal assessment must be performed to determine the amount of cervical effacement, cervical dilation, and position of the presenting part. A cervix that is 100% effaced should feel paper-thin. A fully dilated cervix measures 10 cm. Position refers to the position of the fetus in the birth canal and the subsequent presenting part. The most common position is occiput anterior. In 95% of deliveries, the presenting part is the occiput.[8]

The information obtained during physical examination and vaginal assessment can help gauge the likelihood of an imminent delivery and determine if there is time to transfer a patient to an L&D unit. If the fetus is visibly emerging (crowning), there is not time to transfer and the patient should be delivered in the ED. If a patient is fully dilated and effaced, delivery probably should occur in the ED unless the L&D unit is close (onsite). Any other scenario requires clinical judgment and consideration of the risk and benefits of transfer.

The Emergency Medical Treatment and Active Labor Act (EMTALA) is a law governing the transfer of patients and requires that any patient with an emergency condition receive stabilizing treatment. According to EMTALA, patients in active labor are considered unstable until both baby and placenta have been delivered. Patients in labor, however, still can be transferred if there is adequate time to transfer before delivery or if there is a concern that delivering at the original department poses a greater risk to the mother or the unborn baby. The emergency physician must obtain consent for transfer, including a discussion of the risk and benefits, and must have an accepting physician.[9] It is possible for labor to significantly progress during the time transfer is arranged. It is prudent to repeat the vaginal assessment just before the patient leaves the ED to ensure delivery is still not imminent.

NORMAL VAGINAL DELIVERY
Preparation

If delivery is imminent, the ED team should prepare by heating a radiant infant warmer and obtaining supplies. At a minimum, supplies include sterile gloves, gown, mask with face shield, 2 umbilical clamps or hemostats, surgical scissors, bulb suction, towels, suture material, and fetal resuscitation equipment. It is helpful to have the necessary equipment collected in advance and stored as a readily accessible ED delivery kit. Obstetric and pediatric colleagues should be immediately notified of the impending delivery. Place the patient in the dorsal lithotomy position on her back with her hips and knees flexed and legs abducted. If time permits, the perineum should be cleansed with mild soap or povidone-iodine. Importantly, the delivering physician should be sure to wear personal protective equipment.[10]

Maneuvers and Management of Nuchal Cord

There are 7 cardinal movements of fetal descent during a normal delivery: engagement, flexion, descent, internal rotation, extension, external rotation, and expulsion.[8] As the fetus descends, the perineum stretches to accommodate the fetal head. Physicians can perform firm digital stretching of the perineum to help prevent tears. Episiotomies are not routinely performed but may be needed in cases of fetal distress or shoulder dystocia. An episiotomy can be performed by injecting local anesthetic to the area and then making a 2-cm to 3-cm cut with scissors either midline or 45° from the midline while protecting the fetal head. Median incisions carry a greater risk of extension to the anal sphincter.[10]

As the fetal head emerges from the introitus, control delivery by supporting the inferior perineum with 1 hand and the fetal head the other hand. It is important to control the delivery of the head as it emerges to help prevent perineal tears from a rapid delivery. As the fetal head emerges, the inferior hand supports the fetal chin while the superior hand remains on the fetal crown. As the head delivers, palpate the fetal neck to assess for the presence of a nuchal cord. Nuchal cord is defined as the umbilical cord wrapped around the fetal neck 360°. Nuchal cords are common, occurring in up to 29% of fetuses.[11] Although they are perceived as high-risk situations, the cord is usually is loose and does not cause harm.[12] A long and loose cord rarely impedes delivery of the body and can simply be unwound immediately after delivery. A loose cord also may be reduced prior to delivery of the body by bringing the loop over the baby's head.[13] Rarely, the cord is wrapped tightly, constricting the umbilical vessels or impeding delivery. A tight nuchal cord that cannot be reduced may be clamped in 2 places with hemostats and cut in-between. Cutting the umbilical cord prior to birth only be considered should as a last resort, because this intervention has been associated with serious fetal complications, such as hypovolemia, anemia, shock, hypoxemic-ischemic encephalopathy, and cerebral palsy.[14]

After the head delivers, it turns to 1 side (now facing maternal thigh). As the fetal head rotates, the physician should move hands to either side of the fetal head with small fingers to the perineum, while providing gentle downward traction to help deliver the anterior shoulder. After the anterior shoulder is delivered, the physician applies gentle upward traction to deliver the posterior shoulder and remainder of the fetus[10] (**Fig. 1**).

After delivery, suction the infant's mouth and nose, then wrap the infant in a warm blanket and stimulate the baby by rubbing the blanket. The umbilical cord should be double-clamped approximately 3 cm distal to the insertion, placed 4 cm to 5 cm apart and cut with sterile scissors. If infant and mother are both stable, place the baby on the maternal chest. If the infant is unstable, it should be taken directly to the warmer for further assessment and treatment.[10]

The third stage of labor is defined as the time between fetal delivery and placenta delivery and usually lasts for 10 minutes to 30 minutes. To deliver the placenta, use gentle traction on the umbilical cord to help minimize umbilical cord tearing, placental injury, and uterine inversion. Active management of the placental delivery reduces the length of this third stage and decreases the risk of postpartum hemorrhage.[7] Signs of placental separation include spontaneous umbilical cord lengthening, firming of the uterus, and sudden gush of blood.[6] Once the placenta is delivered, it should be examined to assess whether it appears intact, because the lack of an intact placental should alert the clinician to possible retained placenta or invasive placenta (ie, placenta accreta, placenta percreta, or placenta increta). Next the uterus should be vigorously massaged at the level of the fundus to help promote contractions. Additionally,

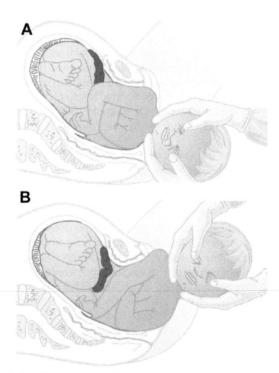

Fig. 1. Delivery of the shoulders. Gentle downward traction on the head is applied to deliver the anterior shoulder (*A*). Gentle upward traction is applied to deliver the posterior shoulder (*B*). (*From* In: Hacker NF, editor. Essential obstetrics and gynecology. Philadelphia: Elsevier Saunders; 2016; with permission.)

oxytocin can be administered to aid in uterine contraction.[10] The vagina and cervix should be examined for lacerations, which may require repair.

SHOULDER DYSTOCIA

Shoulder dystocia is a rare, unpredictable obstetric emergency that is associated with increased risk of maternal and fetal morbidity and mortality.[15] Shoulder dystocia is defined as failure of the fetal anterior shoulder to deliver following the usual downward traction on the fetal head or when additional obstetric maneuvers are necessary to deliver the fetal shoulders.[16] It is estimated to occur in 0.3% to 3% of vaginal deliveries.[17] Although several risk factors for shoulder dystocia have been identified, such as maternal diabetes and increased fetal weight, a majority of cases occur without major risk factors.[15,18]

Complications

Shoulder dystocia is associated with a variety of maternal and fetal complications. Postpartum hemorrhage, vaginal lacerations and tears, and uterine rupture are possible maternal complications. The most common fetal injuries include brachial plexus palsies (4%–40%), humeral and/or clavicular fractures (10.6%), and hypoxemic ischemic encephalopathy (0.5%–23%).[19] A crucial factor in the development of hypoxemic ischemic injury is the head-to-body delivery interval; the risk increases markedly when the head-to-body delivery interval is greater than 5 minutes.[20]

Management

Because management of shoulder dystocia is time sensitive, early recognition is critical. The turtle sign may herald shoulder dystocia: the head delivers but does not externally rotate and instead retracts against the perineum, indicating the anterior shoulder is impacted on the pubic bone.[18] Once shoulder dystocia is recognized, announce the problem and call for help. Obstetric, neonatal, and anesthesia colleagues should be alerted, and the team should prepare for the delivery of a distressed infant. Similar to codes, 1 staff member should be assigned to monitor time intervals and record the order of events for the delivering physician.

Maneuvers

Several different maneuvers have been proposed for the management of shoulder dystocia. No 1 sequence of maneuvers has proved the most effective. If a particular maneuver is not successful after 30 seconds, another maneuver should be attempted until delivery is accomplished. The American College of Obstetricians and Gynecologists advises that McRoberts maneuver is a reasonable initial maneuver.[21] McRoberts maneuver is technically easy, noninvasive, and, when combined with suprapubic pressure, alleviates a majority of cases of shoulder dystocia.[22] Ideally, McRoberts maneuver is performed with the help of 2 assistants—each holding a maternal leg and hyperflexing the mother's thighs toward her abdomen. This straightens/flattens the sacrum, allowing cephalad rotation of the pubis symphysis over the impacted anterior shoulder.[23] One assistant then applies suprapubic pressure with the heel of a hand or with a fist over the fetal anterior shoulder just proximal to the maternal pubic bone (**Figs. 2** and **3**). Pressure can be continuous or in a pulsatile motion similar to chest compressions. Fundal pressure should never be applied and only worsens the impaction.[24]

Additional maneuvers to consider include internal rotational maneuvers, such as the Rubin II and Woods corkscrew maneuvers. The Rubin II maneuver is performed by

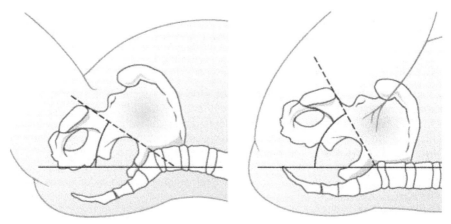

Fig. 2. The McRoberts maneuver does not change the actual dimension of the maternal pelvis. Rather, the maneuver straightens the sacrum relative to the lumbar spine, allowing cephalic rotation of the symphysis pubis sliding over the fetal shoulder. *Left panel* is before McRoberts maneuver applied, *right panel* is after McRoberts maneuver applied. (*Reprinted with permission from* the American College of Obstetricians and Gynecologists. From Gottlieb AG, Galan HL. Shoulder dystocia: An update. Obstet Gynecol Clin N Am. 2007;34:501–31, with permission from the Foreign Policy Research Institute.)

placing fingers on the posterior aspect of the anterior shoulder and pushing the shoulder toward the fetal chest. This reduces the diameter of the shoulders, allowing the anterior shoulder to be dislodged from behind the pubic bone. To perform the Woods corkscrew maneuver, place fingers on the anterior aspect of the posterior fetal shoulder and push the shoulder toward the fetal back. The Rubin II and Woods corkscrew maneuvers can be attempted simultaneously and may be performed with the mother in McRoberts position. If Rubin II and/or Woods corkscrew maneuvers fail, the physician may attempt rotating the fetus in the opposite direction by placing fingers on the back of the posterior shoulder (reverse Woods corkscrew) **(Fig. 4)**.

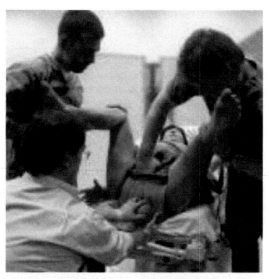

Fig. 3. McRoberts maneuver performed with 2 assistants. Assistant on patient's left applies suprapubic pressure. (*Courtesy of* CAE Healthcare, Sarasota, Florida, USA; with permission.)

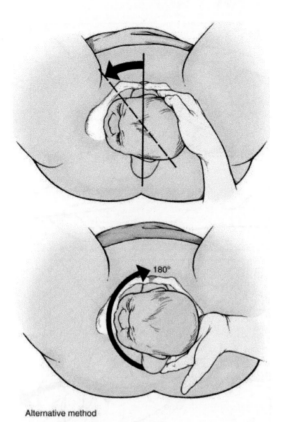

Alternative method

Fig. 4. Rubin II rotation of the anterior shoulder forward into the fetal chest (*top*). Reverse Woods corkscrew maneuver place fingers behind posterior shoulder and rotate fetus in the opposite direction of Rubin II (*bottom*). (*From* In: Gabbe SG, editor. Obstetrics: normal and problem pregnancies, 7th edition. Philadelphia: Elsevier; 2017. Figures 17–30; with permission.)

If internal rotational maneuvers are unsuccessful, delivery of the posterior arm can be attempted. Place 1 hand behind the posterior fetal shoulder, move hand down the fetal arm to the elbow, and grasp the forearm. Sweep the forearm across the fetal chest to deliver the arm hand-first (**Fig. 5**). Delivery of the posterior arm reduces the diameter of the shoulders and allows the anterior shoulder to drop below the pubic bone.

Another maneuver that may be attempted is the Gaskin maneuver or all-fours position, where the mother is assisted onto her hands and knees. This repositioning increases the pelvic outlet by up to 20 mm.[25] The additional space combined with gravity often is enough to relieve the dystocia; if not, the rotational maneuvers may be repeated with the mother in this position (**Fig. 6**). If all other maneuvers have failed, several heroic maneuvers may be considered, including the Zavanelli maneuver (cephalic replacement), followed by immediate cesarean section or symphysiotomy.

BREECH PRESENTATION

Breech presentation is the presentation of the fetal buttocks or feet and is the most common malpresentation.[26] The incidence of breech delivery depends on gestational age. At less than 28 weeks, 25% of fetuses are in breech position; by term, most have

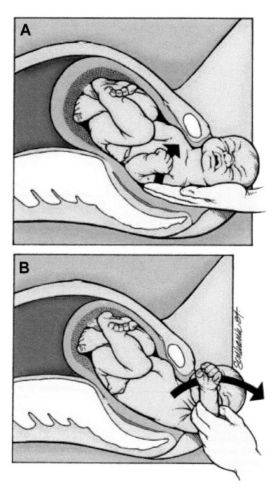

Fig. 5. Delivery of the posterior arm. The operator inserts a hand (*A*) and sweeps the posterior arm across the chest and over the perineum (*B*). Care should be taken to distribute the pressure evenly across the humerus to avoid unnecessary fracture. (*From* In: Gabbe SG, editor. Obstetrics: normal and problem pregnancies, 7th edition. Philadelphia: Elsevier; 2017; with permission.)

rotated to cephalic presentation and only 3% to 4% remain in breech position.[27] Significant risks of vaginal breech delivery include umbilical cord prolapse, prolonged cord compression, head entrapment, and birth trauma.[28,29] In a normal delivery, the large fetal head maximally dilates the cervix, allowing for smooth passage of the rest of the body. The fetal buttocks, trunk, and feet have a smaller diameter than the head and may not adequately dilate the cervix, resulting in head entrapment after delivery of the body. Further trauma, such as brachial plexus and cervical spine injuries, can be sustained when delivery of the head is attempted, especially if traction is inappropriately or excessively applied.[30]

Types of Breech Presentation

There are 3 types of breech presentation. Frank breech is the most common and is when the fetal hips are fully flexed and knees fully extended (feet by ears—pike

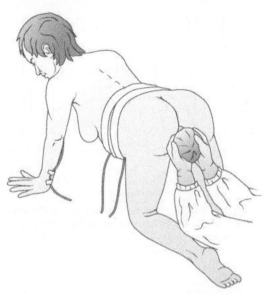

Fig. 6. The Gaskin position. The all-fours position exploits the effects of gravity and increased space in the hollow of the sacrum to facilitate delivery of the posterior shoulder and arm. (*Reprinted with permission from* the American College of Obstetricians and Gynecologists. From Gottlieb AG, Galan HL. Shoulder dystocia: An update. Obstet Gynecol Clin N Am. 2007;34:501–31, with permission from the Foreign Policy Research Institute.)

position). This is the most favorable breech position because the presenting part fits snuggly in the pelvic outlet preventing cord prolapse and maximally dilating the cervix. Complete breech is when the fetal hips and knees are flexed, so the feet are at the same level as the buttocks. The third type is incomplete or footling breech. In this position, 1 foot or both feet are pointing downward and deliver before the rest of the body (**Fig. 7**). Incomplete breech carries the highest risk of cord prolapse and head entrapment.[31–33]

Management

If breech presentation is recognized and delivery is not in progress or imminent, patients should be taken to an operating room to facilitate cesarean delivery by an obstetrician. If a patient cannot be transferred, immediately call for help from obstetric, anesthesia, and pediatric colleagues. Place the patient in lithotomy position. If possible, delay maternal pushing until an obstetrician arrives. In the event an obstetrician is not immediately available, an emergency physician should be prepared to assist the breech delivery.

The single most important rule for assisted breech delivery is to maintain hands off the breech. If, on initial vaginal examination, anything other than a head is the presenting part, the physician should step back and await events. Premature intervention can adversely affect the delivery by causing cervical retraction and head entrapment. Rushed delivery also can increase the chance of a fetal arm or arms becoming trapped behind the head above the pelvic inlet.[34] Be patient and encourage the mother to push until the fetal feet, legs, trunk, and umbilicus are visible. The physician may gently support the fetal body outside the birth canal but should never pull on the breech. Any traction by the physician can result in extension of the fetal neck and cause head entrapment.[34]

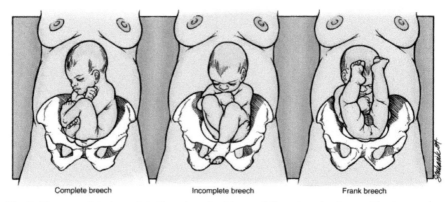

| Complete breech | Incomplete breech | Frank breech |

Fig. 7. The complete breech is flexed at the hips and flexed at the knees. The incomplete breech shows incomplete flexion of 1 or both knees or hips. The frank breech is flexed at the hips and extended at the knees. (*From* In: Gabbe SG, editor. Obstetrics: normal and problem pregnancies, 7th edition. Philadelphia: Churchill Livingston; 2017. Figures 17–14; with permission.)

Once the baby has spontaneously delivered to the level of the umbilicus, gently grasp the fetal bony pelvis using a sterile towel to improve grip. Avoid grabbing or squeezing the fetal abdomen. Aim to keep the fetal back in the anterior position, because this facilitates performing the maneuvers to assist delivery if necessary. In frank breech presentation, assistance often is required for delivery of the extended legs. Place 2 or 3 fingers under the fetal femur, slightly abduct and flex the hip, and then flex the knee to release the leg. Repeat maneuver on the other side.[30] Maternal effort alone usually is sufficient to deliver the remaining lower abdomen and fetal trunk. If the arms do not deliver spontaneously, gently rotate the fetus 90° to 1 side, pass 1 or 2 fingers over the anterior fetal shoulder, slide fingers down along the humerus, and sweep the arm across the chest to deliver the elbow and forearm. A 180o rotation of the fetus is then performed to repeat the maneuver on the other side. Once the nape of the infant's neck is visible under the pubic arch, it is time to assist delivery of the head. The Mauriceau-Smellie-Veit maneuver involves physicians placing a forearm under the fetal body with a fetal leg on either side. The second and middle fingers of this hand are placed on the fetal maxilla on either side of the nose. The other hand is placed on the fetal back with the middle finger flexing the head down and the other fingers resting on the fetal shoulders. Apply gentle downward traction on the shoulders, while lifting the body of the fetus upward and outward.[30]

SUMMARY

Precipitous ED delivery is an uncommon but stressful event. A vast majority of ED deliveries are cephalic (head-first) fetal presentation and result in good outcomes for mother and baby with adequate preparation. Nuchal cords are common, usually loose, and easily reducible and do not cause fetal harm. The combination of McRoberts maneuver and suprapubic pressure alleviates a majority of cases of shoulder dystocia, but physicians should be prepared to progress quickly through additional maneuvers. When encountering breech presentation, maintain hands off the breech as much as possible, and never pull on the breech from below.

REFERENCES

1. Suzuki S. Clinical significance of precipitous labor. J Clin Med Res 2015;7:150–3.
2. Cunningham FG, Leveno KJ, Bloom SL, et al. Abnormal labor. In: Cunningham FG, Leveno KJ, Bloom SL, et al, editors. Williams obstetrics. 23rd edition. New York: McGraw-Hill; 2009. p. 464–89.
3. Brunette D, Sterner S. Prehospital and emergency department delivery: a review of eight years experience. Ann Emerg Med 1989;18:1116–8.
4. Rodie V, Thomson A, Norman J. Accidental out-of-hospital deliveries: an obstetric and neonatal case control study. Acta Obstet Gynecol Scand 2002;81:50–4.
5. Sheiner E, Levy A, Mazor M. Precipitate labor: higher rates of maternal complications. Eur J Obstet Gynecol Reprod Biol 2004;116:43–7.
6. Vasquez V, Desai S. Labor and delivery and their complications. In: Walls RM, Hockberger RS, Gausche-Hill M, editors. Rosen's emergency medicine: concepts and clinical practice. 9th edition. Philadelphia: Elsevier; 2018. p. 2296–312.
7. Hobel CJ, Zakowski M. Normal labor, delivery, and postpartum care: anatomic considerations, obstetric analgesia and anesthesia, and resuscitation of the newborn. In: Hacker NF, Gambone JC, Hobel CJ, editors. Essentials of obstetrics and gynecology. 6th edition. Philadelphia: Elsevier; 2016. p. 96–124.
8. Kilpatrick S, Garrison E. Normal labor and delivery. In: Gabbe EG, Niebyl JR, Simpson JL, et al, editors. Obstetrics: normal and problem pregnancies. 7th edition. Philadelphia: Elsevier; 2017. p. 368–94.
9. What are the provisions for a pregnant woman in labor? In: frequently asked questions on EMTALA. 2011. Available at: www.emtala.com/faq.htm. Accessed July 1, 2018.
10. VanRooyen M, Scott J. Emergency delivery. In: Stapczynski JS, Tintinalli JE, editors. Tintinalli's emergency medicine: a comprehensive study guide. 7th edition. New York: McGraw-Hill; 2011. p. 703–11.
11. Peesay M. Nuchal cord and its implications. Matern Health Neonatol Perinatol 2017;3:28–39.
12. Vasa R, Dimitrov R, Patel S. Nuchal cord at delivery and perinatal outcomes: single-center retrospective study with emphasis on fetal acid-base balance. Pediatr Neonatol 2018;59:439–47.
13. Hutchon DJR. Management of nuchal cord at birth. J Midwifery Reprod Health 2013;1(1):4–6.
14. Mercer JS, Skovgaard RL, Peareara-Eaves J, et al. Nuchal cord management and nurse midwifery practice. J Midwifery Womens Health 2005;50:373–9.
15. Mehta SH, Sokol RJ. Shoulder dystocia: risk factors, predictability, and preventability. Semin Perinatol 2014;38:189–93.
16. Grobman W. Shoulder dystocia. Obstet Gynecol Clin N Am 2013;40:59–67.
17. Gherman RB. Shoulder dystocia: an evidence-based evaluation of the obstetric nightmare. Clin Obstet Gynecol 2002;45(2):345–62.
18. Anderson J. Complications of labor and delivery: shoulder dystocia. Prim Care 2012;39:135–44.
19. Dajani NK, Magann EF. Complications of shoulder dystocia. Semin Perinatol 2014;38:201–4.
20. Leung TY, Stuart O, Shaota DS, et al. Head-to-body delivery interval and risk of fetal acidosis and hypoxic ischaemic encephalopathy in shoulder dystocia: a retrospective review. Br J Obstet Gynaecol 2011;118:474–9.
21. ACOG Committee on Practice Bulletins—Gynecology, The American College of Obstetrician and Gynecologists. ACOG practice bulletin clinical management

guidelines for obstetrician-gynecologists. Number 40, November 2002. Obstet Gynecol 2002;100(5 Pt 1):1045–50.

22. Gherman RB, Chauhan S, Ouzounian JG, et al. Shoulder dystocia: the unpreventable obstetric emergency with empiric management guidelines. Am J Obstet Gynecol 2006;195:657–72.

23. Gherman RB, Tramont J, Muffley P, et al. Analysis of McRoberts' maneuver by x-ray pelvimetry. Obstet Gynecol 2000;95(1):43–7.

24. Gross SJ, Shime J, Farine D. Shoulder dystocia: predictors and outcome. Am J Obstet Gynecol 1987;156:334–6.

25. Baxley E, Gobbo R. Shoulder dystocia. Am Fam Physician 2004;6917:1707–14.

26. Hofmeyr GJ, Kulier R, West HM. Expedited versus conservative approaches for vaginal delivery in breech presentation. Cochrane Database Syst Rev 2015;(7):CD000082.

27. Collea JV. Current management of breech presentation. Clin Obstet Gynecol 1980;23:525–31.

28. Pradhan P, Mohajer M, Deshpande S. Outcome of term breech births: 10-year experience at a district general hospital. BJOG 2005;112(2):218–22.

29. Rietberg CC, Elferink-Stinkens PM, Brand R, et al. Term breech presentation in the Netherlands from 1995 to 1999: mortality and morbidity in relation to the mode of delivery of 33824 infants. BJOG 2003;110(6):604–9.

30. Baskett TF. Breech delivery. In: Basket TF, Calder AA, Arulkumaran S, editors. Munro Kerr's Operative Obstetrics. 12th edition. Philadelphia: Elsevier; 2014. p. 157–68.

31. Collea JV, Chein C, Quilligan EJ. The randomized management of term frank breech presentation: a study of 208 cases. Am J Obstet Gynecol 1980;137: 235–44.

32. Gimovsky ML, Wallace RL, Schifrin BS, et al. Randomized management of the nonfrank breech presentation at term: a preliminary report. Am J Obstet Gynecol 1983;146:34–40.

33. Brown L, Karrison T, Cibils LA. Mode of delivery and perinatal results in breech presentation. Am J Obstet Gynecol 1994;171:28–34.

34. Lanni SM, Gherman R, Gonik B. Malpresentations. In: Gabbe EG, Niebyl JR, et al, editors. Obstetrics: normal and problem pregnancies. 7th edition. Philadelphia: Elsevier; 2017. p. 368–94.

Late Pregnancy and Postpartum Emergencies

Natasha Wheaton, MD*, A. Al-Abdullah, MD, Tyler Haertlein, MD

KEYWORDS

- Late pregnancy complications • Postpartum complications
- Postpartum hemorrhage • Postpartum depression • Amniotic fluid embolism
- Mastitis • Endometritis • Postpartum headache

KEY POINTS

- Late pregnancy and the postpartum period is a high-risk time for women with associated morbidity and mortality.
- There are differences in the United States in pregnancy complication rates across socio-economic and racial groups with minority women suffering from much higher rates.
- Late pregnancy and postpartum complications are commonly encountered by emergency physicians and one should be comfortable diagnosing and stabilizing these pathologies.
- Pregnancy-related depression is common but often difficult to detect, EPs should consider screening all postpartum women they come in contact with.

INTRODUCTION

The period just after delivery is a high-risk period for women with associated morbidity and even mortality; more than 60% of maternal deaths across the globe, including within the United States, occur in the postpartum period.[1] There are large variations in complication rates across various groups in the United States with black women having a three times higher pregnancy-related mortality than white women.[2] Additionally, in contrast to many other industrialized countries where women receive more intensive care post birth, most women in the United States have only a single postpartum visit scheduled at 6 weeks.[3] This means that many women seek care in the emergency department (ED) for routine and more serious postpartum pathologies. Emergency physicians (EPs) should be well versed in common and life-threatening postpartum pathologies. The specific pathologies discussed in this article include peripartum depression; peripartum cardiomyopathy (PPCM); and a common but complicated complaint, the late pregnancy or postpartum headache.

Disclosure Statement: The authors have no financial interests to disclose.
UCLA Ronald Reagan-Olive View Emergency Medicine Residency, Ronald Reagan Medical Center, 924 Westwood Boulevard, Suite 300, Los Angeles, CA 90095, USA
* Corresponding author.
E-mail address: nwheaton@mednet.ucla.edu

PERIPARTUM DEPRESSION
Introduction and Epidemiology

Peripartum depression is defined as an episode of major depression that occurs during pregnancy, usually at the later end, or within 4 weeks following delivery.[4] The prevalence of postpartum depression varies widely among studies and across socioeconomic groups and geographic locations. In the United States, the strongest studies estimate that postpartum depression affects between 10% and 15% of pregnancies.[5] Thankfully, the most feared adverse events associated with postpartum depression, suicide and infanticide, are rare, with rates in the United States estimated at approximately 1 per 100,000 live births.[6] Nevertheless, postpartum depression and subsequent suicide is a significant cause of death in postnatal women. Emergency medicine providers should have a high clinical index of suspicion for postpartum depression and consider screening all postpartum women they come into contact with in the ED regardless of chief complaint. Women may present with unrelated complaints, or complaints related to their infant, hoping the medical team uncovers their true mental health concerns.

Clinical Features

Aside from the temporal association to pregnancy, the clinical features of postpartum depression are similar to those of any other major depressive episode. Specifically, patients must exhibit at least five out of the nine cardinal symptoms of depression (see the Diagnostic and Statistical Manual of Mental Disorders, Fifth Edition, criteria for major depressive episode). Of the features present, at least one must be either depressed mood or anhedonia. Furthermore, these symptoms must result in a significant degree of distress or change in functional status and not be attributable to an underlying medical condition or medication. To classify as a purely depressive episode, the EP must ensure that concomitant manic or psychotic features do not exist.[4] In postpartum patients, depressive symptoms may manifest as anxiety about the infant's health; concern about their ability to care for the infant; or conversely, a lack of interest in the infant.[7] Of note, many of the somatic symptoms of depression (including sleep, energy level, and appetite changes) may overlap with normal observed changes in postpartum women.[8] Therefore, additional care should be taken to evaluate these features in the context of the normal postpartum experience. Given this overlap, and a mother's potential reluctance to discuss any psychological distress, postpartum depression may go undiagnosed and therefore untreated.[9] EPs must have a low threshold for screening women and then involving mental health professionals in the care of postpartum patients that exhibit these sometimes subtle signs of depression.

Risk Factors

Postpartum depression shares many of the same risk factors as nonperinatal depression. Of all the factors that have been identified, a history of prior perinatal or no nonperinatal depression has been demonstrated to have the strongest association with the development of postpartum depression. Additional risk factors include intimate partner violence, poor socioeconomic support, young age, and unwanted pregnancy. **Box 1** provides a more comprehensive list of risk factors for postpartum depression.[5]

Differential Diagnosis

Normal postpartum changes and postpartum "blues" may share clinical features with postpartum depression. New mothers often have abnormal sleep-wake cycles because they typically mirror the sleep patterns of their infant. Consequently, it is

Box 1
Risk factors for postpartum depression
History of depression (perinatal or nonperinatal)
Intimate partner violence
Poor socioeconomic support
Young age
Undesired pregnancy
Single marital status
Multiparity
Body image dissatisfaction
Substance abuse

not unusual to find new mothers with fatigue, decreased energy levels, and associated appetite changes. The differences between these normal changes and true depressive symptoms may be subtle. For example, although insomnia is common postpartum, a mother who is unable to sleep even when their infant is sleeping may be exhibiting signs of postpartum depression. Other examples include appetite changes that are also associated with rapid weight loss or decreased energy beyond what would be expected from normal postpartum sleep deprivation. Excessive (or conversely limited) concern over the child's well-being is also concerning for postpartum depression. Thyroid disorders are also common postpartum and the EP should be on the lookout for this depression mimic.

By definition, postpartum "blues" shares many of the same features as postpartum depression; the two are only distinguished by the number of features exhibited by a patient and the duration of symptoms. Patients exhibiting less than five of the cardinal features of depression fall into the category of postpartum "blues." In addition, symptoms of postpartum "blues" tend to be mild and typically resolve within 2 weeks. Features typically develop within 2 to 3 days after delivery and peak within a few days. If symptoms persist longer than 2 weeks after onset, the episode is referred to as postpartum depression rather than postpartum "blues."[10]

Patients with symptoms of mania or hypomania at any point during their depressive episode are typically diagnosed with postpartum bipolar depression. The presence of other psychotic features including but not limited to hallucinations, delusions, paranoia, and disorganized speech is not typical of major depression and should point the clinician toward alternative psychiatric diagnoses, such as postpartum psychosis, a much rarer entity.[4]

Because of the stigma that surrounds mental illness especially in the postpartum period, many patients may require substantial encouragement to discuss symptoms. Involving a mental health care professional to further the conversation and obtain collateral information is prudent when the EP is concerned. Consider screening all postpartum women for depression because their presentations can be subtle, and remember there are generally two lives at risk in these cases.

PERIPARTUM CARDIOMYOPATHY
Introduction and Epidemiology

PPCM refers to new evidence of heart failure near the end of pregnancy or within the first 5 months postpartum.[11] The cause of PPCM is unknown and likely multifactorial.

PPCM is a global phenomenon with varying rates of incidence across socioeconomic statuses, race, and geographic location. For this reason, many experts agree that genetics play at least a part in its pathophysiology. Several risk factors have been identified for the development of PPCM including previous PPCM, multiparity, advanced maternal age (age >40), preeclampsia or eclampsia, and underlying chronic hypertension.[12]

PPCM is a serious illness with a mortality rate approaching 10% across ethnicities and 30% in black patients.[13] Other poor prognostic factors include low socioeconomic status and advanced maternal age. Morbidity is also significant with high rates of major adverse events including thromboembolic complications, fulminant pulmonary edema requiring invasive positive-pressure ventilation, and arrhythmia requiring defibrillation or pacemaker implantation.[14]

Presentation and Risk Factors

Presentation is similar to other forms of systolic heart failure and includes fatigue, shortness of breath, orthopnea, cough, paroxysmal nocturnal dyspnea, and pedal edema. Patients often present later in the disease process because there is significant overlap between symptoms of PPCM and those of normal pregnancy or postpartum periods. Major adverse complications of the disease process, such as thromboembolic cerebrovascular accidents or malignant arrhythmias, often precede the diagnosis of PPCM itself. Physical signs may include cardiac murmurs, pulmonary rales, jugular venous distention, lower extremity edema, hemodynamic instability, and respiratory distress.

Laboratory Testing and Imaging

ED evaluation of PPCM is similar to that of all patients with congestive heart failure and should include laboratory studies (troponin, B-type natriuretic peptide, basic metabolic panel, complete blood count), electrocardiogram, chest radiograph, and bedside echocardiography (if available). The EP should give serious consideration to other underlying etiologies of cardiac dysfunction in the postpartum period including pulmonary embolism, amniotic fluid emboli, preeclampsia/eclampsia, acute myocardial infarction, and spontaneous coronary artery dissection. Pregnant and postpartum women are at a three times higher risk of acute myocardial infarction than their age- and sex-matched cohort[15] and spontaneous coronary artery dissection is a disease process almost entirely limited to pregnancy and the postpartum period.[16]

Management Approach and Prognosis

Generally, the treatment of PPCM is the same as other types of systolic heart failure. The treatment should focus on correction of hypoxia either with supplemental oxygen and/or positive-pressure ventilation as needed, optimization of preload usually with diuresis, and pressor and inotropic support if required.

Breastfeeding can generally be continued in the hemodynamically stable patient with PPCM. Most medications are compatible with nursing but EPs should consult LacMed or other resources as needed. Many patients have a full recovery of their cardiac function and can proceed with a stepwise weaning of their heart failure medications within 6 months of initiation.[17] Finally, given the high rate of PPCM recurrence, women should be counseled regarding their future risk and family planning options.

PREGNANCY HEADACHES AND NEUROLOGIC EMERGENCIES
Introduction

Headaches in the late pregnancy and postpartum period present a unique challenge for clinicians. A woman who has had recent spinal anesthesia, is often sleep deprived, and is experiencing various hormonal fluctuations postdelivery certainly has plenty of reasons to develop a benign headache and up to 39% of women experience a headache in their first week postpartum.[18] However, late pregnancy and postpartum patients are also at increased risk for several neurologic emergencies. This section focuses on the clinical approach to the late pregnant or postpartum patient with headaches and/or neurologic symptoms.

Differential Diagnosis and Warning Signs

Late pregnant or postpartum women with headaches, neurologic symptoms, and even mildly elevated blood pressure should be triaged as emergent cases because of the broad and clinically challenging differential associated with this patient population. The differential diagnosis and warning signs for postpartum headaches are summarized in **Table 1** and **Box 2**, respectively.

Migraine Headaches

Patients with a history of migraine headaches often have a recurrence in the postpartum period. The rise in estrogen levels toward the end of pregnancy seems to have a protective effect and conversely the precipitous drop in estrogen following delivery often results in recurrence of symptoms, with upward of 50% experiencing recurrent migraines by 1 month postpartum.[19] Patients who breastfeed have decreased prevalence of postpartum migraine recurrence compared with mothers who bottle feed their infants, likely caused by more stable estrogen levels in mothers who breastfeed.[20]

The acute management of migraines in the postpartum period is similar to that of other migraine patients. This generally includes ketorolac, prochlorperazine, or metoclopramide, with consideration of diphenhydramine. All of these medications are safe during breastfeeding, although it is important to counsel patients regarding a potential decrease in breast milk production with the administration of diphenhydramine.

Postdural Puncture Headache

Another common cause of postpartum headache in those that received an epidural or spinal anesthesia is a postdural puncture headache. These are benign but are severely limiting in terms of their symptomatology. They are generally described as positional headaches, worse with sitting or standing, and present 72 hours after delivery. These headaches are debilitating and severely limit a mother's ability to care for her newborn.

Table 1	
Differential diagnosis of postpartum headache	
Causes of Postpartum Headaches	
Non–life threatening	Life threatening
Headache syndromes (migraine, tension, cluster)	Intracranial hemorrhage
Sinus headaches	Ischemic stroke
Idiopathic intracranial hypertension	Central venous thrombosis
	Central nervous system tumor
	Meningitis/encephalitis
	Preeclampsia/eclampsia

Box 2
Warning signs in postpartum headache

- New-onset headaches in pregnancy
- Different than prior headaches
- Worst headache of life
- Thunderclap headache
- Focal neurologic deficits
- Altered mental status
- Fevers
- Meningismus
- Elevated blood pressure
- Papilledema or evidence of elevated intracranial pressure
- Hyperreflexia

The incidence of postdural puncture headache ranges significantly in studies, and on the needle type used and the experience of the anesthesiologist, but best estimates place its incidence at 3% to 5%.[21] Many of these headaches self-resolve with rest and time, although if these patients present to the ED they should be treated with intravenous fluids, analgesics, and caffeine (intravenously if available).[22] Blood patches are up to 90% effective and should be offered to women who are refractory to conventional therapy.[23] Finally, although rare after obstetric spinal anesthesia or epidural, the EP should be suspicious of post-procedural meningitis in the febrile postpartum patient presenting with headache.

Intracranial Hemorrhage

Patients who are pregnant, and especially those postpartum, are at increased risk of intracranial hemorrhage (ICH) compared with the general population. This risk extends until about 6 weeks postpartum, with one population-based study assigning a relative risk for ICH of 2.5 during pregnancy and 28.3 during the postpartum period.[24] The most common subclass of ICH in pregnancy is subarachnoid hemorrhage, which despite being a rare maternal complication, accounts for about 4.4% of all maternal deaths and is the third most common cause of nonobstetric maternal death.[25] Risk factors for ICH include hypertension, advanced maternal age, presence of aneurysms or arteriovenous malformations, African American race, and maternal cocaine or alcohol use.

Pregnancy or postpartum state does not alter the presentation of intracranial bleeding. The location and extent of the hemorrhage can result in a variety of different presenting symptoms. Suspect ICH in patients with sudden-onset severe headaches, headaches that are different than prior, headaches in the setting of hypertension, patients with neurologic complaints, or those with altered mental status. Imaging with computed tomography (CT) (or MRI if focal symptoms exist) should be considered, with CT generally being preferred for the diagnosis of acute ICH.[26] Evaluation for an intracranial aneurysm with either a CT angiography or MR angiography should be considered if a subarachnoid hemorrhage is found. As with nonpregnant patients, patients with a high clinical suspicion for subarachnoid hemorrhage and negative neurologic imaging should undergo a lumbar puncture to evaluate for xanthochromia, especially if imaging was obtained greater than 6 hours after symptom onset.

Management principles for ICH are the same as for nonobstetric patients and focus on blood pressure control, correction of coagulopathy, and prompt neurosurgical consultation.

Stroke Syndromes

Physiologic changes in pregnancy result in a hypercoagulable state that places women at an increased risk for cerebral infarct and central venous thrombosis. This risk is greatest during the postpartum period, with an estimated relative risk of 8.7 for cerebral infarction within 6 weeks of delivery.[24]

Similar to ICH, pregnancy does not affect the presenting symptoms of cerebral ischemia. If a stroke is suspected in a pregnant or postpartum patient, initial imaging is typically a CT brain scan without contrast to rule out ICH. With appropriate fetal shielding, the radiation exposure from these studies is generally considered safe, with no evidence of increased risk for fetal complications.[27] If readily available, an MRI of the brain is an appropriate initial imaging modality and is more sensitive for the detection of small or early infarcts and MRI is likely able to evaluate for most ICH.[28] Because there are no safety data on gadolinium administration in pregnancy, it is generally avoided in the United States, although the European Society of Radiology guidelines states that it is safe.[29] Radiology contrast, iodinated and gadolinium, are safe to administer to breastfeeding women and there is no need to recommend cessation of breastfeeding or "pumping and dumping" the breast milk for any period of time.[30]

For patients with radiographically confirmed acute ischemic stroke, treatment consists of anticoagulation with consideration of thrombolysis. Alteplase use in pregnancy is controversial but not absolutely contraindicated. In pregnant patients with moderate to severe stroke symptoms and otherwise no contraindications to its use, alteplase therapy should not be withheld, although it is imperative that a careful discussion of risks and benefits is held.[31] Of note, alteplase does not cross the placenta but there are concerns for maternal and fetal risk from hemorrhagic complications, particularly if the patient goes into labor or cesarean delivery is required.[32] In postpartum patients, management principles are the same as they are for the general population, although their risk of cerebrovascular accidents is much higher. Therefore, EPs should take seriously any new neurologic symptoms in the postpartum period even if subtle or subjective.

Central venous thrombosis is a rare but potentially catastrophic complication of pregnancy and the postpartum period. Presenting symptoms are varied and can range from simple headache, to seizures, to significant altered mental status and focal neurologic findings mimicking an ischemic cerebrovascular accident.[33] In pregnant patients with an abnormal neurologic examination and/or new severe (or progressive) headaches, a noncontrast CT of the brain is often an appropriate initial diagnostic choice to rule out ICH or large acute cerebral infarcts. However, this test is often normal in the setting of central venous thrombosis and a CT venogram (or MR venogram) of the brain is usually needed to make this diagnosis.[34] Consider this in pregnant or postpartum women with daily, worsening, progressive headaches even in the absence of neurologic findings, which occur late in the disease process. Treatment consists of anticoagulation with heparin or low-molecular-weight heparin, regardless of the presence of associated hemorrhagic venous infarction. Early consultation with a neurologist should be obtained in all cases.

Sheehan syndrome, also known as postpartum hypopituitarism, may occur in patients who suffer from postpartum hemorrhage with associated hypovolemic shock. Physiologic changes of pregnancy result in enlargement of the pituitary gland, which can subsequently place the pituitary at risk for subsequent infarction secondary to hypoperfusion. Sheehan syndrome should be suspected in postpartum patients with clinical manifestations of hypopituitarism, including but not limited to hypotension, hyponatremia, hypothyroidism, or lactation failure. Symptom onset varies and may occur anytime postpartum, including several years after delivery. Clinical manifestations may range from mild to life threatening. Although formal diagnosis is typically reserved for the outpatient setting, emergency medicine physicians should consider the diagnosis in postpartum patients with hemorrhage and persistent hypotension despite adequate hemorrhage control and volume resuscitation. These patients should be managed similarly to other patients with adrenal insufficiency and be treated with stress-dose corticosteroids. Severe electrolyte disturbances and hypothyroidism should also be managed according to traditional treatment guidelines.[35]

Preeclampsia, Eclampsia, and HELLP Syndrome

The epidemiology, clinical manifestations, diagnosis, and treatment of eclampsia and HELLP syndromes are discussed in detail elsewhere in this issue. However, it is important to consider these diagnoses not only in pregnant patients but also in postpartum patients because approximately 21% of preeclampsia and eclampsia cases occur during the postpartum period, generally within the first few weeks.[36] These syndromes can have serious neurologic sequela including posterior reversible encephalopathy, seizures, and increased risk of hemorrhagic and ischemic strokes.[37,38]

Summary

Headaches during pregnancy and the postpartum period are extremely common. Most are benign headaches related to pregnancy or the postpartum period itself but remember that postpartum women are at particularly high risk for serious pathology including ICH/subarachnoid hemorrhage, ischemic stroke, and venous sinus thrombosis. Take new neurologic symptoms seriously, even if subtle or subjective. Finally, remember that almost one-quarter of preeclampsia and eclampsia cases occur postpartum, so pay careful attention to blood pressures in postpartum patients.

REFERENCES

1. Li XF, Fortney J, Kotelchuck M, et al. The postpartum period: the key to maternal mortality. Int J Gynecol Obstet 1996;54(1):1–10.
2. CDC. Pregnancy mortality surveillance system. U.S. Department of Health & Human Services, 2018. Available at: https://www.cdc.gov/reproductivehealth/maternalinfanthealth/pregnancy-mortality-surveillance-system.htm.
3. Fogel N. The inadequacies in postnatal health care. Curr Med Res Pract 2017; 7(1):16–7.
4. American Psychiatric Association. Diagnostic and statistical manual of mental disorders, 5th edition (DSM-5). Arlington (VA): American Psychiatric Association; 2013.
5. Gaillard A, Le Strat Y, Mandelbrot L, et al. Predictors of postpartum depression: prospective study of 264 women followed during pregnancy and postpartum. Psychiatry Res 2014;215(2):341–6.
6. Palladino CL, Singh V, Campbell J, et al. Homicide and suicide during the perinatal period: findings from the national violent death reporting system. Obstet Gynecol 2011;118(5):1056–63.
7. Pearlstein T, Howard M, Salisbury A, et al. Postpartum depression. Am J Obstet Gynecol 2009;200(4):357–64.

8. Committee on Obstetric Practice. Committee opinion no. 630: screening for perinatal depression. Obstet Gynecol 2015;125(5):1268–71.

9. Cerimele JM, Vanderlip ER, Croicu CA, et al. Presenting symptoms of women with depression in an obstetrics and gynecology setting. Obstet Gynecol 2013;122(2 Pt 1):313–8.

10. O'Hara MW, Wisner KL. Perinatal mental illness: definition, description and aetiology. Best Pract Res Clin Obstet Gynaecol 2014;28(1):3–12.

11. Sliwa K, Hilfiker-Kleiner D, Petrie MC, et al. Current state of knowledge on aetiology, diagnosis, management, and therapy of peripartum cardiomyopathy: a position statement from the Heart Failure Association of the European Society of Cardiology Working Group on peripartum cardiomyopathy. Eur J Heart Fail 2010;12:767.

12. Bhattacharyya A, Basra SS, Sen P, et al. Peripartum cardiomyopathy: a review. Tex Heart Inst J 2012;39(1):8–16.

13. Elkayam U, Akhter MW, Singh H, et al. Pregnancy-associated cardiomyopathy: clinical characteristics and a comparison between early and late presentation. Circulation 2005;111:2050.

14. Goland S, Modi K, Bitar F, et al. Clinical profile and predictors of complications in peripartum cardiomyopathy. J Card Fail 2009;15(8):645–50.

15. Wuntakal R, Shetty NL, Loannou E, et al. Myocardial infarction and pregnancy. Obstet Gynaecol 2013;15:247–55.

16. Sheikh AS, O'Sullivan M. Pregnancy-related spontaneous coronary artery dissection: two case reports and a comprehensive review of literature. Heart Views 2012;13(2):53–65.

17. Cooper LT, Mather PJ, Alexis JD, et al. Myocardial recovery in peripartum cardiomyopathy: prospective comparison with recent onset cardiomyopathy in men and nonperipartum women. J Card Fail 2012;18(1):28–33.

18. Goldszmidt E, Kern R, Chaput A, et al. The incidence and etiology of postpartum headaches: a prospective cohort study. Can J Anaesth 2005;52:971–7.

19. Sances G, Granella F, Nappi RE, et al. Course of migraine during pregnancy and postpartum: a prospective study. Cephalalgia 2003;23(3):197–205.

20. MacGregor EA. Headache in pregnancy. Neurol Clin 2012;30(3):835–66.

21. Reynolds F. Dural puncture and headache. Br Med J 1993;306:874–6.

22. Gaiser R. Postdural puncture headache. Curr Opin Anaesthesiol 2006;19(3):249–53.

23. Rucklidge OMWM. All patients with a postdural puncture headache should receive an epidural blood patch. Int J Obstet Anesth 2014;23(2):171–4.

24. Kittner SJ, Stern BJ, Feeser BR, et al. Pregnancy and the risk of stroke. N Engl J Med 1996;335(11):768–74.

25. Barno A, Freeman DW. Maternal deaths due to spontaneous subarachnoid hemorrhage. Am J Obstet Gynecol 1976;125(3):384–92.

26. Fairhall JM, Stoodley MA. Intracranial haemorrhage in pregnancy. Obstet Med 2009;2(4):142–8.

27. Brent RL. The effect of embryonic and fetal exposure to x-ray, microwaves, and ultrasound: counseling the pregnant and nonpregnant patient about these risks. Semin Oncol 1989;16(5):347–68.

28. Heit JJ, Iv M, Wintermark M. Imaging of intracranial hemorrhage. J Stroke 2017;19(1):11–27.

29. Gardia-Bournissen F, Shrim A, Koren G. Safety of gadolinium during pregnancy. Can Fam Physician 2006;52(3):309–10.

30. Newman J. Breastfeeding and radiologic procedures. Can Fam Physician 2007; 53(4):630–1.
31. Selim MH, Molina CA. The use of tissue plasminogen-activator in pregnancy: a taboo treatment or a time to think out of the box. Stroke 2013;44(3):868–9.
32. Murugappan A, Coplin WM, Al-Sadat AN, et al. Thrombolytic therapy of acute ischemic stroke during pregnancy. Neurology 2006;66(5):768–70.
33. de Bruijn SFTM, de Haan RJ, Stam J. Clinical features and prognostic factors of cerebral venous sinus thrombosis in a prospective series of 59 patients. J Neurol Neurosurg Psychiatry 2001;70(1):105–8.
34. Fink JN, McAuley DL. Cerebral venous sinus thrombosis: a diagnostic challenge. Intern Med J 2008;31(7):384–90.
35. Schrager S, Sabo L. Sheehan syndrome: a rare complication of postpartum hemorrhage. J Am Board Fam Pract 2001;14(5):389–91.
36. Berhan Y, Berhan A. Should magnesium sulfate be administered to women with mild pre-eclampsia? A systematic review of published reports on eclampsia. J Obstet Gynaecol Res 2015;41:831–42.
37. Martin JN Jr, Thigpen BD, Moore RC, et al. Stroke and severe preeclampsia and eclampsia: a paradigm shift focusing on systolic blood pressure. Obstet Gynecol 2005;105(2):246–54.
38. McDermott M, Miller EC, Rundek T, et al. Preeclampsia: association with posterior reversible encephalopathy syndrome and stroke. Stroke 2018;49:525.

Postdelivery Emergencies

Natasha Wheaton, MD*, Aws Al-Abdullah, MD, Tyler Haertlein, MD

KEYWORDS

- Postdelivery complications • Lactation • Postpartum hemorrhage
- Amniotic fluid embolism • Mastitis • Endometritis

KEY POINTS

- The period just after delivery is a high-risk time for women with associated morbidity and mortality.
- Postpartum women frequently seek care in the emergency department because scheduled follow-up in the United States commonly does not occur until 6 weeks after delivery.
- EPs should remember several late pregnancy complications including preeclampsia can also occur postpartum.
- EPs should support lactation while a postpartum woman is under their care in the ED and should be aware that most medications (and specifically contrast dye both gadolinium and iodinated) are compatible with continued breastfeeding.

INTRODUCTION

The period just after delivery is a high-risk period for women with associated morbidity and even mortality; more than 60% of maternal deaths across the globe, including within the United States, occur in the postpartum period.[1] There are large variations in complication rates across various groups in the United States with black women having a three times higher pregnancy-related mortality than white women.[2] Additionally, in contrast to many other industrialized countries where women receive more intensive care postbirth, most women in the United States have only a single postpartum visit scheduled at 6 weeks.[3] This means that many women seek care in the emergency department (ED) for routine and more serious postpartum pathologies. Emergency physicians (EPs) should be well versed in common and life-threatening complications of delivery. The specific pathologies discussed in this article include postpartum hemorrhage, amniotic fluid embolism (AFE), mastitis, endometritis, and support of the lactating mother in the ED.

Disclosure Statement: The authors have no financial interests to disclose.
UCLA Ronald Reagan-Olive View Emergency Medicine Residency, UCLA Medical Center, 924 Westwood Boulevard, Suite 300, Los Angeles, CA 90095, USA
* Corresponding author.
E-mail address: nwheaton@mednet.ucla.edu

Emerg Med Clin N Am 37 (2019) 287–300
https://doi.org/10.1016/j.emc.2019.01.014
0733-8627/19/© 2019 Elsevier Inc. All rights reserved.

LACTATION IN THE EMERGENCY DEPARTMENT

Before we begin our discussion of postpartum complications, it is worth noting that many postpartum women encountered in the ED are nursing their infants. It is incumbent on the EP to be familiar with the basics of breastfeeding including medication safety profiles and ways to support lactating mothers in the ED. Most commonly used medications in the ED are safe for mothers nursing term newborns; specifically including gadolinium and iodinated contrast.[4] LactMed, a free online resource offered by the National Institutes of Health, is available for further recommendations on medication compatibility with nursing. EPs should also offer support to lactating women during their ED visit in the form of an electric pump or access to their infant to continue nursing. In the early months, most women need to nurse or pump every 2 to 3 hours to maintain milk supply. Even short interruptions in nursing, especially in the early weeks, are detrimental to or even end a nursing relationship. Every effort should be made on the part of the EP to support the nursing dyad and EPs should be aware that the advice to "pump and dump" is almost never evidence based and is harmful to the mother and the infant.

POSTPARTUM HEMORRHAGE
Introduction and Epidemiology

Primary postpartum hemorrhage (PPH) is defined as cumulative postpartum blood loss of greater than 500 mL and/or clinical signs and symptoms of hypovolemia within the first 24 hours after birth, regardless of the route of delivery. Secondary postpartum hemorrhage is not as clearly defined but is generally classified as excessive vaginal bleeding occurring any time between 24 hours and up to 12 weeks postpartum. The incidence of postpartum hemorrhage varies geographically and among different socioeconomic classes; however, it remains the leading direct obstetric cause of maternal death worldwide.[5] Overall rates of PPH in the United States have remained stable over the past 10 years, although severe PPH requiring blood transfusion or other intervention has increased from 2% to almost 5% over the same time period.[6] There are also significant racial disparities in maternal death rates in the United States, overall and those attributable specifically to PPH, with black women having an almost 3.4 times higher risk of death than whites during pregnancy and the postpartum period.[7] A summary of risk factors for all-cause primary and secondary PPH is listed in **Box 1**.

Given that in late pregnancy and the early postpartum period uterine artery blood flow accounts for approximately 15% of cardiac output (approximately 700 mL/min), PPH is quickly fatal.[8] Early diagnosis and aggressive management are paramount to avoid maternal morbidity and mortality.

Etiologies and Risk Factors

Uterine atony is the most common cause of PPH. It occurs when the uterus does not contract after the third stage of labor (delivery of the baby). Uterine atony complicates approximately 1 in 40 births in the United States and accounts for approximately 70% to 80% of PPH.[9] These rates have risen in developed nations over recent years thought to be secondary to an increased use of oxytocin for labor augmentation. In addition to uterotonic drug use, risk factors for uterine atony include the use of tocolytics, preeclampsia, prolonged labor, multiparity, fetal macrosomia, uterine infection, and retained placenta. With diffuse uterine atony, blood loss may be greater than observed because a flaccid uterus may retain a significant volume of blood.

| Box 1 |
Risk factors for postpartum hemorrhage
Prior postpartum hemorrhage
Prior cesarean section
Primiparity or grand multiparity
Eclampsia or preeclampsia
Fetal macrosomia (>4.5 kg)
Abnormal placental implantation
Retained placenta
Labor induction or augmentation
Instrument use during delivery
Intrauterine fetal demise
Prolonged third stage of labor

Lower genital tract lacerations represent another potential cause of PPH. Cervical, vaginal, and perineal lacerations may be consequences of the natural process of delivery; however, provider interventions, such as an episiotomy or surgically assisted vaginal births (ie, vacuum or forceps) increases the risk of postpartum bleeding. A careful history and physical examination are essential in all cases of suspected PPH; this is especially true in cases of birth trauma-related hemorrhage. There is great potential for large-volume hemorrhage from the disruption of vasculature and early identification and intervention are vital to successful resuscitative efforts.

Uterine inversion is a rare complication of vaginal delivery and if unrecognized and untreated, can lead to severe hemorrhage, shock, and maternal death. Uterine inversion occurs when the uterine fundus collapses into the endometrial cavity, essentially turning the organ inside-out. The severity of uterine inversion is classified on a spectrum from first degree (fundus remains within the endometrial cavity) to fourth degree (both the uterus and the vagina are inverted). Most cases occur within the first 24 hours after birth; however, upward of 10% of cases may not occur until a month or more postpartum.[10] Although physical examination may reveal an inverted fundus filling the vagina in severe cases, a transvaginal or transabdominal ultrasound may be necessary to make the diagnosis in more subtle cases.

Secondary PPH is most commonly caused by subinvolution of the placental bed. Uterine subinvolution refers to the failure of blood vessels underlying the placental implantation site to resolve leading to delayed postpartum bleeding. This is most commonly caused by retained placental tissue or infection (ie, endometritis). Subinvolution is identified by visualizing hypoechoic tortuous vessels along the inner third of the myometrium on transvaginal ultrasound in the setting of secondary PPH.

Less common causes of primary and secondary postpartum hemorrhage include placenta accreta (abnormal placental implantation), inherited or acquired coagulopathy, and uterine rupture.

Laboratory Testing

For patients with significant postpartum hemorrhage, initial laboratory testing should include a complete blood count, type and screen, basic metabolic panel, and coagulation studies. Other studies should be directed based on the clinical context. If the patient is febrile or there is concern for uterine infection, one should consider vaginal cultures (discussed later in section on endometritis) and blood cultures should be obtained in all ill-appearing febrile postpartum patients. Finally, patients with significant PPH or concurrent sepsis are at risk for disseminated intravascular coagulation (DIC) so coagulation studies including fibrinogen and D dimer should be considered in these patients.

Management Approach

The management of primary and secondary postpartum hemorrhage should focus on simultaneous volume resuscitation with fluid and/or blood and hemorrhagic source control. As with all causes of hemorrhagic shock, an initial assessment of airway, breathing, and circulation should take precedence and as a part of the assessment of circulation, an attempt should be made to assess the severity of hemorrhage. The Advanced Trauma Life Support manual describes four classes of hemorrhage based on the volume of blood loss and subsequent vital sign changes. Although these classifications may be the most familiar to EPs, these classes were derived from nonpregnant patients and thus may not be fully representative of postpartum physiology. Early vital sign abnormalities indicative of shock may be more difficult to identify in pregnant or early postpartum women because many of these patients exhibit a resting tachycardia and relative hypotension at baseline. The California maternal quality care collaborative hemorrhage protocol outlines four stages of PPH (**Fig. 1**), which may be more clinically applicable in these cases.

All patients with suspected large-volume PPH should be placed on continuous cardiac monitoring and intravenous access should be obtained with two large-bore intravenous lines. Initiation of crystalloid solution should be initiated without delay with early transition to blood products if hemodynamic instability or significant bleeding continues. Uncross-matched emergency blood (type O-) should be considered early if signs of shock exist. Postpartum women often have physiologic changes that make the early identification of shock more difficult. If in doubt, assume the hemorrhage is significant and do not wait for the patient to decompensate. If the EP

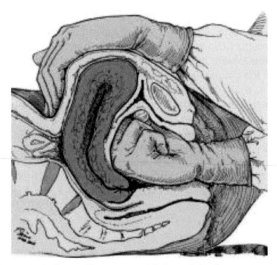

Fig. 1. California maternal quality care collaborative four stages of postpartum hemorrhage.

anticipates needing multiple units of blood, they should consider activating their hospital's massive transfusion protocol if available. If not, they should give platelets and fresh frozen plasma in addition to packed red blood cells per typical hemorrhage resuscitation protocols.

Finally, in addition to the administration of blood products, tranexamic acid (TXA) may be considered as an adjunct in significant PPH. Although limited by some methodologic concerns, the WOMAN trial, an international study of 20,000 women with primary PPH, showed that early TXA administration likely reduced maternal death caused by PPH with a number needed to treat of 267 and no increase in adverse events (primarily thrombosis).[11] This effect was strongest in those given TXA early, similar to the CRASH trial evaluating TXA for hemorrhagic shock in trauma, and thus if considered, TXA should be administered as soon as possible.

Once resuscitation has begun, the physical examination and history (when available) are essential components of PPH management because identification and control of the hemorrhagic source is as important as resuscitative efforts. Before (or simultaneous with) starting an examination, it is important to gather materials, such as suction, ring forceps with gauze, and towels or lap pads to aid in visualization and bleeding source control. In cases of significant PPH, a balloon uterine tamponade device (ie, Bakri) is life-saving. If not available, a condom attached to a Foley catheter (or a condom catheter) is used for tamponade. Finally, double suction may help with visualization for patients with significant bleeding. External and internal gynecologic examination may identify lacerations, show evidence of uterine atony with a large boggy uterus, or demonstrate uterine inversion. Foul smelling lochia, maternal pyrexia, and uterine tenderness may indicate endometritis manifesting as secondary PPH.

If identified, lacerations with active bleeding should be sutured and bleeding vessels should be ligated. Failing that, if the vessel is accessible, local pressure can often temporize bleeding. Based on the location and complexity, it is often necessary to involve an obstetrician for definitive management either bedside or in the operating room.

If uterine inversion is identified, an attempt to restore anatomic position should be made bedside. However, be aware that this is a painful procedure and often requires general anesthesia and tocolytic agents to be successful.

In cases of uterine atony, bimanual uterine massage should be performed as outlined in **Fig. 2**. Uterotonic drugs should be administered as part of first-line therapy, typically starting with oxytocin with transition to further medications as needed (outlined in **Box 2**). If first-line medical interventions fail to establish source control, more invasive techniques may be indicated, including intrauterine balloon tamponade, uterine artery embolization, and in severe cases, even hysterectomy. If available, ED physicians can place intrauterine balloon devices, such as a Bakri. If that is not readily available, a condom filled via a Foley catheter (or a condom catheter knotted off) placed in the uterus can also be effective.[12] Be aware that one Foley balloon is not large enough to tamponade a postpartum uterus and if placed, will likely only obscure the bleeding by obstructing the cervical canal.

Early obstetrics consultation in almost all cases of postpartum hemorrhage is indicated, especially in cases of significant hemorrhage. Given the success of uterine artery embolization,[13] it is also reasonable to consider early consultation with interventional radiology in unstable patients if available.

Pelvic ultrasonography should be considered in all hemodynamically stable patients with PPH, particularly if the source of bleeding is not readily identified on physical

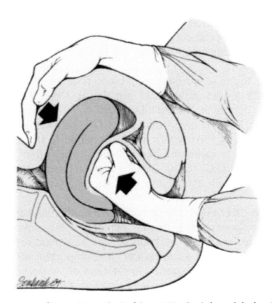

Fig. 2. Uterine massage. (*From* Vora S, Dobiesz VA. Social and behavioral sciences and public health. In: Roberts JR, Custalow CB, Thomsen TW, editors. Roberts and Hedges' clinical procedures in emergency medicine and acute care. 7th edition. Philadelphia: Elsevier; 2019.)

examination. Ultrasound may aid in the diagnosis of retained products of conception, uterine inversion, and subinvolution.

AMNIOTIC FLUID EMBOLUS
Introduction and Epidemiology

AFE occurs when amniotic fluid and fetal cells enter the maternal circulation during the labor, delivery, or the postpartum period.[14] Although rare, estimated to occur in less than 10 cases per 100,000 pregnancies, an AFE can have catastrophic effects on mother and fetus.[15] Most cases (approximately 70%) occur during labor, with the remaining cases occurring within a few hours of delivery.[16] Risk factors for AFE are poorly established but include cesarean delivery, advanced maternal age, eclampsia, and multiparity.[17] Although strong data are lacking regarding prognosis, it is known that maternal mortality rates in those that suffer from AFE are high and those that do survive often suffer from significant neurologic injury secondary to cerebral hypoxia.[16]

Box 2
Uterotonic medications for postpartum hemorrhage

Oxytocin (first line), 10 IU intramuscularly or 20 IU in 500 mL Intravenous fluids at 250 mL/h (dosing may vary per institution)

Methylergonovine, 0.2 mg intramuscularly (avoid in preeclampsia or other hypertension)

Carboprost, 0.25 μg intramuscularly q 15 min up to 2 mg

Misoprostol, 800 μg, 1000 μg rectal (not Food and Drug Administration approved for this use)

Presentation

Patients typically present with respiratory distress, hypoxia, and pulmonary edema with rapid progression toward sudden maternal cardiovascular collapse. This often occurs concomitantly with hemorrhage secondary to DIC, which may manifest as bleeding or bruising from peripheral lines or in some cases, major obstetric hemorrhage. Neurologic manifestations including tonic-clonic seizures or stroke are less common initial presentations of an AFE.[18]

Differential Diagnosis and Laboratory Testing

The differential diagnosis for AFE is broad and varies greatly based on the clinical presentation. For those that present with respiratory distress and cardiovascular instability, it is important to evaluate the patient for pulmonary embolus, acute respiratory distress syndrome, anaphylaxis, or cardiomyopathy, all of which may present postpartum. However, those with neurologic symptoms may require a work-up for eclampsia, intracranial hemorrhage, cerebral vascular event, or primary seizure disorder as clinically indicated. AFE is a diagnosis of exclusion and therefore a broad initial work-up is indicated to help narrow the differential diagnosis. Laboratory analysis should include a complete blood count, comprehensive metabolic panel, coagulation studies, blood gasses, cardiac enzymes, and blood cultures if indicated. Chest radiography, and electrocardiography and bedside ultrasonography (if available) should also be obtained to evaluate for alternative causes of symptoms. Once the patient is stabilized, more thorough investigative studies may be undertaken with computed tomography angiography of the chest and neurologic imaging as indicated.[19]

Management Approach

Treatment of AFE is supportive. Because many cases of AFE present with rapid cardiorespiratory failure and hemorrhage, early airway management and intravascular volume resuscitation are often required. Hypotension in patients is almost always secondary to cardiogenic shock even in the setting of obstetric hemorrhage and DIC. Care should be taken when volume resuscitating these patients because excessive fluid administration may worsen pulmonary edema and respiratory status. Initiation of vasopressor agents, typically norepinephrine or epinephrine, should be considered early in patients that do not respond to initial fluid resuscitation.[20] In patients with postpartum hemorrhage, a thorough examination should be performed to rule out uterine atony, lacerations, or alternative causes of obstetric hemorrhage (discussed previously).

In patients that have not yet delivered, immediate delivery of the fetus should be considered. Particularly in the setting of maternal cardiac arrest, emergency cesarean delivery may be indicated to aid in resuscitative efforts of mother and fetus.[21] In all cases of suspected AFE, it is important to involve a multidisciplinary team early (including critical care, obstetrics, anesthesia, and respiratory therapy) given the dynamic clinical features and need for simultaneous diagnostic and treatment modalities. Finally, in hospitals with the capability, extracorporeal membrane oxygenation may be a life-saving intervention for refractory cases.

LACTATIONAL MASTITIS
Introduction and Epidemiology

Lactational mastitis is an infectious condition of the breast seen in breastfeeding women. It is most common in the first 2 to 3 months postpartum, although it is reported in women up to 1 year after delivery. It is thought that nipple breakdown and poor milk drainage lead to an entry pathway and nidus for bacterial infection from the infant's nasopharynx or the mother's own skin.[22] Pathogens include *Staphylococcus aureus* (methicillin sensitive and methicillin resistant), *Streptococcus pyogenes*, and *Escherichia coli*, although methicillin-sensitive *S aureus* makes up most cases. Other contributing factors include maternal stress or malnutrition; illness in mother or baby; and breast pressure, such as from a bra or seatbelt.

Depending on the study cited, the incidence of lactation mastitis ranges from just less than 10% to more than 17%.[23,24] Thankfully, the number of women with infectious mastitis requiring hospitalization is much lower. In one retrospective analysis of 136,459 women who delivered at a single hospital, only 127 of them were later found to be admitted for puerperal mastitis, an incidence of less than 0.1%.[25]

Presentation and Risk Factors

Most commonly seen in the first 3 months of breastfeeding and more often in primiparous mothers, females with lactational mastitis present with a painful, swollen, and red breast. Before 24 hours of symptoms, in an otherwise well-appearing woman, symptoms are usually attributable to engorgement or a clogged milk duct and often self-resolve.[26] Infectious lactational mastitis occurs once the stagnant breast milk has had time to colonize bacteria, generally requiring 12 to 24 hours of poor milk drainage. During this period, women develop fever and other systemic symptoms including chills, malaise, and myalgias. Physical examination may demonstrate firm, erythematous swelling of the affected breast and reactive axillary lymphadenopathy.

Risk factors include cracked nipples, a known blocked duct, breast pump use, maternal fatigue, primiparity, and most commonly a prior history of mastitis.[27]

Laboratory Testing and Imaging

Mastitis is a clinical diagnosis. Cultures are rarely useful and should be reserved for immunocompromised patients, those with sepsis, and those who have failed outpatient therapy.[28]

Formal breast ultrasound should be considered in mothers with a palpable, fluctuant breast mass and all patients not responsive to initial antibiotic regimens after 48 to 72 hours. Similar to other forms of cellulitis, ultrasound in mastitis demonstrates subcutaneous fat lobules surrounded by hypoechoic fluid (**Fig. 3**). Alternatively, those with breast abscess show a discrete fluid collection as seen in **Fig. 4**.

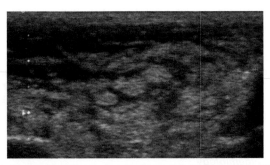

Fig. 3. Ultrasound of cellulitis without abscess. (*From* Teh JL. Disorders of the ankle and foot: forefoot. In: McNally EG, editor. Practical musculoskeletal ultrasound. Philadelphia: Elsevier; 2014. Figure 28.)

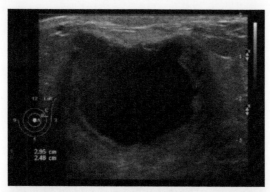

Fig. 4. Ultrasound showing breast abscess. (*From* Mansel RE, Webster DJT, Sweetland HM, et al. Hughes, Mansel & Webster's benign disorders and diseases of the breast. Philadelphia: Elsevier; 2009. p. 227–41.)

Management Approach

Because the pathophysiology of lactational mastitis centers around poor milk drainage, initial management includes frequent emptying of the breast. Emptying is performed by continued breastfeeding, pumping, and/or manual expression. Breastfeeding should be continued and is encouraged because this is the optimal means of emptying the breast. Nonsteroidal inflammatory agents and cold compresses can alleviate symptomatic pain and swelling.

Ultimately, infective mastitis requires early antibiotic therapy to fully resolve and empiric therapy with activity against S aureus should be initiated in all cases with symptoms greater than 24 hours. Hemodynamically stable patients with nonprogressive erythema may be treated as outpatients. Dicloxacillin (500 mg four times a day for 10–14 days) or cephalexin (500 mg four times a day for 10–14 days) are generally first-line treatment. Consider methicillin-resistant S aureus coverage for women with a history of methicillin-resistant S aureus infection and in these cases, clindamycin (300 mg four times a day for 10–14 days) or trimethoprim-sulfamethoxazole (one double-strength tablet orally twice daily) may be used. However, trimethoprim-sulfamethoxazole is safe only for breastfeeding mothers with infants greater than 2 months of age.

In the hemodynamically unstable patient, immunosuppressed patient, and those failing appropriate outpatient oral antibiotics, vancomycin (15–20 mg/kg/dose every 8–12 hours) should be initiated. These patients should be admitted and have milk and blood cultures drawn in addition to consideration of breast ultrasound to rule out an underlying abscess.

Treatment of lactational mastitis complicated by breast abscess includes admission for intravenous antibiotics and surgical drainage of the abscess with either needle aspiration or open incision. As with uncomplicated lactational mastitis, breastfeeding should be continued in patients with breast abscess and antibiotics should be chosen that are compatible with nursing. Breastfeeding should only be interrupted if the infants mouth occludes any abscess incisions made.[29]

Finally, referral for needle aspiration or excisional biopsy may be necessary to differentiate mastitis from galactocele or inflammatory breast cancer in particular cases. Although rare, it is important to keep in mind the possibility of inflammatory breast cancer in patients with recurrent mastitis in the same location, breast skin thickening, and the classic peau d'orange appearance (**Fig. 5**).

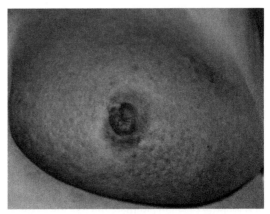

Fig. 5. Inflammatory breast cancer. (*From* Dixon, JM. The breast. In: Garden OJ, Parks RW, editors. Principles and practice of surgery. 7th edition. Philadelphia: Elsevier; 2018.)

POSTPARTUM ENDOMETRITIS
Introduction and Epidemiology

Postpartum endometritis refers specifically to an infection of the postpartum decidua (the endometrium), although it is commonly used to refer to a spectrum of infectious complications that often overlap. These include infections of the myometrium, parametrium, and surgical site (if delivery was performed by cesarean section). The general consensus is that as the infection spreads through the myometrium and into the broad ligaments the more severe the infection is, although all cases of endometritis should be considered serious in nature. Although not particularly well defined, postpartum endometritis specifically refers to endometrial infections within 2 to 10 days after birth. Fever in the first 24 hours is generally excluded because a low-grade fever is common during this time and often spontaneously resolves.[30]

Studies in developed countries have shown rates of maternal mortality from genital and urinary tract sepsis ranging as low as 0.29 deaths per 100,000 pregnancies.[31] Yet the World Health Organization still holds puerperal bacterial infections as a leading factor in maternal death accounting for about one-tenth of maternal deaths globally. Endometritis incidence and uterine instrumentation share a linear relationship as evidenced by the low rate of endometritis after vaginal birth (<3%) compared with the alarmingly high rate after cesarean section delivery (up to 20%).[32] In addition to lowering rates of mortality, early diagnosis and treatment of endometritis may shorten or even prevent hospital stays.[33]

Pathogens seen in endometritis generally involve the genitourinary flora and include gram-positive and gram-negative aerobes and anaerobes. Common microbes include group A and group B streptococci, *Mycoplasma hominis*, *Enterococcus*, *Escherichia*, *Enterobacter*, *Bacteroides*, and *Gardnerella vaginalis*. Postpartum endometritis is uncommonly caused by *Neisseria gonorrhoeae* or *Chlamydia trachomatis* given aggressive screening during pregnancy but outside 10 days postdelivery these microbes should be considered more heavily.[34] When endometritis is complicated by a surgical site infection, methicillin-resistant *S aureus* should also be considered.

Presentation and Risk Factors

The diagnosis is aided by laboratory testing but is largely clinical. In a postpartum woman with fever the diagnosis is a pelvic infection until proven otherwise. Cesarean section is the most significant risk factor for postpartum endometritis. Other risk factors include prolonged labor and membrane rupture, internal fetal monitoring, instrument-assisted delivery, postpartum anemia, lower socioeconomic status, and maternal immunosuppression.[35]

Typically, within the first 2 to 10 days, patients with postpartum endometritis present with fever, foul-smelling lochia, and pelvic pain. On examination, patients exhibit uterine tenderness and can have varying levels of cervical discharge. Importantly, patients can have endometritis without significant discharge. Patients who delivered by cesarean section may present with obvious external wound infections, although they may also have a normal external examination.

Complications of endometritis, and cesarean section wound infection, include surgical site and pelvic abscesses, infected hematomas, and parametrial phlegmons. These wounds can also develop into necrotizing fasciitis, a truly devastating complication.[36]

Laboratory Testing and Imaging

Postpartum endometritis is largely a clinical diagnosis and treatment is primarily antibiotics. However, other emergent infectious etiologies need to be excluded and complications of endometritis need to be considered before safely treating with antibiotics alone.

Cultures are of questionable utility. Vaginal cultures may help support a diagnosis of endometritis but are often contaminated. Certainly, any grossly purulent material on examination should be cultured. Bacteremia is a common complication of endometritis, seen in some studies to range as high as 5%.[37] However, many agree blood cultures should be reserved for patients with sepsis, immunocompromised patients, and for those failing to respond to empiric therapy. Testing for gonorrhea and chlamydia is routine in pregnancy and important in establishing the microbiologic cause especially in cases of endometritis presenting after 10 days postpartum.

Imaging studies in patients with puerperal fever can include pelvic ultrasound and/or computed tomography of the abdomen and pelvis. In endometritis, these studies may show uterine enlargement, endometrial thickening, fluid within the endometrial cavity, and an indistinct endomyometrial junction. Air in the endometrial cavity is nondiagnostic because it is a normal variant for several weeks postpartum. Imaging is not required for the diagnosis of uncomplicated endometritis, although is useful for characterizing potential complications (discussed previously). Imaging should be considered in all patients with sepsis, patients post–cesarean delivery, those with a concerning abdominal examination, and those that fail appropriate outpatient antibiotic therapy.

Management Approach

Therapy for postpartum endometritis varies based on the clinical stability of the patient. A patient with mild illness, stable vital signs, and close follow-up can occasionally be discharged home on oral antibiotics after discussion with the obstetrician on-call. Alternatively, any patient who has a concern for endometritis in the setting of a cesarean section, a concern for complications, has underlying significant comorbidities, or who exhibits hemodynamic instability should be admitted for intravenous antibiotics and evaluated for potential surgical management. When in doubt, the safest option is to admit for intravenous antibiotics.

For the well-appearing patient status-post an uncomplicated vaginal delivery, one should still consult the obstetrician on-call to discuss management and arrange for close follow-up. For patients with the ability to follow up within 24 to 48 hours, common antibiotic recommendations include a 10-day course of clindamycin (300 mg three times per day) or doxycycline (100 mg twice per day) if the mother is not breast feeding.

First Line	First-Line Therapy in Patients with Renal Insufficiency	Second-Line Therapy with Equivalent Efficacy for General Population	Second-Line Therapy in Nonbreastfeeding Women
Table 1 **Antibiotic treatment options for endometritis**			
Clindamycin 900 mg q 8 h plus gentamicin 1.5 mg/kg intravenously q 8 h	Clindamycin 900 mg q 8 h plus cefoxitin or cefotaxime (2 g q 6 h)	Cefoxitin or cefotaxime (2 g q 6 h) and vancomycin (1 g q 12 h)	Metronidazole 500 mg q 8 h plus ampicillin 2 g q 4 h plus gentamicin 1.5 mg/kg intravenously q 8 h

For ill-appearing patients, those with significant comorbidities, those with a concern for complication, and those who have endometritis in the setting of a cesarean section, there are several intravenous regimens available as displayed in **Table 1**. Antibiotic choice is directed by local resistance patterns and compatibility with nursing (if applicable).

REFERENCES

1. Li XF, Fortney J, Kotelchuck M, et al. The postpartum period: the key to maternal mortality. Int J Gynaecol Obstet 1996;54(1):1–10.
2. CDC. Pregnancy Mortality Surveillance System.
3. Fogel N. The inadequacies in postnatal health care. Curr Med Res Pract 2017; 7(1):16–7.
4. Newman J. Breastfeeding and radiologic procedures. Can Fam Physician 2007; 53(4):630–1.
5. Khan KS, Wojdyla D, Say L, et al. WHO analysis of causes of maternal death: a systematic review. Lancet 2006;367(9516):1066–74.
6. Ahmadzia HK, Grotegut CA, James AH. 509: Rates of postpartum hemorrhage and related interventions: United States, 2000-2012. Am J Obstet Gynecol 2016;214(1):S277.
7. Creanga AA, Syverson C, Seed K, et al. Pregnancy-related mortality in the United States, 2011 to 2013. Obstet Anesth Dig 2018;38(1).
8. Hall ME, George EM, Granger JP. The heart during pregnancy. Rev Esp Cardiol 2011;64(11):1045–50.
9. Mousa HA, Blum J, Abou El Senoun G, et al. Treatment for primary postpartum haemorrhage. Cochrane Database Syst Rev 2014;(2):CD003249.
10. Hostetler DR, Bosworth MF. Uterine inversion: a life-threatening obstetric emergency. J Am Board Fam Pract 2000;13(2):120–3.
11. Shakur H, Roberts I, Fawole B, et al. Effect of early tranexamic acid administration on mortality, hysterectomy, and other morbidities in women with post-partum haemorrhage (WOMAN): an international, randomised, double-blind, placebo-controlled trial. Lancet 2017;389(10084):2105–16.
12. Darwish AM, Abdallah MM, Shaaban OM, et al. Bakri balloon versus condom-loaded Foley's catheter for treatment of atonic postpartum hemorrhage secondary to vaginal delivery: a randomized controlled trial. J Matern Fetal Neonatal Med 2018;31(6):747–53.

13. Kim T-H, Lee H-H, Kim J-M, et al. Uterine artery embolization for primary postpartum hemorrhage. Iran J Reprod Med 2013;11(6):511–8.
14. Gist RS, Stafford IP, Leibowitz AB, et al. Amniotic fluid embolism. Anesth Analg 2009;108(5):1599–602.
15. Abenhaim HA, Azoulay L, Kramer MS, et al. Incidence and risk factors of amniotic fluid embolisms: a population-based study on 3 million births in the United States. Am J Obstet Gynecol 2008;199(1):49.e1–8.
16. Clark SL, Hankins GDV, Dudley DA, et al. Amniotic fluid embolism: analysis of the national registry. Am J Obstet Gynecol 1995;172(4):1158–69.
17. Knight M, Tuffnell D, Brocklehurst P, et al. Incidence and risk factors for amniotic-fluid embolism. Obstet Gynecol 2010;115(5):910–7.
18. Conde-Agudelo A, Romero R. Amniotic fluid embolism: an evidence-based review. Am J Obstet Gynecol 2009;201(5):445.e1–13.
19. Gilmore DA, Wakim J, Secrest J, et al. Anaphylactoid syndrome of pregnancy: a review of the literature with latest management and outcome data. AANA J 2003; 71:120.
20. Cheng SH, BM. Management of amniotic fluid embolism. Evidence- Based Crit Care 2017;737–41.
21. Jeejeebhoy FM, Zelop CM, Lipman S, et al. Cardiac arrest in pregnancy: a scientific statement from the American Heart Association. Circulation 2015;132: 1747–73.
22. Olsen CG, Gordon RE Jr. Breast disorders in nursing mothers. Am Fam Physician 1990;41(5):1509–16.
23. Kataria K, Srivastava A, Dhar A. Management of lactational mastitis and breast abscesses: review of current knowledge and practice. Indian J Surg 2013; 75(6):430–5.
24. Vogel A, Hutchison BL, Mitchell EA. Mastitis in the first year postpartum. Birth 2001;26(4):218–25.
25. Stafford I, Hernandez J, Laibl V, et al. Community-acquired methicillin-resistant Staphylococcus aureus among patients with puerperal mastitis requiring hospitalization. Obstet Gynecol 2008;112(3):533–7.
26. Amir LH. ABM clinical protocol #4: mastitis, revised march 2014. Breastfeed Med 2014;9(5):239–43.
27. Jonsson S, Pulkkinen MO. Mastitis today: incidence, prevention and treatment. Ann Chir Gynaecol Suppl 1994;208:84–7.
28. WHO. Baby-friendly hospital initiative. Geneva (Switzerland): World Health Organization; 2009.
29. Prachniak GK. Common breastfeeding problems. Obstet Gynecol Clin North Am 2002;29(1):77–88.
30. Filker R, Monif GR. The significance of temperature during the first 24 hours postpartum. Obstet Gynecol 1979;53:358.
31. NPEU. NPEU Perinatal Mortality Registry. 2016.
32. WHO. WHO recommendations for prevention and treatment of maternal peripartum infections. Geneva (Switzerland): World Health Organization.
33. Chaim W, Bashiri A, Bar-David J, et al. Prevalence and clinical significance of postpartum endometritis and wound infection. Infect Dis Obstet Gynecol 2000; 8:77–82.
34. Hoyme UB, Kiviat N, Eschenbach DA. Microbiology and treatment of late postpartum endometritis. Obstet Gynecol 1986;68:226.
35. Newton ER, Prihoda TJ, Gibbs RS. A clinical and microbiologic analysis of risk factors for puerperal endometritis. Obstet Gynecol 1990;75(3 Pt 1):402–6.

36. Manning-Geist B, Rimawi BH. Severe infections in obstetrics and gynecology: how early surgical intervention saves lives. J Clin Gynecol Obstet 2016;5(1).
37. Kankuri E, Kurki T, Carlson P, et al. Incidence, treatment and outcome of peripartum sepsis. Acta Obstet Gynecol Scand 2003;82(8):730–5.

Hypertensive Disorders of Pregnancy

R. Gentry Wilkerson, MD[a],*, Adeolu C. Ogunbodede, MD[a,b]

KEYWORDS

- Preeclampsia • Eclampsia • Gestational hypertension • HELLP

KEY POINTS

- In the United States, 1 of every 9 pregnancies is complicated by a hypertensive disorder and 3% to 5% are complicated by preeclampsia.
- Hemolysis, elevated liver enzymes, low platelets (HELLP) syndrome is considered a severe form of preeclampsia.
- Proteinuria is no longer required to make the diagnosis of preeclampsia as some women will already have advanced disease by the time proteinuria is detectable.
- Intravenous magnesium sulfate is the initial treatment of eclampsia and preeclampsia with severe features. The initial loading dose of magnesium is 4 to 6 g intravenously (IV) over 15 to 20 minutes followed by an infusion rate of 1 to 2 g/h.
- First-line agents for the acute lowering of elevated blood pressure in pregnancy include intravenous labetalol, intravenous hydralazine, and oral nifedipine.

INTRODUCTION

The hypertensive disorders of pregnancy are among the leading causes of maternal and fetal morbidity and mortality. Differentiating these disorders requires careful evaluation of the patient's history with a thorough physical examination and appropriate laboratory testing. The 4 categories of hypertensive disorders of pregnancy are chronic hypertension, gestational hypertension, preeclampsia-eclampsia, and chronic hypertension with superimposed preeclampsia. Proper diagnosis in the emergency department is crucial to initiate appropriate treatment to reduce the potential harm to the mother and the fetus. In recent years, updates to the diagnostic criteria for preeclampsia have removed the requirement for proteinuria. In the emergency department, it is important to recognize the severe features of preeclampsia, which include

Disclosure Statement: Both authors have no disclosures to declare.
[a] Department of Emergency Medicine, University of Maryland School of Medicine, 110 South Paca Street, Suite 200; 6th Floor, Baltimore, MD 21201, USA; [b] Department of Internal Medicine, University of Maryland School of Medicine, 110 South Paca Street, Suite 200; 6th Floor, Baltimore, MD 21201, USA
* Corresponding author.
E-mail address: gwilkerson@som.umaryland.edu

Emerg Med Clin N Am 37 (2019) 301–316
https://doi.org/10.1016/j.emc.2019.01.008
0733-8627/19/© 2019 Elsevier Inc. All rights reserved.

blood pressure greater than 160/110 mm Hg, acute kidney injury, elevated liver function tests, severe abdominal pain, pulmonary edema, and central nervous system disturbances. The presence of any of these features mandates initiation of rapid treatment to reduce the risk of eclampsia. Publication of the results of recent studies led to updated recommendations regarding blood pressure thresholds for initiation of antihypertensives, dosing of aspirin in patients at high risk for preeclampsia, and gestational ages for corticosteroid administration in anticipated premature deliveries. This article reviews each of the disorders of hypertension in pregnancy as well as how to evaluate and manage these high-risk patients.

CLASSIFICATION OF HYPERTENSIVE DISORDERS OF PREGNANCY
Chronic Hypertension

Chronic hypertension during pregnancy is defined as the presence of hypertension before conception, the development of elevated blood pressure before 20 weeks' gestational age, or the persistence of hypertension beyond 12 weeks after delivery.[1] The 2017 report by the American College of Cardiology/American Heart Association (ACC/AHA) Task Force on Clinical Practice Guidelines defines elevated blood pressure as a systolic blood pressure (BP) of 120 to 129 mm Hg, with diastolic BP of less than 80 mm Hg. Hypertension is present when the systolic BP is ≥130 mm Hg and the diastolic BP is ≥80 mm Hg. To make the diagnosis of hypertension, the average of 2 or more readings obtained on 2 or more occasions should be used.[2] The lowering of the diagnostic cutoff for hypertension by the ACC/AHA Task Force is not reflected in the criteria used to define hypertensive disorders of pregnancy. In pregnant women, mild hypertension is present when the systolic BP is 140 to 159 mm Hg and the diastolic BP is between 90 and 109 mm Hg. Severe hypertension is present when the systolic BP is ≥160 mm Hg and/or the diastolic BP is >110 mm Hg.[3] (Table 1) Approximately 1% to 5% of pregnancies are affected by chronic hypertension, and that percentage is expected to increase.[4] The increase in the age of pregnant women in addition to the rising prevalence of obesity is contributing to a rise in the prevalence of chronic hypertension during pregnancy.[5–7] Between 2000 and 2014, the mean age of first-time mothers increased from 24.9 to 26.3 years.[8]

Chronic hypertension can be divided into 2 types based on underlying pathophysiology. In essential hypertension, also known as primary hypertension, there is no obvious cause. In secondary hypertension, which accounts for 10% to 15% of cases of chronic hypertension, the elevation in blood pressure is due to an underlying

Table 1				
Diagnostic parameters for hypertension				
		SBP (mm Hg)		**DBP (mm Hg)**
AHA/ACC (2017)				
Non-pregnant	Normal	<120	and	<80
	Elevated	120–129	and	<80
	Stage 1	130–139	or	80–89
	Stage 2	≥140	or	≥90
ACOG (2013) and ISSHP (2018)				
Pregnant	Normal	<140	and	<90
	Mild	140–159	or	90–110
	Severe	≥160	or	≥110

Abbreviations: DBP, diastolic blood pressure; SBP, systolic blood pressure.

process. Processes that cause elevated blood pressure include renal disease (glomerular, renal artery stenosis, nephritis), aortic disease (coarctation), collagen or vascular disease (lupus, scleroderma), and endocrinopathies (pheochromocytoma, Cushing's syndrome, thyrotoxicosis, hyperaldosteronism).[9] Renal parenchymal disease, renovascular disease, primary hyperaldosteronism, and obstructive sleep apnea are the most common causes of secondary hypertension in the general population.[2]

Chronic hypertension differs from gestational hypertension in regard to the time at which elevated blood pressure is detected. In gestational hypertension, elevated pressure develops after 20 weeks of gestation in a woman without preexisting hypertension. In women presenting after 20 weeks of gestation who have no previously documented blood pressures or had limited prenatal care, it can be difficult to distinguish between the 2 diagnoses.[10,11] In addition, recognition of chronic hypertension can be challenging due to the normal physiologic changes that occur during pregnancy. These changes include reduced vascular tone of the maternal arteries, leading to reduced peripheral vascular resistance and an associated drop in blood pressure.[12] This process occurs by 16 weeks of gestation to accommodate increased circulating blood volume. If this normally occurring reduction in blood pressure results in readings below the threshold for diagnosis of elevated blood pressure, then the diagnosis of chronic hypertension can be masked.

Chronic hypertension in pregnancy is associated with an increased risk of maternal and fetal complications. The risk is related to the severity of the blood pressure elevation. During pregnancy, mild-to-moderate hypertension is usually regarded as systolic BP of 140 to 159 mm Hg, diastolic BP of 90 to 109 mm Hg, or both. Severe maternal hypertension is present when the systolic pressure is 160 mm Hg or higher or the diastolic is 110 mm Hg or higher.[1] Between 13% and 40% of pregnant women with chronic hypertension will go on to develop superimposed preeclampsia.[1,13–15] In those with severe hypertension, the rate of developing superimposed preeclampsia can be as high as 78%.[16] The presence of chronic hypertension without superimposed preeclampsia is an independent risk factor for perinatal death and small-for-gestational-age births.[13,17]

Gestational Hypertension

Gestational hypertension, formerly called pregnancy-induced hypertension, is the development of de novo hypertension after 20 weeks of gestation in the absence of diagnostic criteria for preeclampsia. It is a provisional diagnosis that can change to chronic hypertension if the blood pressure remains elevated beyond 12 weeks postpartum. If the blood pressure normalizes after 12 weeks, then the diagnosis is changed to transient hypertension of pregnancy. Gestational hypertension develops in 6% to 17% of healthy nulliparous women and 2% to 4% of multiparous women.[18] Of women initially diagnosed with gestational hypertension, 15% to 46% will develop preeclampsia.[19,20] The risk of progression to preeclampsia is inversely related to the gestational age at which gestational hypertension is diagnosed. In a study by Saudan and colleagues,[19] the risk was 36% to 42% for gestational ages before 34 weeks and 7% to 20% for gestational ages 34 weeks and higher. As with chronic hypertension in pregnancy, gestational hypertension can be categorized as mild or severe. In mild gestational hypertension, the systolic BP is 140 to 159 mm Hg and/or the diastolic BP is 90 to 109 mm Hg on 2 separate occasions at least 4 hours apart and no more than 1 week apart. In severe gestational hypertension, the systolic BP is >160 mm Hg and/or the diastolic BP is greater than 110 mm Hg.[18] Lack of prenatal care complicates the diagnosis of gestational hypertension versus other hypertensive disorders of pregnancy. In the emergency department, a few factors can contribute to blood pressure elevation after 20 weeks of gestation: pain, anxiety, acute illness, and "white coat" hypertension.

Pregnancy outcomes in women with mild versus severe gestational hypertension are significantly different. Non-severe gestational hypertension is typically associated with favorable outcomes.[18,20,21] Severe gestational hypertension is associated with a much worse prognosis for the mother and fetus. A secondary analysis of data from a prospective interventional trial involving pregnant women with a history of preeclampsia found that outcomes of severe gestational hypertension were worse than for mild preeclampsia. There were higher rates of preterm delivery at less than 37 weeks of gestation (54.2% versus 17.8% [$P = .001$]) and less than 35 weeks of gestation (25.0% versus 8.4% [$P = .016$]) and delivery of small-for-gestational-age infants (20.8% versus 6.5% [$P = .024$]).[22]

When the diagnosis of gestational hypertension is considered in a pregnant woman presenting with elevated blood pressure, she should be screened for preeclampsia and other signs of end-organ dysfunction. This assessment includes careful review of systems, physical examination, ultrasound to assess fetal growth, urinalysis, blood analysis, and tocodynamometry monitoring for fetal distress, if appropriate. The American College of Obstetrics and Gynecology (ACOG) Task Force on Hypertension in Pregnancy recommends close monitoring of blood pressure twice weekly along with weekly assessment of platelet count, liver enzymes, and proteinuria in women identified with gestational hypertension. The Task Force does not recommend routine prescription of bed rest, a low-salt diet, or weight loss,[1] treatment modalities that have little effect on end-organ dysfunction and progression to preeclampsia.[23,24]

Preeclampsia-Eclampsia

Preeclampsia is defined as new-onset hypertension that develops after 20 weeks of gestation and is accompanied by proteinuria or evidence of end-organ dysfunction. Before 2013, the presence of proteinuria was a required element for the diagnosis of preeclampsia. It was later recognized that some patients have advanced disease before protein becomes detectable in the urine. This was removed in the 2013 report from ACOG Task Force on Hypertension in Pregnancy.[1] Features of end-organ dysfunction include thrombocytopenia, liver or renal impairment, pulmonary edema, and neurologic or visual dysfunction. Proteinuria is the presence of 300 mg or more of protein in a 24-hour urine collection. A urine dipstick protein of 1+ is often used as a surrogate marker of this level of protein in the urine.[25] A meta-analysis performed in 2003 found that visual detection of 1+ protein on a urine dipstick was 55% sensitive and 84% specific for $\geq$300 mg/24-h urine protein.[26] Despite the high incidence of lower-extremity edema in preeclampsia, it is not used as a diagnostic criterion because of its high prevalence during normal pregnancy.[27] Preeclampsia can be classified as early onset if it occurs before 34 weeks of gestation or late onset if it develops at 34 weeks of gestation or later.[28] One retrospective study demonstrated that late-onset preeclampsia was associated with a significantly higher incidence of perinatal death and severe neonatal morbidity compared with early-onset disease.[29] Preeclampsia is also classified as to the presence or absence of severe features (**Table 2**). They include blood pressure greater than 160 mm Hg systolic or 100 mm Hg diastolic, acute kidney injury with a creatinine greater than 1.1 or an increase greater than 2-fold above the baseline, doubling of liver function tests, persistent or severe central nervous system symptoms, platelet count less than 100 × 10⁹/L, and the presence of pulmonary edema. Severe proteinuria ($\geq$5 g in a 24-h urine collection) is no longer used as a severe feature of preeclampsia, as the level of proteinuria does not correlate with outcome.[30] Hemolysis, elevated liver enzymes, and low platelets

Table 2 Risk factors for preeclampsia	
Risk Level	Risk Factor
High	History of preeclampsia Multiple gestation Chronic hypertension Diabetes, type 1 or 2 Renal disease Autoimmune disorder
Moderate	Nulliparity Body mass index >30 kg/m² Family history of preeclampsia (first degree relative) Sociodemographic characteristics (African American, low socioeconomic status) Age ≥35 y Personal history factors (prior low birth weight or small-for-gestational-age delivery, prior adverse pregnancy outcome, >10 y interval since previous pregnancy)
Low	Previous uncomplicated full-term delivery

Reprinted with permission from the American College of Obstetricians and Gynecologists. From Sutton ALM, Harper LM, Tita ATN. Hypertensive Disorders in Pregnancy. Obstet Gynecol Clin N Am. 2018;45(2):333–47, with permission from the Foreign Policy Research Institute.

(HELLP) syndrome is considered by ACOG to be a variant of preeclampsia with severe features, not a distinct entity.

The mechanism underlying the development of preeclampsia seems to be abnormal placentation. During normal pregnancy, fetal cytotrophoblasts migrate into the maternal uterus, where they penetrate and remodel the spiral arteries of the endometrium, which are the terminal branches of the uterine artery supplying blood to the placenta.[31] Preeclampsia is thought to develop as a result of a 2-stage process: abnormal placentation followed by a dysfunctional maternal immune response.[32] During the first stage, invasion of the fetal cytotrophoblasts is inadequate, leading to insufficient remodeling of the spiral arteries and eventually to reduced perfusion of the placenta.[33] During the second (maternal) stage, a systemic inflammatory response is launched.[34] Ischemia caused by hypoperfusion of the placenta leads to release of numerous mediators, causing endothelial dysfunction and a cascade of systemic disturbances—the hypertension, edema, proteinuria, and platelet aggregation seen in preeclampsia. Activation of platelets and the coagulation cascade lead to development of microthrombi, further worsening blood flow to the uterus.[35] Immunologic factors can also play a key role in the development of preeclampsia. The underlying pathophysiology of preeclampsia is similar to that of graft-versus-host disease.[36]

Multiple factors increase the risk of preeclampsia (**Table 3**). A history of preeclampsia during a previous pregnancy is associated with an 8-fold increased risk of developing preeclampsia during the current one. Other factors that increase the risk are antiphospholipid antibody syndrome, chronic hypertension, pregestational diabetes mellitus, prepregnancy body mass index greater than 30, and assisted reproductive technology.[37] In the United States, clear racial differences in the incidence and level of severity of preeclampsia have been documented: African American women have a higher incidence of preeclampsia than white women and a 3-fold higher rate of maternal fatality. This increase could be related to disparities in access to health care as well as differences in co-morbid conditions.[38]

Table 3
Severe features of preeclampsia

Elevated blood pressure	• SBP ≥160 mm Hg • DBP ≥110 mm Hg • 2 measurements 4 h apart at rest
CNS symptoms	• Persistent headache • Visual changes
Thrombocytopenia	• Platelet count <100,000/mL
Renal insufficiency	• Elevated creatinine >1.1 mg/dL • Doubling of baseline creatinine
Liver dysfunction	• Transaminase levels ≥2× upper limit of normal • Persistent severe RUQ or epigastric tenderness
Pulmonary edema	• Diagnosed on physical examination

Abbreviations: CNS, central nervous system; DBP, diastolic blood pressure; RUQ, right upper quatrant; SBP, systolic blood pressure.

Hemolysis, elevated liver enzymes, and low platelets syndrome is associated with hemolysis, elevated liver function tests, and low platelet count. Most experts consider HELLP syndrome a manifestation of preeclampsia rather than a distinct hypertensive disorder of pregnancy.[1,39] In contrast to preeclampsia, nulliparity is not a risk factor for HELLP syndrome. More than 50% of patients who develop HELLP syndrome are multiparous. Other risk factors include a prior history of preeclampsia or HELLP syndrome, obesity, and extremes of age. The underlying pathophysiology of the syndrome is similar to that of preeclampsia but with a greater degree of hepatic inflammation and activation of the complement and coagulation cascades.[40] Hemolysis, elevated liver enzymes, and low platelets syndrome is characterized by microangiopathic hemolytic anemia, which develops in response to destructive forces that act on red blood cells in small blood vessels, resulting in the formation of schistocytes.[41] Typical symptoms of HELLP syndrome include right upper quadrant abdominal pain, nausea, and vomiting. Because HELLP syndrome is often associated with preeclampsia with severe features, headache, visual changes, and pulmonary edema might be present.

The Tennessee Classification System for HELLP syndrome uses the following diagnostic criteria: hemolysis with increased lactate dehydrogenase (>600 U/L), increased aspartate aminotransferase (≥70 U/L), and low platelet count (<100 × 10⁹/L). Complete expression of the disease is the presence of all 3 variables; partial expression is the presence of 2 of them.[42] The Mississippi Triple-Class HELLP System further classifies the severity of the syndrome based on the platelet count, with the most severe form, class I, having platelet counts less than 50 × 10⁹/L.[43] (**Table 4**)

Eclampsia is defined as seizures in a pregnant woman with preeclampsia with no other identifiable cause. The mechanism underlying the development of seizures is not well understood. There is evidence that elevated blood pressure causes breakdown of the autoregulatory function of the cerebral circulatory system, resulting in either hypoperfusion or hyperperfusion of the brain, endothelial dysfunction, and edema.[44] Eclampsia can occur during the antepartum period, during delivery, or in the postpartum period. More than 90% of cases occur at 28 weeks gestation or later. Up to 44% of cases of eclampsia occur during the postpartum period.[45] Before the development of seizure, the most common signs and symptoms are elevated blood pressure, headache, visual changes, and right upper quadrant and epigastric pain. No preceding symptoms are reported by up to 25% of women with eclampsia.[46]

Table 4
Classification systems for HELLP syndrome

Tennessee Classification System for HELLP Syndrome	
Complete	• Platelets <100 × 10^9/L • LDH >600 U/L • AST ≥70 U/L
Partial	• Having 2 of the 3 above variables
Mississippi Triple-Class HELLP System	
Class 1	• Platelets <50 × 10^9/L • AST or ALT ≥70 U/L • LDH ≥600 U/L
Class 2	• Platelets 50–100 × 10^9/L • AST or ALT ≥70 U/L • LDH ≥600 U/L
Class 3	• Platelets 100–150 × 10^9/L • AST or ALT ≥40 U/L • LDH ≥600 U/L

Abbreviations: AST, aspartate aminotransferase; LDH, lactate dehydrogenase.
Data from Audibert F, Friedman SA, Frangieh AY, et al. Clinical utility of strict diagnostic criteria for the HELLP (hemolysis, elevated liver enzymes, and low platelets) syndrome. Am J Obstet Gynecol 1996;175(2):460–64; and Martin JN Jr, Owens MY, Keiser SD, et al. Standardized Mississippi Protocol treatment of 190 patients with HELLP syndrome: slowing disease progression and preventing new major maternal morbidity. Hypertens Pregnancy 2010;31(1):79–90.

Seizures are typically generalized tonic-clonic, lasting 60 to 90 seconds and followed by a post-ictal phase.[47]

Both preeclampsia and eclampsia may be associated with the development of posterior reversible encephalopathy syndrome (PRES), that is, the development of vasogenic cerebral edema and focal neurologic deficits. The signs and symptoms of PRES are reversible with treatment, although permanent deficits can occur.[48] Because the changes of PRES almost always involve the occipital lobe of the brain, visual changes are common. They include scotomata, hallucinations, diplopia, and blurred vision. The changes of PRES are seen as hyperintense signals on T2 and fluid-attenuated inversion recovery sequences on brain MRI.[49]

Chronic Hypertension with Superimposed Preeclampsia

Preeclampsia in a pregnant patient with known chronic hypertension after 20 weeks' gestation[1] is the hypertensive disorder of pregnancy with the highest rate of maternal and fetal complications, higher than with either condition alone. Diagnosis of preeclampsia in a patient with chronic hypertension can be challenging because her blood pressure is already elevated and chronic hypertension might already have induced proteinuria. The diagnosis should be suspected if the blood pressure increases, if the blood pressure becomes resistant to treatment, or if the level of proteinuria increases.[10]

EPIDEMIOLOGY

In the United States, hypertensive disorders of pregnancy complicate approximately 1 of every 9 pregnancies.[50] The incidence of chronic hypertension among women of childbearing age is increasing in the United States, largely due to obesity, diabetes, and poor diet. The National Health and Nutrition Examination Survey detected a

10% prevalence of chronic hypertension in women aged 20 to 44 years using a systolic BP/diastolic BP threshold of ≥140/90 mm Hg.[2] Chronic hypertension complicates 1% to 2% of deliveries in the United States,[51] whereas gestational hypertension develops in 2% to 3% of pregnancies.[52] Preeclampsia affects 3% to 5% of pregnancies in the United States.[53] Eclampsia will develop in 0.6% of pregnant women with preeclampsia without severe features and in 2% to 3% of those with severe features.[54]

PATIENT EVALUATION

The approach to pregnant patient with elevated blood pressure in the emergency department begins with determining, if possible, if the elevation antedated or developed during the pregnancy. Preeclampsia can develop in patients with or without chronic hypertension. As discussed earlier, it is a disorder associated with dysfunctional placentation and therefore does not occur until after the 20th week of gestation.

The history should include queries regarding complaints that would suggest preeclampsia with severe features, such as headache, visual changes, right upper quadrant abdominal pain, and lower-extremity edema. The mother should be placed on a cardiac monitor and her blood pressure should be measured frequently. For patients with newly diagnosed preeclampsia or any evidence of worsening preeclampsia, fetal monitoring should be used to confirm fetal well-being.

The physical examination should assess for the presence of end-organ damage. All patients with visual complaints should have an assessment of their visual acuity and visual fields. The fundoscopic examination might demonstrate findings in up to half of patients with a hypertensive disorder of pregnancy. The most common finding is arterial attenuation; retinal hemorrhages, retinal edema, and retinal detachment, and papilledema also could be noted.[55] The cardiopulmonary system should be examined to assess for the presence congestive heart failure and pulmonary edema. Examination of the abdomen might demonstrate tenderness, especially in the right upper quadrant secondary to liver involvement. Lower-extremity edema is seen frequently in normal pregnancies and those complicated by preeclampsia. Documentation of severity of edema is important because a rapid increase in peripheral edema could be a sign of the development of preeclampsia. A thorough neurologic examination should be performed. Hyperreflexia with or without clonus is an indicator of central nervous system excitability.

Laboratory evaluations include urinalysis to assess for protein, serum chemistry to evaluate electrolytes, liver function tests, complete blood count with platelet count, and a baseline magnesium level. Uric acid levels are often sought but the utility of this test is not clear. Two systematic reviews published in 2006 concluded that uric acid level has poor accuracy as a predictor of preeclampsia.[56,57] A secondary analysis of data collected during the Preeclampsia Integrated Estimate of Risk study demonstrated that a gestational age-corrected uric acid level was associated with adverse perinatal but not maternal outcomes.[58] Coagulation studies can be requested if the patient appears to be sick and if there is concern about disseminated intravascular coagulation.

MANAGEMENT

The goals of evaluation and management of a pregnant patient with elevated blood pressure in the emergency department are to identify the presence of any complications, treat presenting symptoms, and reduce the risk of progression to eclampsia.

Urgent or emergent lowering of the blood pressure might be required based on the presenting blood pressure and the presence of signs of end-organ dysfunction. For women with gestational hypertension or preeclampsia without severe features, the ACOG guidelines recommend outpatient treatment with antihypertensive medications once the systolic BP is >160 mm Hg or the diastolic BP is >110 mm Hg. When emergent lowering of blood pressure is required, the goal is to keep the systolic BP between 140 and 150 mm Hg, and the diastolic BP between 90 and 100 mm Hg, to prevent hypoperfusion of the maternal organs and the fetus.[59] The Control of Hypertension in Pregnancy Study demonstrated similar outcomes in women who had blood pressure tightly controlled and those whose pressure was less tightly controlled.[60] In contrast to the ACOG guidelines of 2013, recommendations from the International Society for the Study of Hypertension in Pregnancy (ISSHP), published in 2018, advocate the treatment of any type of hypertensive disorder of pregnancy when the blood pressure is greater than 140/90 mm Hg in the clinic or office or greater than 135/85 mm Hg at home.

Magnesium

The benefit of magnesium sulfate infusion in reducing the risk of eclampsia in women with preeclampsia was confirmed in the Magnesium Sulfate for Prevention of Eclampsia Trial.[61] Magnesium works as a vasodilator through its antagonism of calcium receptors on vascular smooth muscle cells. Reduction in blood pressure as a result of magnesium administration has not been shown clearly.[62] The anti-seizure benefit of magnesium may be the result of antagonism at the N-methyl-D-aspartate receptors.[63] Parenteral magnesium is indicated in women with severe preeclampsia or evidence of pending eclampsia, such as severe headache, altered mental status, and clonus. The ACOG guidelines recommend against universal treatment of women with preeclampsia without severe features because the low incidence of progression to eclampsia would require treatment of thousands of patients to prevent 1 case of preeclampsia. In addition, the guidelines cite only 2 studies addressing this issue, showing no reduction in progression to preeclampsia with severe features.[1] The initial loading dose of magnesium is 4 to 6 g intravenously (IV) over 15 to 20 minutes followed by an infusion rate of 1 to 2 g/h. Women receiving a magnesium infusion should have their respiratory rate and blood pressure evaluated every 30 minutes, their pulse and urine output evaluated every hour, and their reflexes checked at the end of the loading dose and every 2 hours during infusion. Continued magnesium infusion is based on physical examination findings, not serum magnesium levels.

Aspirin

Low-dose aspirin has a moderate effect in the prevention of preeclampsia in women identified as high risk. ACOG recommends initiation of aspirin at a dose of 60 to 80 mg late in the first trimester in women at high risk for preeclampsia.[1] The mechanism by which aspirin prevents preeclampsia is thought to be through restoration of the prostacyclin-thromboxane A2 balance through acetylation of cyclooxygenase, which limits the formation of thromboxane A2.[64] In the Aspirin versus Placebo in Pregnancies at High Risk for Preeclampsia Study, aspirin at a dose of 150 mg daily was compared with placebo in 1620 subjects. For women receiving aspirin, the incidence of preeclampsia was 1.6% compared with 4.3% for the placebo group.[65] The results of this study led the ISSHP to recommend initiation of aspirin at a dose of 150 mg daily for women at high risk for preeclampsia before 20 weeks' gestational age (ideally, before 16 weeks).

Timing of Delivery

The timing of delivery must allow as much fetal development while minimizing the risk of harm to the mother or the fetus by prolonging the pregnancy. The definitive treatment of eclampsia is delivery. Before delivery, the patient is stabilized, with focus on protection of the airway and control of blood pressure. Fetal monitoring should be initiated to assess for signs of distress. Consultation with an obstetrician should be initiated immediately. Intravenous magnesium sulfate is used to prevent recurrent seizure.[45] For women with mild gestational hypertension or preeclampsia without severe features and with no indication for delivery at less than 37 weeks of gestation, expectant management with maternal and fetal monitoring is suggested. For women beyond 37 weeks of gestation, delivery rather than continued observation is suggested. One retrospective study of women diagnosed with mild gestational hypertension who underwent elective delivery found that waiting until the gestational age was greater than 38 weeks was associated with lower rates of low birth weight, small-for-gestational age delivery, neonatal intensive care unit admission, and respiratory distress syndrome.[66] Blood pressures are typically monitored for at least 72 hours postpartum and again 7 to 10 days after delivery, with continued assessment for symptoms of end-organ dysfunction. In severe gestational hypertension, time to delivery is the biggest mitigating factor for reducing morbidity and mortality in the peripartum setting. The decision to deliver is individualized, taking into consideration maternal factors of disease progression and fetal considerations, such as gestational age and results of serial ultrasonographic testing during pregnancy (umbilical artery pressure, amniotic fluid volume, gestational age).

For deliveries that are expected within the subsequent 72 hours and the gestational age is less than 32 weeks, magnesium sulfate should be administered to reduce the

Table 5
Oral medications for blood pressure control in pregnancy

Drug	FDA Pregnancy Category[a]	Mechanism of Action	Dose	Side Effects
Labetalol	C	Non-selective β-blocker	200–1200 mg/d in 2–3 divided doses	Bronchospasm (caution in asthma & COPD), hypotension, fetal bradycardia
Nifedipine XL	C	Calcium channel blocker	30–120 mg/d	Headache, flushing, peripheral edema
Methyldopa	B	α-2 agonist	500 mg-3 g/d in 2 divided doses	Increased LFTs, depression
HCTZ	C	Diuretic	12.5–25 mg/d	Volume depletion, hypokalemia
Metoprolol	C	Selective β-1 blocker	25–200 mg/d in 2 divided doses	Same as for labetalol
Hydralazine	C	Peripheral vasodilator	50–300 mg/d in 2–4 divided doses	Hypotension, fetal thrombocytopenia

Abbreviations: COPD, chronic obstructive pulmonary disease; d, day; FDA, US Food and Drug Administration; HCTZ, hydrochlorothiazide; LFTs, liver function tests; mg, milligrams.
  [a] Category A, controlled studies show no risk; category B, no evidence of risk in humans; category C, risk cannot be ruled out; category D, positive evidence of risk; category X, contraindicated in pregnancy.

risk of moderate or severe cerebral palsy.[67] If delivery is anticipated within the subsequent 7 days and the gestational age is between 24 and 34 weeks, corticosteroids should be given to promote fetal lung maturity. An updated ACOG committee opinion, in 2016, expanded antenatal corticosteroid recommendations to support betamethasone administration to women at high risk for late preterm birth (34 0/7–36 6/7 weeks). Dexamethasone and betamethasone are the most widely studied corticosteroids used for this indication. Suggested regimens are 2 doses of betamethasone (12 mg administered intramuscularly [IM] or IV, given 24 hours apart) or 4 doses of dexamethasone (6 mg administered IM every 12 hours).[68]

PHARMACOLOGIC TREATMENT OF BLOOD PRESSURE

First-line long-term pharmacologic treatment of pregnant women with hypertension includes labetalol, nifedipine, and methyldopa (**Table 5**). Labetalol is a non-selective

Labetalol Algorithm

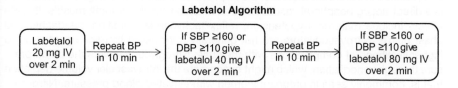

* Continuous infusion dosing is 1–2 mg/min
* Max cumulative dose 220 mg in 24 h
* Caution in history of asthma or COPD due to possible bronchoconstriction
* May cause neonatal bradycardia
* FDA Class C

Hydralazine Algorithm

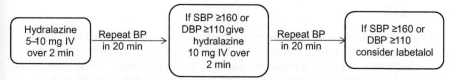

* Continuous infusion dosing is 0.5–10 mg/hr
* Max cumulative dose 25 mg in 24 h
* May cause disproportionate hypotension
* FDA Class C

Oral Nifedipine Algorithm

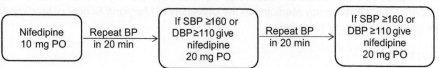

* May cause headache, maternal reflex tachycardia, GI transit slowing
* May cause abrupt hypotension if given with intravenous magnesium
* FDA Class C

Fig. 1. Medications for acute blood pressure management for severe preeclampsia/eclampsia.

β-blocker with vascular α-blockade properties. It can be used for immediate and long-term control of blood pressure. One maternal side effect is bronchoconstriction; therefore, labetalol should be avoided in patients with asthma as well as those with bradycardia. Other side effects of labetalol include fatigue and orthostatic hypotension. There is some concern about intrauterine growth retardation; the evidence is inconclusive.[3] Nifedipine is a dihydropyridine calcium channel blocker that can be associated with flushing, peripheral edema, reflex tachycardia, and headache. Caution is advised regarding the concomitant administration of magnesium and nifedipine due to reports of hypotension and neuromuscular blockade.[69] Methyldopa is a centrally acting α_2-adrenergic agonist. It is considered safe to the fetus; adverse maternal effects include liver damage and hemolytic anemia.[70] Thiazide diuretics are generally avoided due to the risk of volume depletion.

Rapid reduction of blood pressure is frequently accomplished with the use of intravenous labetalol or hydralazine. Oral nifedipine is also considered a first-line therapy for reduction in severe elevations of blood pressure in pregnancy (**Fig. 1**). Hydralazine is a direct-acting peripheral vasodilator that relaxes vascular smooth muscle. Its side effects include maternal hypotension, reflex tachycardia, vomiting, headache, and chest pain.[59] Nitrovasodilators are not generally considered first-line agents due to higher likelihood of complications with their use. Nitroglycerin lowers the blood pressure through venodilation, which might exacerbate the intravascular volume depletion that is, commonly seen in pregnant women with elevated blood pressure. Nitroprusside, an intravenous agent, is used uncommonly in the emergency setting for blood pressure control. Its very short half-life makes it very effective for rapid titration, but there is concern for cyanide accumulation in the mother and fetus if used longer than 4 hours. Nitroprusside is thus generally viewed as an agent to use if the agents named above fail to achieve adequate blood pressure control.[71] Agents that should be avoided in pregnancy include angiotensin-converting enzyme inhibitors and angiotensin receptor blockers because of the risk of teratogenicity.

SUMMARY

The hypertensive disorders of pregnancy continue to cause a substantial amount of maternal and fetal morbidity and mortality despite efforts to promote proper diagnosis and treatment. Current guidelines provide evidence-based recommendations regarding the care of pregnant patients with hypertension. Although the body of evidence supporting these recommendations has grown over the years, areas of research remain. Additional evidence will help to refine treatment strategies and promote both maternal and fetal well-being.

ACKNOWLEDGMENTS

The authors thank Linda J. Kesselring, MS, ELS, the technical editor/writer in the Department of Emergency Medicine at the University of Maryland School of Medicine, for her copyediting of the article.

REFERENCES

1. American College of Obstetricians and Gynecologists. Task force on hypertension in pregnancy. ACOG hypertension in pregnancy task force. Washington, DC: American College of Obstetricians and Gynecologists; 2013.
2. Whelton PK, Carey RM, Aronow WS, et al. 2017 ACC/AHA/AAPA/ABC/ACPM/AGS/APhA/ASH/ASPC/NMA/PCNA Guideline for the Prevention, Detection,

Evaluation, and Management of High Blood Pressure in Adults: a report of the American College of Cardiology/American Heart Association Task Force on Clinical Practice Guidelines. J Am Coll Cardiol 2018;71(19):e127–248.

3. Chahine KM, Sibai BM. Chronic hypertension in pregnancy: new concepts for classification and management. Am J Perinatol 2018. https://doi.org/10.1055/s-0038-1666976.

4. National High Blood Pressure Education Program Working Group. National high blood pressure education program working group report on high blood pressure in pregnancy. Am J Obstet Gynecol 2000;183:S1.

5. Seely EW, Ecker J. Chronic hypertension in pregnancy. N Engl J Med 2011; 365(5):439–46.

6. O'Brien TE, Ray JG, Chan W-S. Maternal body mass index and the risk of pre-eclampsia: a systematic overview. Epidemiology 2003;14(3):368–74.

7. Sibai BM, Koch MA, Freire S, et al. The impact of prior preeclampsia on the risk of superimposed preeclampsia and other adverse pregnancy outcomes in patients with chronic hypertension. Am J Obstet Gynecol 2011;204(4). 345.e1-6.

8. Mathews TJ, Hamilton BE. Mean age of mothers is on the rise: United States, 2000-2014. NCHS Data Brief 2016;(232):1–8.

9. Malha L, August P. Secondary hypertension in pregnancy. Curr Hypertens Rep 2015;17(7):53.

10. Seely EW, Ecker J. Chronic hypertension in pregnancy. Circulation 2014;129(11): 1254–61.

11. Redman CWG. Hypertension in pregnancy: the NICE guidelines. Heart 2011; 97(23):1967–9.

12. Goulopoulou S. Maternal vascular physiology in preeclampsia. Hypertension 2017;70(6):1066–73.

13. Khosravi S, Dabiran S, Lotfi M, et al. Study of the prevalence of hypertension and complications of hypertensive disorders in pregnancy. Open J Prev Med 2014; 04(11):860–7.

14. Spinnato JA, Freire S, Pinto e Silva JL, et al. Antioxidant therapy to prevent pre-eclampsia: a randomized controlled trial. Obstet Gynecol 2007;110(6):1311–8.

15. Poston L, Briley AL, Seed PT, et al, Vitamins in Pre-eclampsia (VIP) Trial Consortium. Vitamin C and vitamin E in pregnant women at risk for pre-eclampsia (VIP trial): randomised placebo-controlled trial. Lancet 2006;367(9517):1145–54.

16. Vigil-De Gracia P, Lasso M, Montufar-Rueda C. Perinatal outcome in women with severe chronic hypertension during the second half of pregnancy. Int J Gynaecol Obstet 2004;85(2):139–44.

17. Rey E, Couturier A. The prognosis of pregnancy in women with chronic hypertension. Am J Obstet Gynecol 1994;171(2):410–6.

18. Sibai BM. Diagnosis and management of gestational hypertension and pre-eclampsia. Obstet Gynecol 2003;102(1):181–92.

19. Saudan P, Brown MA, Buddle ML, et al. Does gestational hypertension become pre-eclampsia? Br J Obstet Gynaecol 1998;105(11):1177–84.

20. Barton JR, O'Brien JM, Bergauer NK, et al. Mild gestational hypertension remote from term: progression and outcome. Am J Obstet Gynecol 2001;184(5):979–83.

21. Cruz MO, Gao W, Hibbard JU. Obstetrical and perinatal outcomes among women with gestational hypertension, mild preeclampsia, and mild chronic hypertension. Am J Obstet Gynecol 2011;205(3):260.e1-9.

22. Buchbinder A, Sibai BM, Caritis S, et al. Adverse perinatal outcomes are significantly higher in severe gestational hypertension than in mild preeclampsia. Am J Obstet Gynecol 2002;186(1):66–71.

23. Duley L, Henderson-Smart D, Meher S. Altered dietary salt for preventing pre-eclampsia, and its complications. Cochrane Database Syst Rev 2005;(4):CD005548.
24. Meher S, Abalos E, Carroli G. Bed rest with or without hospitalisation for hypertension during pregnancy. Cochrane Database Syst Rev 2005;(4):CD003514.
25. Airoldi J, Weinstein L. Clinical significance of proteinuria in pregnancy. Obstet Gynecol Surv 2007;62(2):117–24.
26. Waugh JJS, Clark TJ, Divakaran TG, et al. Accuracy of urinalysis dipstick techniques in predicting significant proteinuria in pregnancy. Obstet Gynecol 2004; 103(4):769–77.
27. Thomson AM, Hytten FE, Billewicz WZ. The epidemiology of oedema during pregnancy. J Obstet Gynaecol Br Commonw 1967;74(1):1–10.
28. von Dadelszen P, Magee LA, Roberts JM. Subclassification of preeclampsia. Hypertens Pregnancy 2003;22(2):143–8.
29. Lisonkova S, Joseph KS. Incidence of preeclampsia: risk factors and outcomes associated with early- versus late-onset disease. Am J Obstet Gynecol 2013; 209(6):544, e1-544.e12.
30. Newman MG, Robichaux AG, Stedman CM, et al. Perinatal outcomes in preeclampsia that is complicated by massive proteinuria. Am J Obstet Gynecol 2003;188(1):264–8.
31. Brosens JJ, Pijnenborg R, Brosens IA. The myometrial junctional zone spiral arteries in normal and abnormal pregnancies: a review of the literature. Am J Obstet Gynecol 2002;187(5):1416–23.
32. Roberts JM, Hubel CA. The two stage model of preeclampsia: variations on the theme. Placenta 2009;30(Suppl A):S32–7.
33. Sheppard BL, Bonnar J. Ultrastructural abnormalities of placental villi in placentae from pregnancies complicated by intrauterine fetal growth retardation: their relationship to decidual spiral arterial lesions. Placenta 1980;1(2):145–56.
34. Redman CWG, Sargent IL. Placental stress and pre-eclampsia: a revised view. Placenta 2009;30(Suppl A):S38–42.
35. Roberts JM, Taylor RN, Musci TJ, et al. Preeclampsia: an endothelial cell disorder. Am J Obstet Gynecol 1989;161(5):1200–4.
36. Gleicher N. Why much of the pathophysiology of preeclampsia-eclampsia must be of an autoimmune nature. Am J Obstet Gynecol 2007;196(1):5.e1-7.
37. Bartsch E, Medcalf KE, Park AL, et al, High Risk of Pre-eclampsia Identification Group. Clinical risk factors for pre-eclampsia determined in early pregnancy: systematic review and meta-analysis of large cohort studies. BMJ 2016;353:i1753. https://doi.org/10.1136/bmj.i1753.
38. US Preventive Services Task Force, Bibbins-Domingo K, Grossman DC, Curry SJ, et al. Screening for preeclampsia: US preventive services task force Recommendation statement. JAMA 2017;317(16):1661–7.
39. Brown MA, Magee LA, Kenny LC, et al. Hypertensive disorders of pregnancy: ISSHP classification, diagnosis, and management recommendations for international practice. Hypertension 2018;72(1):24–43.
40. Abildgaard U, Heimdal K. Pathogenesis of the syndrome of hemolysis, elevated liver enzymes, and low platelet count (HELLP): a review. Eur J Obstet Gynecol 2013;166(2):117–23.
41. Haram K, Svendsen E, Abildgaard U. The HELLP syndrome: clinical issues and management. A review. BMC Pregnancy Childbirth 2009;9:8.
42. Audibert F, Friedman SA, Frangieh AY, et al. Clinical utility of strict diagnostic criteria for the HELLP (hemolysis, elevated liver enzymes, and low platelets) syndrome. Am J Obstet Gynecol 1996;175(2):460–4.

43. Martin JN Jr, Owens MY, Keiser SD, et al. Standardized Mississippi Protocol treatment of 190 patients with HELLP syndrome: slowing disease progression and preventing new major maternal morbidity. Hypertens Pregnancy 2010;31(1):79–90.
44. Cipolla MJ. Cerebrovascular function in pregnancy and eclampsia. Hypertension 2007;50:14–24.
45. Sibai BM. Diagnosis, prevention, and management of eclampsia. Obstet Gynecol 2005;105(2):402–10.
46. Berhan Y, Berhan A. Should magnesium sulfate be administered to women with mild pre-eclampsia? A systematic review of published reports on eclampsia. J Obstet Gynaecol Res 2015;41(6):831–42.
47. Leeman L, Dresang LT, Fontaine P. Hypertensive disorders of pregnancy. Am Fam Physician 2016;93(2):121–7.
48. McDermott M, Miller EC, Rundek T, et al. Preeclampsia: association with posterior reversible encephalopathy syndrome and stroke. Stroke 2018;49(3). https://doi.org/10.1161/STROKEAHA.117.018416.
49. Raman R, Devaramane R, Mukunda Jagadish G, et al. Various imaging manifestations of posterior reversible encephalopathy syndrome (PRES) on magnetic resonance imaging (MRI). Pol J Radiol 2017;82:64–70.
50. Mogos MF, Salemi JL, Spooner KK, et al. Hypertensive disorders of pregnancy and postpartum readmission in the United States: national surveillance of the revolving door. J Hypertens 2018;36(3):608–18.
51. Bateman BT, Bansil P, Hernandez-Diaz S, et al. Prevalence, trends, and outcomes of chronic hypertension: a nationwide sample of delivery admissions. Am J Obstet Gynecol 2012;206(2):134.e1-8.
52. Wallis AB, Saftlas AF, Hsia J, et al. Secular trends in the rates of pre-eclampsia, eclampsia, and gestational hypertension, United States, 1987–2004. Am J Hypertens 2008;21:521–6.
53. Ananth CV, Keyes KM, Wapner RJ. Pre-eclampsia rates in the United States, 1980-2010: age-period-cohort analysis. BMJ 2013;347:f6564.
54. Sibai BM. Magnesium sulfate prophylaxis in preeclampsia: lessons learned from recent trials. Am J Obstet Gynecol 2004;190(6):1520–6.
55. Bakhda RN. Clinical study of fundus findings in pregnancy induced hypertension. J Family Med Prim Care 2016;5(2):424–9.
56. Cnossen JS, de Ruyter-Hanhijärvi H, van der Post JAM, et al. Accuracy of serum uric acid determination in predicting pre-eclampsia: a systematic review. Acta Obstet Gynecol Scand 2006;85(5):519–25.
57. Thangaratinam S, Ismail KMK, Sharp S, et al, Tests in Prediction of Pre-eclampsia Severity Review Group. Accuracy of serum uric acid in predicting complications of pre-eclampsia: a systematic review. BJOG 2006;113(4):369–78.
58. Livingston JR, Payne B, Brown M, et al. Uric acid as a predictor of adverse maternal and perinatal outcomes in women hospitalized with preeclampsia. J Obstet Gynaecol Can 2014;36(10):870–7.
59. ElFarra J, Bean C, Martin JN. Management of hypertensive crisis for the obstetrician/gynecologist. Obstet Gynecol Clin North Am 2016;43(4):623–37.
60. Magee LA, Dadelszen von P, Rey E, et al. Less-tight versus tight control of hypertension in pregnancy. N Engl J Med 2015;372(5):407–17.
61. Altman D, Carroli G, Duley L, et al. Do women with pre-eclampsia, and their babies, benefit from magnesium sulphate? The Magpie Trial: a randomised placebo-controlled trial. Lancet 2002;359(9321):1877–90.

62. Abalos E, Duley L, Steyn DW. Antihypertensive drug therapy for mild to moderate hypertension during pregnancy. Cochrane Database Syst Rev 2014;(2):CD002252.
63. Lambert G, Brichant JF, Hartstein G, et al. Preeclampsia: an update. Acta Anaesthesiol Belg 2014;65(4):137–49.
64. Cadavid AP. Aspirin: the mechanism of action revisited in the context of pregnancy complications. Front Immunol 2017;8:261.
65. Rolnik DL, Wright D, Poon LC, et al. Aspirin versus placebo in pregnancies at high risk for preterm preeclampsia. N Engl J Med 2017;377(7):613–22.
66. Barton JR, Barton LA, Istwan NB, et al. Elective delivery at $34^0(/)^7$ to $36^6(/)^7$ weeks' gestation and its impact on neonatal outcomes in women with stable mild gestational hypertension. Am J Obstet Gynecol 2011;204(1):44.e1-5.
67. Committee Opinion No. 652. magnesium sulfate use in obstetrics. Obstet Gynecol 2016;127(1):e52–3.
68. Committee Opinion No. 713. Antenatal corticosteroid therapy for fetal maturation. Obstet Gynecol 2017;130(2):e102–9.
69. Ben-Ami M, Giladi Y, Shalev E. The combination of magnesium sulphate and nifedipine: a cause of neuromuscular blockade. Br J Obstet Gynaecol 1994; 101(3):262–3.
70. Arndt PA. Drug-induced immune hemolytic anemia: the last 30 years of changes. Immunohematology 2014;30(2):44–54.
71. Magee LA, Abalos E, Dadelszen von P, et al. How to manage hypertension in pregnancy effectively. Br J Clin Pharmacol 2011;72(3):394–401.

Trauma in Pregnancy

Jeffrey Sakamoto, MD[a], Collin Michels, MD[a], Bryn Eisfelder, MD[a],
Nikita Joshi, MD[b],*

KEYWORDS

- Trauma in pregnancy • Blunt trauma • Penetrating trauma

KEY POINTS

- Trauma in pregnancy is challenging because there are two patients to consider during resuscitation. It may not be clear based on history or physical that a patient is pregnant, and the physician should assess for pregnancy in patients of child-bearing age.
- Prioritization of maternal resuscitation is important to ensure optimal outcome for mother and fetus, which includes proceeding with medications and radiology examinations because they are indicated without delay.
- Trauma management in pregnancy requires coordination between multiple specialties including emergency medicine, trauma surgery, obstetrics, and neonatology.
- Pregnant trauma patients often require prolonged observation in labor and delivery units after initial stabilization in the emergency department. This may require transfer to another facility for higher level of care.

INTRODUCTION

Although pregnant trauma patients present infrequently to the emergency department (ED), it is one of the most common contributors to maternal and fetal morbidity and mortality.[1–8] Up to 1.5% of women admitted for traumatic injuries are pregnant[4]; however, immediate recognition of pregnancy is not always possible, especially in cases of first-trimester pregnancy, morbid obesity, or in critically injured patients. Additional to the rarity of presentation and complicated pathophysiology, there is the cognitive load of resuscitating two patients, mother and fetus; working with multiple specialties including trauma, obstetrics, and neonatology; and processing emotional and social issues that can arise. Furthermore, the clinical course is difficult to predict because of a lack of correlation between the degree of trauma and clinical outcome.[2] Unique challenges in pregnant trauma patients are listed in **Box 1**.

Disclosure Statement: None of the authors have any relationship with a commercial company that has a direct financial interest in subject matter or materials discussed in article or with a company making a competing product. The authors acknowledge the contribution of Dr Kimberly S. Harney, Clinical Professor, Obstetrics, Stanford University, to this article.
[a] Department of Emergency Medicine, Stanford University, 900 Welch Road, Suite 350, Palo Alto, CA 94304, USA; [b] Alameda Health Systems, 490 Grand Avenue, Oakland, CA 94610, USA
* Corresponding author.
E-mail address: njoshi8@gmail.com

Emerg Med Clin N Am 37 (2019) 317–338
https://doi.org/10.1016/j.emc.2019.01.009
0733-8627/19/© 2019 Elsevier Inc. All rights reserved.

emed.theclinics.com

Box 1
Unique challenges in pregnant trauma patients

Complex physiologic adaptations of the pregnant patient throughout pregnancy

Need for multidisciplinary approach with multiple specialties

Mitigation of exposure to radiation and other teratogens

Management of pregnancy-specific related condition (ie, Rhesus factor isoimmunization, placental abruption)

Management of two patients concurrently

BACKGROUND AND EPIDEMIOLOGY

Trauma has been found to be the leading nonobstetric cause of maternal death during pregnancy, and is associated with up to 20% of maternal deaths in the United States.[1,9] Traumatic injuries are estimated to complicate up to 1 in 12 pregnancies.[2–4] In 2017, a study involving 1148 pregnant trauma patients found that pregnant women had significantly higher mortality compared with nonpregnant women, with a relative risk (RR) of 1.6.[1]

Risk factors commonly associated with trauma in pregnancy include[1,2,4,9]:

- Age less than 26 years
- African-American or Hispanic ethnicity
- Medicaid insurance
- Lower socioeconomic status
- Minimal or no prenatal care in the first trimester

Risk stratification and identification of potential maternal and fetal complications are also difficult. Even minor injuries as evaluated by the Injury Severity Score,[10] a validated tool in predicting mortality in nonpregnant populations,[11,12] is not predictive of fetal morbidity and mortality, and can still be associated with adverse pregnancy outcomes.[2,8]

Mechanism of Injury

Unintentional or nonviolent trauma accounts for the largest portion of trauma in pregnancy, including motor vehicle accidents (MVAs) and falls.[8] Intentional or violent trauma accounts for approximately 16% of traumatic injuries in pregnant women, and includes suicide, gunshot wounds, stab wounds, sexual assault, strangulation, and domestic violent (DV). Blunt trauma including MVAs and falls accounts for 88% to 92% of injuries, penetrating trauma including gun shot wounds (GSWs) and stab wounds account for approximately 2% to 7%, and burn injuries up to 4%. Although most traumas are nonviolent in cause, pregnant patients are nearly twice as likely to experience violent trauma compared with nonpregnant patients with increased mortality and a RR of 3.14.[1,2,13–17]

ANATOMY AND PHYSIOLOGY OF PREGNANT PATIENTS

As seen in **Fig. 1**, the uterus remains within the pelvis until approximately 12 weeks gestational age (GA), reaching the umbilicus by 20 weeks GA, and the costal margins by 34 weeks GA.[18] By the end of the third trimester, the uterus size significantly alters anatomic location and function of abdominal and pelvic structures. **Tables 1** and **2** summarize pertinent anatomic and physiologic changes as it relates

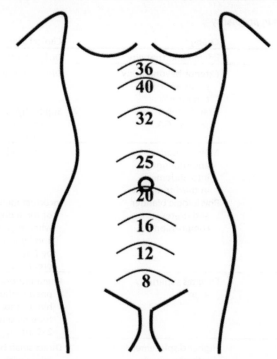

Fig. 1. Approximate location of uterine fundus at different gestational ages.

to trauma management.[18–24] Understanding the clinical impact of these changes is important because it affects symptoms and manifestations of traumatic injuries.

Cardiovascular Changes

Cardiovascular adaptations allow for optimal oxygen (O_2) delivery to maternal and fetal tissues. Plasma volume begins to expand by 6 to 8 weeks GA, increasing cardiac output up to 45%.[6,18,21,24] Blood pressure decreases throughout pregnancy with average diastolic blood pressure decrement of 10 to 15 mm Hg, and average systolic blood pressure decrement of 5 to 10 mm Hg.[19] After 20 weeks GA, the uterus rises to the level of the inferior vena cava (IVC), causing compression of the IVC in the supine position, decreasing cardiac preload and cardiac output by 10% to 30%.[20,21] The changes can cause difficulty in identification of maternal hemorrhagic shock with up to 30% to 35% of circulating blood volume (almost 2000 mL) lost before exhibiting hypotension. Increased blood flow to the uterus and injuries is a significant source of hemorrhage. There may also be marked venous congestion throughout the pelvis and lower extremities increasing the risk of retroperitoneal hemorrhage with pelvic injuries.[18,22,25]

Pulmonary Changes

Respiratory changes to optimize fetal oxygenation lead to 40% increase (approximately 200 mL) in tidal volume leading to increased minute ventilation[26] and lower arterial $Paco_2$ (mean value of 30 mm Hg in pregnancy). The diaphragm rises up to 4 cm during pregnancy, resulting in perceived penetrating chest trauma to actually be intra-abdominal.[27]

Structure	Change	Clinical Significance
Table 1		
Anatomic changes in pregnancy		
Airway	Edema and friability	Difficult intubation
Uterus	Extends beyond bony pelvis after first trimester	Direct uterine injury
	Gravid uterus >20 wk GA	Supine hypotension secondary to IVC compression
Bladder	Moves anteriorly and superiorly into abdomen in third trimester	Direct bladder injury
	Physiologic bladder and ureter compression	Incorrect identification of renal obstruction, when hydronephrosis and hydroureter can be physiologic in pregnancy
Diaphragm	Elevates superiorly 4 cm	Pneumothorax, tension pneumothorax requiring higher thoracostomy tube placement 2–3 interspaces superiorly
Small bowel	Higher displacement into abdomen	Direct small bowel injury with penetrating trauma to upper abdomen
Peritoneum	Abdominal wall stretches as pregnancy progresses	Underestimation of intra-abdominal bleeding or organ injury because of blunted response to peritoneal irritation
Ligaments of PS and SI joints	Loosening	Incorrect identification of pelvic disruption on radiograph because of baseline diastasis

Abbreviations: IVC, inferior vena cava; PS, pubic symphysis; SI, sacroiliac.

Renal Changes

By 26 weeks GA, the renal plasma blood flow and glomerular filtration rate increase resulting in decreased serum levels of creatinine and blood urea nitrogen.[26] Renal excretion of bicarbonate compensates for respiratory alkalosis resulting in decreased levels of serum sodium bicarbonate to 19 to 20 mEq/L.[26] The bladder may be displaced anteriorly and superiorly, causing susceptibility to injury.[22] Physiologic hydronephrosis and hydroureter may be seen on radiology imaging.[21,24]

Gastrointestinal Changes

Progesterone mediates delays in gastric emptying, decreased intestinal motility, and decreased lower esophageal sphincter tone, which increases the risk of aspiration.[22,23] Early gastric decompression should be considered in gravid women greater

Table 2
Physiologic changes in pregnancy

System	Physiologic Change	Clinical Significance
Airway		
Pulm	Airway edema	Difficulty airway, may require smaller ETT (6.0 and 6.5) and additional airway adjuncts
	↑ O$_2$ consumption, ↓ RV, and ↓ FRC	Requires preoxygenation with high flow O$_2$ before induction
GI	↓ Gastric emptying, ↓ LES tone	↑ Risk of aspiration
Breathing		
Pulm	↑ TV and ↑ MV	Compensated respiratory alkalosis, maintain Etco$_2$ 30–35 mm Hg
	Elevation of diaphragm	Place chest tubes 1–2 intercostal spaces above fifth interspace
Circulation		
CV	↑ Plasma volume	Delayed recognition of hemorrhagic shock with large-volume blood loss; physiologic anemia
	↑ HR and ↓ BP	Vital signs poor marker of hemodynamic stability
	↑ Uterine and bladder blood flow	↑ Risk of maternal hemorrhage with direct injury
	↑ Vascular congestion	↑ Risk of retroperitoneal hemorrhage or lower extremity brisk bleed
Miscellaneous		
Renal	↑ rPBF, ↑ GFR, and ↓ Serum Cr	Caution with drugs excreted through renal system
	↑ Bicarb excretion	↓ HCO$_3$ on ABG (19–20 mEq/L), increased susceptibility to acidosis
Heme	↑ Fibrinogen, ↑ D dimer, ↓ PT, PTT, ↓ PLTs	Propensity to develop DIC

Abbreviations: ABG, arterial blood gas; BP, blood pressure; Cr, creatinine; CV, cardiovascular; DIC, disseminated intravascular coagulation, ETT, endotracheal tube; FRC, functional residual capacity; GFR, glomerular filtration rate; GI, gastrointestinal; HR, heart rate; LES, lower esophageal sphincter; MV, minute ventilation; PT, prothrombin time; PLT, platelet; PTT, partial thromboplastin time; Pulm, pulmonary; rPBF, renal plasma blood flow; RV, residual volume; TV, tidal volume.

than 16 weeks GA with altered mental status, especially if undergoing intubation.[18] The most common cause of abdominal hemorrhage is secondary to splenic injury.[22]

Hematopoietic Changes

Beyond the increase in plasma volume, other hematopoietic changes that gradually occur are summarized in **Table 3**.[18,21,23,24] These alterations make it challenging to detect hemorrhage and shock.

ANATOMY AND PHYSIOLOGY OF FETUS

Fetal O$_2$ requirements lead to increased blood flow to the uterus at the end of the third trimester. Uterine blood flow is directly proportional to maternal mean arterial

Table 3
Summary of hematopoietic differences in pregnancy

Laboratory Studies (Units)	Nonpregnant Women Range	Pregnant Women	
		Change	Range
Hemoglobin (g/dL)	12–15.8	↓	9–11
Hematocrit (%)	36–47	↓	31–35
White blood cell count ($\times 10^3/mm^3$)	3.5–9.1	↑	14–16[a]
Platelets ($\times 10^9/L$)	250[b]	↓	213[b]
Fibrinogen (mg/dL)	256[b]	↑	473[b]
Factor VII (%)	99.3[b]	↑	181.4[b]
Factor X (%)	97.7[b]	↑	144.5[b]

[a] Peak of 25 during labor.
[b] Mean value.

pressure, and inversely proportional to the resistance of the uterine vasculature.[20,22] This makes uteroplacental perfusion sensitive to decrease in maternal blood pressure during resuscitation and maternal hemorrhage.[25] The placenta creates a large, inelastic, and vascular conduit through which mother and fetus can exsanguinate during placental abruption without obvious external signs. In the event of uterine laceration or rupture, rapid maternal exsanguination with significant impact to the fetus can occur.[24] Fetal hemoglobin and relative acidemia compared with mother causes slight preservation of fetal oxygenation regardless of maternal Pa_{O_2} levels.[22] However, these factors are not fully protective during prolonged maternal hypoxia.[18,20,22]

MATERNAL TRAUMA RESUSCITATION

As with nonpregnant patients, the trauma evaluation of a pregnant patient starts with airway, breathing, and circulation. All women should be considered pregnant until proven otherwise, because it was found that 3% of women admitted to a trauma center were pregnant and of those, 11% were incidental findings.[28]

Primary Survey

Airway
Advanced airway intubation is an independent risk factor of trauma-related mortality in pregnant trauma patients, with an RR of 6.0.[1] Anatomic and physiologic changes make the pregnant airway more challenging with a greater risk of airway management problems than nonpregnant patients, with up to 1 in 250 failed intubations found in a surgical setting.[29] Pregnant women may have decreased ability to maintain a patent airway and sufficient ventilation, resulting in fetal distress. Maternal hyperventilation and alkalosis can reduce uterine blood flow via uterine vasoconstriction, also leading to fetal distress.[30] Airway edema, hyperemia, and landmark distortion can cause difficult visualization during laryngoscopy.[31]

It is reasonable to have a lower threshold for advanced airway management given the low maternal oxygen reserve and exaggerated fetal response to maternal hypoxia. Preoxygenation and apneic oxygenation is critical to prevent maternal and fetal hypoxia throughout the procedure.[32] Specific patient positioning beyond the sniffing position is essential to maintain preload from left uterine displacement either manually (**Fig. 2**) or with a wedge under the right hip to 30° to reduce aortocaval compression, if GA is 20 weeks.[33] Rapid sequence induction and anesthesia maintenance

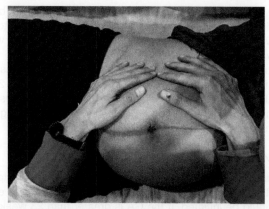

Fig. 2. Manual left uterine displacement. (*Courtesy of* Christie Sun, MD, La Jolla, CA.)

medications, such as volatile agents, depolarizing and nondepolarizing neuromuscular blockers, fentanyl, and morphine, are safe to administer during pregnancy.[33] Cricoid pressure should be used to decrease the risk of aspiration of gastric contents. Blind nasotracheal intubation is not advised because of engorgement and friability of nasal mucosa from increased estrogen.

The ED provider should have the following equipment on hand for intubation:[20]

- Adjunctive airway equipment, such as laryngeal mask airway and videolaryngoscope
- Smaller size endotracheal tube (6.0–6.5) and stylets
- Gum elastic bougie
- Short laryngoscope handles

The initial ventilator settings should be similar to nonpregnant women with goals of P_{CO_2} of 28 to 35 mm Hg and should avoid respiratory alkalosis to prevent decrease in uteroplacental flow.[20] Early nasogastric tube placement is warranted because of the increased risk of gastroesophageal reflux.[23,33]

Breathing

The physiologic changes to the pulmonary system cause a significantly reduced oxygen reserve. This impairs compensation during respiratory compromise, and can result in rapid development of maternal hypoxia.[22] In trauma, supplemental O_2 is indicated with pregnant women, with pulse oximetry goal of greater than 95% to maintain Pa_{O_2} greater than 70 mm Hg.[20,27] Physiologic changes in pregnancy also cause a lower Pa_{CO_2}.[26] Therefore, Pa_{CO_2} of 35 to 40 mm Hg may indicate inadequate ventilation and impending respiratory decompensation in a pregnant woman. Additionally, the superior displacement of the diaphragm should be considered before needle decompression or tube or catheter thoracostomy.[24]

Circulation

Access with two large-bore intravenous (IV) lines should be placed to facilitate rapid crystalloid infusion, volume expansion, and blood transfusions.[27] Femoral and lower extremity access should be avoided because of vascular congestion in the pelvis and lower extremities secondary to IVC compression by the uterus.[22] Patients who show signs of hypovolemia, such as tachycardia, hypotension, or abnormal fetal heart tracings, should receive IV fluid resuscitation. If the patient is thought to be hemorrhaging or in hemorrhagic shock, blood products should be administered instead of crystalloid. Active hemorrhage should be controlled with tourniquet, direct pressure, or pelvic binders. Massive transfusion protocol (MTP) with emergency release O-negative blood should be activated in shock.[27,34]

Proper positioning, as discussed previously, with left uterine displacement (see **Fig. 2**) is critical for maternal hypotension in patients greater than 20 weeks GA to improve maternal venous return and cardiac output.[35] Decompression is accomplished by either turning the patient into a left lateral position, placing a wedge under the right hip, or manual displacement (**Fig. 3**).[27]

Secondary Survey

The secondary survey follows the primary survey, and consists of history, physical examination, and ultrasound to identify maternal injuries. Concomitant evaluation of the fetal heart rate should be initiated. If the GA is greater than 23 weeks, external fetal monitoring (EFM) should be used to assess fetal heart tones (FHTs) and uterine contractions. If the GA is less than 23 weeks, or if EFM is unavailable, M-mode on bedside ultrasound is used to ensure viability and fetal heart rate (normal range is 120–160 beats per minute). Often abnormal fetal heart tracings or heart rates are the first signs of instability. For example, the first manifestation of maternal hypovolemic shock is often uteroplacental insufficiency causing decreased variability and possible late decelerations on FHT.[27,36] This finding may be missed if there is delay in obtaining FHT.

History
History should be obtained regarding mechanism and severity of injury. Additional questions include presence of vaginal bleeding, leakage of fluid, contractions, and fetal movement especially if the fetus is viable and GA greater than 23 weeks. Further

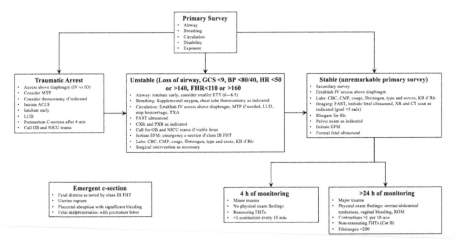

Fig. 3. Proposed algorithm for management of trauma in patients greater than 23 weeks GA. If less than 23 GA, consider focusing all resuscitation efforts on mother. ACLS, advanced cardiac life support; BP, blood pressure; CBC, complete blood count; CMP, complete metabolic panel; CT, computed tomography; CXR, chest radiograph; EFM, external fetal monitoring; ETT, endotracheal tube; FAST, focused assessment with sonography for trauma; FHR, fetal heart rate; FHT, fetal heart tole; GCS, glasgow coma score; HR, heart rate; IO, intra-osseous; KB, Kleihauer-Betke; LUD, lateral uterine displacement; NICU, neonatal intensive care unit; OB, obstetric; PXR, pelvic xray; Rh, rhesus factor; ROM, rupture of membranes; TXA, tranexamic acid; XR, xray.

obstetric history should be acquired including estimated delivery date, and complications affecting current pregnancy, such as diagnosis of preeclampsia, gestational diabetes, placenta previa, and oligohydramnios.

Physical examination

Physical examination of the pregnant trauma patient is similar to the nonpregnant patient and involves full exposure and thorough inspection and palpation of the entire body.[35] Key differences include physiologic vital sign alterations, abdominal examination, gravid uterus, pelvic examination, and fetal evaluation.[37] The abdominal examination can be unreliable in the pregnant patient because of gravid uterus and may mask peritonitis or an acute abdomen.[38] Abdominal contents are displaced superiorly, and penetrating injuries as high as the tip of the scapula posteriorly or the fourth intercostal space anteriorly may involve intra-abdominal organs. Bruising or ecchymosis of the abdomen or persistent pain on examination may indicate visceral injury.[27,39] Uterine tenderness is a sign of rupture or placental abruption.[40]

Pelvic examination

In the pregnant patient with GA greater than 23 weeks, it is important to evaluate for vaginal bleeding or leakage of fluid. The differential for vaginal bleeding includes placental previa, vasa previa, placental abruption, bloody show from cervical dilation with preterm labor, or uterine rupture. External physical examination may suffice if there is no vaginal bleeding, leakage of fluid, uterine tenderness, or contractions present. If there is concern, sterile speculum and digital examination should be performed to identify cause of bleeding, presence of tissue, cervical dilation and effacement, and fetal station. Ultrasound should be performed before examination to rule-out placenta previa. If there is concern for rupture of membranes, sterile speculum examination should be performed to assess for vaginal pooling of amniotic fluid or leakage of fluid from the cervical os.[41] Defer digital examination if high concern for preterm rupture of membranes to reduce infection risk. Ideally these examinations are performed in conjunction with obstetrics.

Bedside ultrasound

Bedside ultrasound is an important part of the secondary survey. Focused assessment with sonography for trauma (FAST) examination is pertinent in the hemodynamically unstable patient to exclude intra-abdominal hemorrhage. In three small studies, the sensitivity and specificity of FAST for detecting intra-abdominal hemorrhage were similar to nonpregnant patients at 80% to 85% and 98% to 100%, respectively.[42–44] One study had a lower sensitivity of 61%.[45] FAST should not be used to exclude intra-abdominal hemorrhage, but may save radiation and time in the setting of positive findings. If the patient is hemodynamically unstable and FAST positive, exploratory laparotomy should be performed. If the patient is stable with a positive FAST, computed tomography (CT) scan may still be necessary to determine whether intra-abdominal injury necessitates emergency surgery. Once the patient is stabilized, formal obstetric ultrasound is obtained.

Laboratory Tests

In general, indicated laboratory tests are similar to the nonpregnant patient. Physiologic changes in normal range for pregnant patients include leukocytosis, anemia, decreased creatinine, and increased clotting markers including fibrinogen and D dimer.[46] In addition to standard trauma laboratory studies, consider obtaining a type and screen, coagulation profile, fibrinogen, and Kleihauer-Betke (KB) test.

Type and screen

It is important to determine Rhesus factor (Rh) status because Rh-negative patients may develop alloimmunization if the fetus is Rh positive, which may lead to hemolytic disease of the fetus and newborn. This process can happen at 4 weeks in pregnancy.[47]

Kleihauer-Betke

Fetal-maternal hemorrhage can occur in up to 30% of pregnant patients.[48] The KB test uses a blood smear to quantify the amount of fetal hemoglobin in the maternal circulation. Because many fetal-maternal hemorrhage are subclinical, the American College of Obstetricians and Gynecologists (ACOG) guidelines advocate for KB testing in all pregnant trauma patients who are Rh negative because of concern for alloimmunization, which can happen at 4 weeks in pregnancy.[47] The KB test helps to correctly dose Rh immunoglobulin.[27,47,49,50]

Imaging Studies

Radiology plays an important role in trauma resuscitations, and it is no different in the pregnant trauma patient. Practitioners may grapple with this because of the perceived fetal risk of teratogenicity and carcinogenesis. In general, imaging should be performed as clinically indicated regardless of pregnancy status, including studies with ionizing radiation, especially in settings of maternal instability.

Per ACOG, Society of Obstetricians and Gynecologists of Canada, and Eastern Association of the Surgery of Trauma (EAST), radiation less than 5 rad (50 mGy) poses little to no risk of teratogenicity or fetal loss. Imaging is generally well below this threshold.[27,49,51,52] The fetus is at highest risk of teratogenicity at less than 12 weeks.[51] If necessary radiation exceeds 5 rad, discussing the risks and benefits of imaging studies and shared decision making with the patient should be done. Conflicting studies exist whether or not fetal exposure to ionized radiation is associated with carcinogenesis.[52–56]

Table 4 lists fetal radiation dose per imaging study. Strategies should be used to limit the amount of fetal radiation exposure when feasible, such as using lead protection over the gravid abdomen, selecting alternative protocols, and imaging with less radiation when it is feasible without compromising resuscitation.

Table 4 Fetal radiation doses of common trauma imaging	
Imaging Study	Fetal Dose (mGy)
Head or neck CT	0.001–0.01
Radiography of any extremity	<0.001
Chest radiography (two views)	0.0005–0.01
Abdominal/pelvic radiography	0.1–3.0
Chest CT	0.01–0.66
Lumbar spine radiography	1.0–10
Abdominal CT	1.3–35
Pelvic CT	10–50

Abbreviation: CT, computed tomography.
Adapted from Committee on Obstetric Practice. Committee opinion no. 723: guidelines for diagnostic imaging during pregnancy and lactation. Obstet Gynecol 2017;130(4):e210–6.

Ultrasound

Ultrasound is generally safe and is easily repeated without harm if the clinical situation requires it. Although B-mode and M-mode are generally safe, there is a theoretic risk of increasing temperature with higher intensity ultrasound transduction through Doppler, use of which should be minimized or reserved only for obstetric ultrasounds.[51,57]

Radiographs

Radiographs of the chest, extremities, and spine generally expose the fetus to low levels of radiation and should be performed as indicated. Pelvic radiograph has a higher dose of radiation (up to 0.3 rad or 3 mGy). The treating physician may consider foregoing pelvic radiograph if abdominal and pelvic CT or MRI will be obtained.[51] Radiation exposure during image acquisition is reduced through such techniques as fluoroscopy, use of mini C-arm, strategic shielding of the fetus, and real-time dosimetry.[58,59]

Computed tomography

CT scans of the head, neck, and chest expose the fetus to low to moderate levels of radiation. CT of the abdomen and pelvis has a higher dose of radiation (up to 5 rad or 50 mGy) and but should be obtained if there is concern for intra-abdominal injury. Ultimately, given the potential risk of tetratogenesis and carcinogenesis, albeit low, radiation exposure should be limited to as low as reasonably possible, without compromising maternal resuscitation.[27,49,51] Iodinated contrast is generally safe in pregnancy and is considered a category B drug by the Food and Drug Administration (FDA).[51,60]

Magnetic resonance imaging

ACOG recommends no special considerations or restrictions for MRI in pregnant patients, whereas the 2010 EAST guidelines do not recommend MRI in the first trimester of pregnancy.[49,51] Gadolinium is no longer recommended in pregnant patients because there is increased risk in inflammatory skin conditions, stillbirth, and neonatal death.[51,61] In the setting of a stable patient with a low suspicion of injury, MRI may be a reasonable alternative to CT scan.[51,60] MRI may also be a superior method of imaging for follow-up studies to avoid additional radiation exposure. However, MRI should not be the initial diagnostic imaging choice if there is high suspicion for injury or instability.[60]

Treatment of Shock

Critical interventions, such as intubation, chest tube thoracostomy, venous access, and IV fluid administration, should all be performed as indicated with appropriate modifications for the pregnant patient. Shock, usually from life-threatening hemorrhage, is critically important to recognize and treat. The end goal should be balanced resuscitation, because overresuscitation with fluids can lead to pulmonary edema and worsened hemorrhage.[62,63] However, permissive hypotension as advocated by current trauma guidelines may be detrimental to fetal well-being, therefore resuscitation strategies should include real-time fetal heart tracing in reassessments and determining next steps in resuscitation.[27] Abnormal FHT can be the first sign of significant maternal hemorrhage.

Hemorrhage control

Controlling hemorrhage is an important part of managing shock. Tourniquets should be placed for exsanguinating extremities, pelvic binders for open book pelvic fractures, and pressure should be placed on bleeding lacerations. If there are signs of intra-abdominal fluid on FAST in the setting of shock, emergent surgical intervention may be necessary.[49]

Massive transfusion protocol

Blood and blood products should be administered to all pregnant patients with hemorrhage and hemodynamic instability or signs of fetal distress. O-negative blood should be used as emergency release if cross-matched blood is not available.[27] MTP should be activated if necessary as per trauma guidelines in a 1:1:1 ratio of packed red blood cells to fresh frozen plasma (FFP) to platelets.[64] Most guidelines on obstetric hemorrhage are based on postpartum hemorrhage and also recommend similar 1:1:1 MTPs.[65–67]

Coagulopathy

FFP, platelets, and cryoprecipitate and fibrinogen are administered if there are signs of coagulopathy. If elevated international normalized ratio is persistent, it may be reasonable to give additional FFP (2–4 units) with a goal international normalized ratio less than 1.5.[67] FFP has an FDA category C rating. Prothrombin complex concentrate is also used to reverse coagulopathy.[68] Platelets may be transfused for goal platelet count greater than 50×10^9/L.[63,68] If fibrinogen is less than 2 g/L in the setting of life-threatening hemorrhage, fibrinogen (1–2 g) or cryoprecipitate (10 units) may be given.[63,66,68] No data exist on the safety of prothrombin complex concentrate, fibrinogen, or cryoprecipitate in pregnancy, but these products should be administered if life-threatening hemorrhage is present with evidence of coagulopathy.

Tranexamic acid

There are no studies evaluating tranexamic acid in the pregnant trauma patient, but it has been shown to reduce mortality in nonpregnant trauma and postpartum hemorrhage patients without increased incidence of venous thromboembolic events.[69,70] Therefore, it is reasonable to give tranexamic acid in the pregnant trauma patient with significant hemorrhage. Tranexamic acid is a category B medication per the FDA.

Vasopressors

In general, traumatic patients are hypotensive because of hypovolemia and hemorrhage and should be treated with volume rather than vasopressors initially. Vasopressors may also cause uteroplacental insufficiency because of effect on uterine tone and vasculature.[27] During cardiac arrest vasopressors should be used per advanced cardiac life support (ACLS) guidelines.[62,71] In specific situations, such as peri-intubation hypotension, it may be reasonable to use phenylephrine for vasoconstriction because this has been shown to be safe in pregnant patients experiencing hypotension from spinal epidural anesthesia.[72]

Other Interventions

Tocolytics/β-methasone

If the fetus is viable with GA greater than 23 weeks but less than 34 weeks, and the patient is in early preterm labor with cervical change, consider using tocolytics. Contraindications to tocolysis in the trauma patient include nonreassuring FHT and hemodynamically instability. Options include betamimetics (terbutaline), magnesium sulfate, or calcium antagonist (nifedipine).[73] If GA is greater than 24 weeks but less than 37 weeks, also consider the use of β-methasone to help with fetal lung maturity.[74,75]

Rhogam

Prophylactic Rho(D) immunoglobulin (Rhogam) should be given to all Rh-negative pregnant trauma patients within 72 hours.[27,47,49] One dose (300 mg) covers 30 mL of fetal blood.[27,47,76] If KB test estimates fetal blood within maternal to be greater than 30 mL, additional Rhogam doses should be given.[27]

Traumatic Arrest

In the event of traumatic arrest, ACLS should be initiated with primary focus on securing the airway, administering adequate oxygenation and ventilation, obtaining sufficient IV access with large-bore catheters above the diaphragm, and providing circulation with chest compressions and left uterine displacement, as well as balanced resuscitation with blood products.[62] If available, trauma, obstetric, anesthesia, and neonatal teams should arrive immediately to the bedside to aid in resuscitation.[77] Equipment for perimortem cesarean delivery (PMCD), thoracotomy, and other resuscitative interventions should immediately be brought to the bedside as indicated.

The focus of resuscitation should be on identifying and treating the underlying cause of traumatic arrest, such as hypovolemia or hemorrhage; tension pneumothorax; cardiac tamponade; hypoxia; or medical etiologies that may have occurred, such as seizure. Indications for thoracotomy should remain similar to the nonpregnant patient given the paucity of data in the pregnant patient.[62,78] Defibrillation, epinephrine, and other ACLS drugs should be administered without altering the dose, timing, or joules.[71,77,79]

Perimortem cesarean delivery

If maternal resuscitation is unsuccessful, the American Heart Association, ACOG, and EAST guidelines recommend emergency PMCD.[27,49,77,79,80] Indications for this procedure include[79,81–84]:

- Unsuccessful maternal resuscitation after 4 minutes
- GA at or greater than 23 weeks or fundal height above umbilicus

A case series by Katz and colleagues[81] identified 38 PMCDs in the setting of maternal cardiac arrest, eight involving trauma. Thirty of the 38 procedures resulted in the delivery of a viable infant, with 7 out of 38 involving fetus delivery greater than 15 minutes from maternal cardiac arrest. Twelve out of 20 cardiac arrests achieved return of spontaneous circulation after PMCD, although none involved traumatic arrest.[81]

FETAL EVALUATION AND RESUSCITATION

It is important to evaluate fetal well-being in parallel with maternal resuscitation, but not at the expense of maternal resuscitation. Strategies to evaluate the fetus include ultrasound, FHT, tocometry, and early involvement of obstetrics. If the fetus is previable, interventions are limited and resuscitation should focus on the mother.[27] In cases of viability, it is important to quickly assess FHTs for signs of distress. Emergency delivery or intervention is indicated in the setting of such injuries as placental abruption, uterine rupture, and maternal hemorrhage.[27] Fetal mortality in the setting of trauma is 61% in major trauma, and between 1.3% and 19% in all trauma based on other cohort studies.[39,85–87]

Ultrasound

Early involvement of obstetrics can allow for ultrasound evaluation beyond beside ultrasound to examine the fetus, placenta, amniotic fluid, and fetal position.[27] Signs of placental abruption may be identified through ultrasound in the hands of an experienced user, although ultrasound is not sensitive for this diagnosis.[6,42,88,89]

Fetal Heart Monitoring and Tocometry

It is important to obtain FHTs and tocometry early and continuously in pregnant trauma patients. All pregnant trauma patients with GA 20 weeks should have minimum of 6 hours EFM observation, and longer if clinically warranted.[49] This provides surrogate information for fetal well-being, fetal acid-base status, and fetal perfusion.[90] Maternal hemorrhage, fetal hemorrhage, fetal hypoxia, placental abruption, and uterine rupture should be considered if FHTs shows signs of fetal distress.[27,87] In the setting of extreme fetal distress, urgent or emergent cesarean should be considered in consultation with neonatology and obstetrics.[27,36] Interventions for nonreassuring FHTs include continuing maternal resuscitation, supplemental oxygen, and left lateral decubitus positioning.[27] Tocometry is the external monitoring of maternal uterine contractions and should take place concurrently with fetal heart monitoring with GA greater than 23 weeks. In the case of contractions causing intense pain and regular contractions less than 10 minutes apart, consider placental abruption or preterm labor.[6,27]

Duration of External Fetal Monitoring

The duration of fetal monitoring is a topic of controversy. Studies have failed to observe reliable predictable factors for fetal demise, preterm delivery, or adverse outcome.[6,91] EAST guidelines suggest a minimum of 6 hours, ACOG guidelines do not give specific time but suggest a minimum of 6 hours.[49,80] Society of Obstetricians and Gynecologists of Canada recommends 4 hours if normal FHT and physical examination, but prolonged monitoring (24 hours) if there are any of the following present: uterine or abdominal tenderness, vaginal bleeding, contraction frequency of more than once per 10 minutes, rupture of membranes, nonreassuring FHTs, serum fibrinogen less than 200 g/L, and high-risk mechanism.[27]

Indications for Emergency Cesarean Section

Indications for emergency cesarean section in the operating room are determined with the consulting obstetrician. Obstetrics should immediately be consulted if there are signs of maternal instability, uteroplacental compromise, and decreased fetal well-being.[27,36] During traumatic cardiac arrest, PMCD should be initiated at 4 minutes and performed at the bedside without delay.

OBSTETRIC PATHOLOGY
Placental Abruption

Placental abruption is the leading cause of fetal death following blunt trauma.[49] A study involving 372 pregnant trauma patients (84% blunt, 16% penetrating) in the third trimester showed placental abruption as the most common complication at 3.5% with 54% mortality. Other studies have indicated a placental abruption rate between 5% and 50%.[89] The time course of presentation is usually delayed between 2 and 6 hours from initial trauma, up to 24 hours. Concerning symptoms include nonreassuring FHTs, vaginal bleeding, uterine tenderness, and contractions. Severe placental abruption can result in hemorrhagic shock and signs of disseminated intravascular coagulation.[49] Although the diagnosis is primarily clinical, CT scan and ultrasound may aid in decision making.[6,27,42,88,89,92–94] Immediate obstetric consultation should take place if there are any signs of placental abruption.

Uterine Injury

Uterine injuries in trauma include uterine contractions, serosal hemorrhage, abrasions, and complete uterine rupture.[27] Uterine contractions are the most common complication associated with maternal trauma.[18] Uterine rupture is rare with an incidence of approximately 0.7% and should be suspected in the setting of direct abdominal injury.[27,58,95]

Signs or symptoms of severe uterine injury and uterine rupture include peritoneal abdominal examination, maternal hemodynamic instability, irregular uterine contractions, palpable fetal parts, and sudden abnormal fetal heart rate pattern.[27] A FAST ultrasound examination will likely show free fluid in the abdomen in uterine rupture.[58] Unfortunately, fetal mortality with traumatic uterine rupture is almost universal. Early recognition is key with obstetric consultation for laparotomy to control hemorrhage, repair the uterus, and evaluate for fetal viability.[27]

Preterm Labor

Evaluation for preterm labor should be done in every injured pregnant patient. There is an associated higher risk of preterm delivery after trauma (RR, 2), increasing with injury severity and earlier GA.[96] Placental abruption may result in preterm labor in up to 20% of cases.[97] EFM should be used to monitor for any contractions, frequency, and regularity of contractions. If preterm labor is suspected and the patient is stable, transfer should be initiated to obstetric services is appropriate for further evaluation.

SPECIFIC MATERNAL INJURIES
Motor Vehicle Accidents

The overall incidence of MVAs during pregnancy has been estimated at 207 cases per 100,000 live births, and is the most common cause of traumatic injury.[85] The presence of illicit drugs or alcohol is significant with pregnancy-related traumas (19.6% and 12.9%, respectively), and is found present in up to 45% of pregnant women involved in MVAs.[4] Pregnant women involved in MVAs are also unrestrained up to 79% of the time. Not wearing a seatbelt is associated with more severe injuries, higher frequency of surgical interventions, and adverse fetal outcome.[98] Seatbelt placement also is an issue with nearly 50% of fetal losses associated with improper strap placement.[99] Seatbelts should be worn below the abdomen, touching the against thighs.[99] Airbag deployment has not been found to significantly increase likelihood of placental abruption or fetal loss.[13]

Up to 89% of pregnant women who are involved in MVAs can present with maternal or fetal complications requiring medical care, with most admissions occurring at greater than 20 weeks GA.[100] Among severely injured women in MVAs, placental abruption can occur in up to 40% of cases with maternal mortality rate of 13.7%.[13,86] However, even nonseverely injured pregnant women have an increased risk of preterm labor, placental abruption, and cesarean delivery.[7] Even minor accidents can create enough force to distort the uterine wall causing the placenta to shear leading to abruption.[6] The fetal mortality rate secondary to MVAs overall has been found to be 10.7%,[13] with an estimated 1300 to 3900 fetal losses per year in the United States secondary to MVAs.[101]

Falls

Falls are the second most common cause of blunt trauma in pregnant women, with an incidence of 48.9 cases per 100,000 live births.[102] Approximately one in four pregnant women fall at least once in pregnancy.[15] Falls are most common in the second and third trimesters,[102] likely caused by anatomic changes occurring in pregnancy leading to a predisposition to falls.[103] Most falls occur from standing height and indoors, with 39% involving stairs.[15,102] Adverse events associated with falling include increase in rates of preterm labor (RR, 4.4), placental abruption (RR, 8), fetal distress (RR, 2.1), fetal hypoxia (RR, 2.9), and stillbirth (RR, 2).[102]

Penetrating Injuries

Penetrating trauma including GSWs in pregnancy is uncommon and incidence is estimated at 3.3 cases per 100,000 live births.[14,16,17,104] Maternal mortality is not significantly different in penetrating trauma mechanisms as compared with blunt; however, there are significant increases in maternal morbidity (66% vs 10%, respectively).[14] Common maternal complications include uterine injury and ileus.[14] Direct fetal injury and mortality in the third trimester is more common with penetrating trauma especially GSWs (up to 70%).[13,34,105]

Domestic Violence

DV or intimate partner violence is the most common form of intentional trauma, with up to 20.1% of women reporting physical or sexual abuse while pregnant.[106,107] The incidence of DV is estimated to be at 8307 cases per 100,000 live births.[108] Most often the domestic partner is identified as the aggressor in DV cases.[107] Risk factors for DV include substance abuse (maternal or partner), unintended pregnancy, history of DV before pregnancy, and unmarried status.[109,110] Adverse outcomes associated with DV include increased risk for spontaneous abortion and preterm birth (1.7), and increased risk for low birth weight, fetal distress, and fetal death (RR, 2).[109] The risk of fetal death has been found to be directly and significantly correlated to severity of maternal injuries.[111] At times, victims may present with a plausible story of injury and therefore DV may be overlooked, making it imperative to screen all pregnant trauma patients.

Burns

Burn injuries in pregnancy are rare, estimated at 0.17 cases per 100,000 live births.[112] Multiple studies have shown the overall maternal and fetal mortality to be high (up to 66%) regardless of total body surface area involved or GA.[113,114] Maternal and fetal mortality rates approach 100% if total body surface area exceeds 55%.[112,113,115] Therefore, urgent obstetric consultation for cesarean delivery is recommended in cases with total body surface area burn greater than 55%.[115] Burns during the first trimester have also been associated with spontaneous abortions,[116] which typically occur within 10 days after the burn.[117] Inhalation injury may also occur with burns making an already difficult airway even more challenging.[58] Co-oximetry and cyanide toxicity should also be considered because carbon monoxide and cyanide can transfer to the fetus.[58,115,116] Treatment is similar to nonpregnant patients with oxygen and hydrocobalamine.[58,112,115]

DISPOSITION

After stabilization, disposition from the ED is generally to labor and delivery for extended monitoring. If labor and delivery is not present at the hospital of the treating ED, transfer for higher level of care is warranted especially if there are signs of fetal distress or abnormalities on maternal physical examination.

Stable patients may be discharged following an appropriate period of observation. This includes at least 4 to 6 hours of observation for low-risk patients with normal physical examination and reassuring FHT, and at least 24 hours for high-risk patients with abnormal physical examination, frequent contractions, or any signs of nonreassuring FHT. Patient should have close obstetric follow-up and strict return precautions including decreased fetal movement, vaginal bleeding, contractions, rupture of membranes, and severe pain.[27]

SUMMARY

The resuscitation and management of pregnant trauma patients is difficult because the provider must consider maternal physiologic changes during pregnancy; fetal well-being; and unique pathologies, such as placental abruption and preterm labor. Prioritization of maternal resuscitation is critical to ensure optimal outcome for the mother and fetus. Trauma in pregnancy, a rare event, also requires close communication and teamwork with multiple specialties.

REFERENCES

1. Deshpande NA, Kucirka LM, Smith RN, et al. Pregnant trauma victims experience nearly 2-fold higher mortality compared to their nonpregnant counterparts. Am J Obstet Gynecol 2017;217(5):590.e1-9.
2. El-Kady D, Gilbert WM, Anderson J, et al. Trauma during pregnancy: an analysis of maternal and fetal outcomes in a large population. Am J Obstet Gynecol 2004;190(6):1661-8.
3. Hill CC, Pickinpaugh J. Trauma and surgical emergencies in the obstetric patient. Surg Clin North Am 2008;88(2):421-40, viii.
4. Ikossi DG, Lazar AA, Morabito D, et al. Profile of mothers at risk: an analysis of injury and pregnancy loss in 1,195 trauma patients. J Am Coll Surg 2005;200(1): 49-56.
5. Pak LL, Reece EA, Chan L. Is adverse pregnancy outcome predictable after blunt abdominal trauma? Am J Obstet Gynecol 1998;179(5):1140-4.
6. Pearlman MD, Tintinallli JE, Lorenz RP. A prospective controlled study of outcome after trauma during pregnancy. Am J Obstet Gynecol 1990;162(6): 1502-7 [discussion: 1507-10].
7. Schiff MA, Holt VL. Pregnancy outcomes following hospitalization for motor vehicle crashes in Washington State from 1989 to 2001. Am J Epidemiol 2005;161(6):503-10.
8. Schiff MA, Holt VL, Daling JR. Maternal and infant outcomes after injury during pregnancy in Washington State from 1989 to 1997. J Trauma 2002;53(5):939-45.
9. Mattox KL, Goetzl L. Trauma in pregnancy. Crit Care Med 2005;33(10 Suppl): S385-9.
10. Senkowski CK, McKenney MG. Trauma scoring systems: a review. J Am Coll Surg 1999;189(5):491-503.
11. Copes WS, Champion HR, Sacco WJ, et al. The injury severity score revisited. J Trauma 1988;28(1):69-77.
12. El Kady D, Gilbert WM, Xing G, et al. Association of maternal fractures with adverse perinatal outcomes. Am J Obstet Gynecol 2006;195(3):711-6.
13. Petrone P, Jimenez-Morillas P, Axelrad A, et al. Traumatic injuries to the pregnant patient: a critical literature review. Eur J Trauma Emerg Surg 2017. [Epub ahead of print].
14. Petrone P, Talving P, Browder T, et al. Abdominal injuries in pregnancy: a 155-month study at two level 1 trauma centers. Injury 2011;42(1):47-9.
15. Dunning K, LeMasters G, Bhattacharya A. A major public health issue: the high incidence of falls during pregnancy. Matern Child Health J 2010;14(5):720-5.

16. Wall SL, Figueiredo F, Laing GL, et al. The spectrum and outcome of pregnant trauma patients in a metropolitan trauma service in South Africa. Injury 2014; 45(8):1220–3.
17. Zangene M, Ebrahimi B, Najafi F. Trauma in pregnancy and its consequences in Kermanshah, Iran from 2007 to 2010. Glob J Health Sci 2014;7(2):304–9.
18. Walls RM, Hockberger RS, Gausche-Hill M. Rosen's emergency medicine: concepts and clinical practice. 9th edition. Philadelphia: Elsevier; 2018.
19. Bardsley CEH. Chapter 103. Normal pregnancy. In: Tintinalli JE, Stapczynski JS, Ma OJ, et al, editors. Tintinalli's emergency medicine: a comprehensive study guide, 7e. New York: The McGraw-Hill Companies; 2011.
20. Burns B. Resuscitation in pregnancy. In: Tintinalli JE, Stapczynski JS, Ma OJ, et al, editors. Tintinalli's emergency medicine: a comprehensive study guide, 8e. New York: McGraw-Hill Education; 2016.
21. Cunningham FG, Leveno KJ, Bloom SL, et al. Maternal physiology. In: Williams obstetrics, 24e. New York: McGraw-Hill Education; 2013.
22. Delorio NM. Trauma in pregnancy. In: Tintinalli JE, editor. Tintinalli's emergency medicine: a comprehensive study guide, 8e. New York: McGraw-Hill Education; 2016.
23. Brown S, Mozurkewich E. Trauma during pregnancy. Obstet Gynecol Clin North Am 2013;40(1):47–57.
24. Petrone P, Marini CP. Trauma in pregnant patients. Curr Probl Surg 2015;52(8): 330–51.
25. Hill CC, Pickinpaugh J. Physiologic changes in pregnancy. Surg Clin North Am 2008;88(2):391–401, vii.
26. Yeomans ER, Gilstrap LC 3rd. Physiologic changes in pregnancy and their impact on critical care. Crit Care Med 2005;33(10 Suppl):S256–8.
27. Jain V, Chari R, Maslovitz S, et al. Guidelines for the management of a pregnant trauma patient. J Obstet Gynaecol Can 2015;37(6):553–71.
28. Bochicchio GV, Napolitano LM, Haan J, et al. Incidental pregnancy in trauma patients. J Am Coll Surg 2001;192(5):566–9.
29. Barnardo PD, Jenkins JG. Failed tracheal intubation in obstetrics: a 6-year review in a UK region. Anaesthesia 2000;55(7):690–4.
30. Meroz Y, Elchalal U, Ginosar Y. Initial trauma management in advanced pregnancy. Anesthesiol Clin 2007;25(1):117–29, x.
31. McKeen DM, George RB, O'Connell CM, et al. Difficult and failed intubation: incident rates and maternal, obstetrical, and anesthetic predictors. Can J Anaesth 2011;58(6):514–24.
32. Weingart SD, Levitan RM. Preoxygenation and prevention of desaturation during emergency airway management. Ann Emerg Med 2012;59(3):165–75.e1.
33. Moaveni DM, Varon AJ. Anesthetic management of the pregnant trauma patient. In: Varon AJ, Smith CE, editors. Essentials of trauma anesthesia. 2nd edition. Cambridge (United Kingdom): Cambridge University Press; 2017. p. 304–16.
34. Shah KH, Simons RK, Holbrook T, et al. Trauma in pregnancy: maternal and fetal outcomes. J Trauma 1998;45(1):83–6.
35. ATLS Subcommittee, American College of Surgeons' Committee on Trauma, International ATLS working group. Advanced trauma life support (ATLS(R)): the ninth edition. J Trauma Acute Care Surg 2013;74(5):1363–6.
36. Morris JA Jr, Rosenbower TJ, Jurkovich GJ, et al. Infant survival after cesarean section for trauma. Ann Surg 1996;223(5):481–8 [discussion: 488–91].
37. Smith KA, Bryce S. Trauma in the pregnant patient: an evidence-based approach to management. Emerg Med Pract 2013;15(4):1–18 [quiz: 18–9].

38. Cappell MS, Friedel D. Abdominal pain during pregnancy. Gastroenterol Clin North Am 2003;32(1):1–58.
39. Rothenberger D, Quattlebaum FW, Perry JF Jr, et al. Blunt maternal trauma: a review of 103 cases. J Trauma 1978;18(3):173–9.
40. Neilson JP. Interventions for treating placental abruption. Cochrane Database Syst Rev 2003;(1):CD003247.
41. Lee SE, Park JS, Norwitz ER, et al. Measurement of placental alpha-microglobulin-1 in cervicovaginal discharge to diagnose rupture of membranes. Obstet Gynecol 2007;109(3):634–40.
42. Goodwin H, Holmes JF, Wisner DH. Abdominal ultrasound examination in pregnant blunt trauma patients. J Trauma 2001;50(4):689–93 [discussion: 694].
43. Brown MA, Sirlin CB, Farahmand N, et al. Screening sonography in pregnant patients with blunt abdominal trauma. J Ultrasound Med 2005;24(2):175–81 [quiz: 183–4].
44. Meisinger QC, Brown MA, Dehqanzada ZA, et al. A 10-year retrospective evaluation of ultrasound in pregnant abdominal trauma patients. Emerg Radiol 2016; 23(2):105–9.
45. Richards JR, Ormsby EL, Romo MV, et al. Blunt abdominal injury in the pregnant patient: detection with US. Radiology 2004;233(2):463–70.
46. Hellgren M, Blomback M. Studies on blood coagulation and fibrinolysis in pregnancy, during delivery and in the puerperium. I. Normal condition. Gynecol Obstet Invest 1981;12(3):141–54.
47. Practice bulletin no. 181 summary: prevention of Rh D alloimmunization. Obstet Gynecol 2017;130(2):481–3.
48. Rose PG, Strohm PL, Zuspan FP. Fetomaternal hemorrhage following trauma. Am J Obstet Gynecol 1985;153(8):844–7.
49. Barraco RD, Chiu WC, Clancy TV, et al. Practice management guidelines for the diagnosis and management of injury in the pregnant patient: the EAST practice management guidelines work group. J Trauma 2010;69(1):211–4.
50. Cunningham FG, Leveno KJ, Bloom SL, et al. Williams obstetrics. 24th edition. New York: McGraw-Hill Education; 2014. Available at: https://getitatduke.library. duke.edu/?sid=sersol&SS_jc=TC0001481193&title=Williams%20obstetrics%20 study%20guide.
51. Committee on Obstetric Practice. Committee opinion no. 723: guidelines for diagnostic imaging during pregnancy and lactation. Obstet Gynecol 2017; 130(4):e210–6.
52. Gjelsteen AC, Ching BH, Meyermann MW, et al. CT, MRI, PET, PET/CT, and ultrasound in the evaluation of obstetric and gynecologic patients. Surg Clin North Am 2008;88(2):361–90, vii.
53. Donnelly EH, Smith JM, Farfan EB, et al. Prenatal radiation exposure: background material for counseling pregnant patients following exposure to radiation. Disaster Med Public Health Prep 2011;5(1):62–8.
54. Ray JG, Schull MJ, Urquia ML, et al. Major radiodiagnostic imaging in pregnancy and the risk of childhood malignancy: a population-based cohort study in Ontario. PLoS Med 2010;7(9):e1000337.
55. Lowe SA. Diagnostic radiography in pregnancy: risks and reality. Aust N Z J Obstet Gynaecol 2004;44(3):191–6.
56. Doll R, Wakeford R. Risk of childhood cancer from fetal irradiation. Br J Radiol 1997;70:130–9.
57. American College of Obstetricians and Gynecologists. ACOG Practice Bulletin No. 101: ultrasonography in pregnancy. Obstet Gynecol 2009;113(2 Pt 1):451–61.

58. Huls CK, Detlefs C. Trauma in pregnancy. Semin Perinatol 2018;42(1):13–20.

59. Tejwani NKK, Looze C, Klifto CS. Treatment of pregnant patients with orthopaedic trauma. J Am Acad Orthop Surg 2017;25:e90–101.

60. Raptis CA, Mellnick VM, Raptis DA, et al. Imaging of trauma in the pregnant patient. Radiographics 2014;34(3):748–63.

61. Ray JG, Vermeulen MJ, Bharatha A, et al. Association between MRI exposure during pregnancy and fetal and childhood outcomes. JAMA 2016;316(9):952–61.

62. Part 10.7: cardiac arrest associated with trauma. Circulation 2005; 112(24_suppl). IV-146–IV-149. Available at: https://www.ahajournals.org/doi/pdf/10.1161/CIRCULATIONAHA.105.166569.

63. Cantle PM, Cotton BA. Balanced resuscitation in trauma management. Surg Clin North Am 2017;97(5):999–1014.

64. Spinella PC, Holcomb JB. Resuscitation and transfusion principles for traumatic hemorrhagic shock. Blood Rev 2009;23(6):231–40.

65. American College of Obstetricians and Gynecologists. ACOG practice bulletin: clinical management guidelines for obstetrician-gynecologists number 76, October 2006: postpartum hemorrhage. Obstet Gynecol 2006;108(4):1039–47.

66. Dacus JV, Dellinger EH, Keiser SD, et al. Preventing maternal death: 10 clinical diamonds. Obstet Gynecol 2012;120(1):179–80 [author reply: 180].

67. Butwick AJ, Goodnough LT. Transfusion and coagulation management in major obstetric hemorrhage. Curr Opin Anaesthesiol 2015;28(3):275–84.

68. Rossaint R, Bouillon B, Cerny V, et al. The European guideline on management of major bleeding and coagulopathy following trauma: fourth edition. Crit Care 2016;20:100.

69. Roberts I, Shakur H, Coats T, et al. The CRASH-2 trial: a randomised controlled trial and economic evaluation of the effects of tranexamic acid on death, vascular occlusive events and transfusion requirement in bleeding trauma patients. Health Technol Assess 2013;17(10):1–79.

70. Pacheco LD, Hankins GDV, Saad AF, et al. Tranexamic acid for the management of obstetric hemorrhage. Obstet Gynecol 2017;130(4):765–9.

71. Kikuchi J, Deering S. Cardiac arrest in pregnancy. Semin Perinatol 2018;42(1): 33–8.

72. Kee WDN. The use of vasopressors during spinal anaesthesia for caesarean section. Curr Opin Anaesthesiol 2017;30(3):319–25.

73. Haas DM, Benjamin T, Sawyer R, et al. Short-term tocolytics for preterm delivery: current perspectives. Int J Womens Health 2014;6:343–9.

74. American College of Obstetricians and Gynecologists' Committee on Practice Bulletins—Obstetrics. Practice bulletin no. 171: management of preterm labor. Obstet Gynecol 2016;128(4):e155–64.

75. Gyamfi-Bannerman C, Thom EA. Antenatal betamethasone for women at risk for late preterm delivery. N Engl J Med 2016;375(5):486–7.

76. American College of Emergency Physicians Clinical Policies Subcommittee on Early Pregnancy, Hahn SA, Promes SB, Brown MD. Clinical policy: critical issues in the initial evaluation and management of patients presenting to the emergency department in early pregnancy. Ann Emerg Med 2017;69(2):241–50.e20.

77. Hui D, Morrison LJ, Windrim R, et al. The American Heart Association 2010 guidelines for the management of cardiac arrest in pregnancy: consensus recommendations on implementation strategies. J Obstet Gynaecol Can 2011; 33(8):858–63.

78. Seamon MJ, Haut ER, Van Arendonk K, et al. An evidence-based approach to patient selection for emergency department thoracotomy: a practice

management guideline from the Eastern Association for the Surgery of Trauma. J Trauma Acute Care Surg 2015;79(1):159–73.

79. Jeejeebhoy FM, Zelop CM, Lipman S, et al. Cardiac arrest in pregnancy: a scientific statement from the American Heart Association. Circulation 2015; 132(18):1747–73.

80. Trauma during pregnancy. ACOG technical bulletin number 161–November 1991. Int J Gynaecol Obstet 1993;40(2):165–70.

81. Katz V, Balderston K, DeFreest M. Perimortem cesarean delivery: were our assumptions correct? Am J Obstet Gynecol 2005;192(6):1916–20 [discussion: 1920–1].

82. Katz VL. Perimortem cesarean delivery: its role in maternal mortality. Semin Perinatol 2012;36(1):68–72.

83. Katz VL, Dotters DJ, Droegemueller W. Perimortem cesarean delivery. Obstet Gynecol 1986;68(4):571–6.

84. Whitten M, Irvine LM. Postmortem and perimortem caesarean section: what are the indications? J R Soc Med 2000;93(1):6–9.

85. Kvarnstrand L, Milsom I, Lekander T, et al. Maternal fatalities, fetal and neonatal deaths related to motor vehicle crashes during pregnancy: a national population-based study. Acta Obstet Gynecol Scand 2008;87(9):946–52.

86. Ali J, Yeo A, Gana TJ, et al. Predictors of fetal mortality in pregnant trauma patients. J Trauma 1997;42(5):782–5.

87. Hoff WS, D'Amelio LF, Tinkoff GH, et al. Maternal predictors of fetal demise in trauma during pregnancy. Surg Gynecol Obstet 1991;172(3):175–80.

88. Dahmus MA, Sibai BM. Blunt abdominal trauma: are there any predictive factors for abruptio placentae or maternal-fetal distress? Am J Obstet Gynecol 1993; 169(4):1054–9.

89. Goodwin TM, Breen MT. Pregnancy outcome and fetomaternal hemorrhage after noncatastrophic trauma. Am J Obstet Gynecol 1990;162(3):665–71.

90. American College of Obstetricians and Gynecologists. ACOG Practice Bulletin No. 106: intrapartum fetal heart rate monitoring: nomenclature, interpretation, and general management principles. Obstet Gynecol 2009;114(1):192–202.

91. Weiner E, Gluck O, Levy M, et al. Obstetric and neonatal outcome following minor trauma in pregnancy. Is hospitalization warranted? Eur J Obstet Gynecol Reprod Biol 2016;203:78–81.

92. Shinde GR, Vaswani BP, Patange RP, et al. Diagnostic performance of ultrasonography for detection of abruption and its clinical correlation and maternal and foetal outcome. J Clin Diagn Res 2016;10(8):QC04–7.

93. Kopelman TR, Bogert JN, Walters JW, et al. Computed tomographic imaging interpretation improves fetal outcomes after maternal trauma. J Trauma Acute Care Surg 2016;81(6):1131–5.

94. Saphier NB, Kopelman TR. Traumatic Abruptio Placenta Scale (TAPS): a proposed grading system of computed tomography evaluation of placental abruption in the trauma patient. Emerg Radiol 2014;21(1):17–22.

95. EL Kady D, Gilbert WM, Xing G, et al. Maternal and neonatal outcomes of assaults during pregnancy. Obstet Gynecol 2005;105(2):357–63.

96. Sperry JL, Casey BM, McIntire DD, et al. Long-term fetal outcomes in pregnant trauma patients. Am J Surg 2006;192:715–21.

97. Wolf EJ, Mallozzi A, Rodis JF, et al. The principal pregnancy complications resulting in preterm birth in singleton and twin gestations. J Matern Fetal Med 1992;14: 2016–212.

98. Luley T, Fitzpatrick CB, Grotegut CA, et al. Perinatal implications of motor vehicle accident trauma during pregnancy: identifying populations at risk. Am J Obstet Gynecol 2013;208(6):466.e1-5.

99. Klinich KD, Flannagan CA, Rupp JD, et al. Fetal outcome in motor-vehicle crashes: effects of crash characteristics and maternal restraint. Am J Obstet Gynecol 2008;198(4):450.e1-9.

100. Vivian-Taylor J, Roberts CL, Chen JS, et al. Motor vehicle accidents during pregnancy: a population-based study. BJOG 2012;119(4):499–503.

101. Weiss HB, Lawrence B, Miller T. Prevalence and risk of hospitalized pregnant occupants in car crashes. Annu Proc Assoc Adv Automot Med 2002;46:355–66.

102. Schiff MA. Pregnancy outcomes following hospitalisation for a fall in Washington State from 1987 to 2004. BJOG 2008;115(13):1648–54.

103. McCrory JL, Chambers AJ, Daftary A, et al. Dynamic postural stability during advancing pregnancy. J Biomech 2010;43(12):2434–9.

104. Mendez-Figueroa H, Dahlke JD, Vrees RA, et al. Trauma in pregnancy: an updated systematic review. Am J Obstet Gynecol 2013;209(1):1–10.

105. Oxford CM, Ludmir J. Trauma in pregnancy. Clin Obstet Gynecol 2009;52(4):611–29.

106. Beydoun HA, Tamim H, Lincoln AM, et al. Association of physical violence by an intimate partner around the time of pregnancy with inadequate gestational weight gain. Soc Sci Med 2011;72(6):867–73.

107. Tinker SC, Reefhuis J, Dellinger AM, et al. Epidemiology of maternal injuries during pregnancy in a population-based study, 1997-2005. J Womens Health (Larchmt) 2010;19(12):2211–8.

108. Gazmararian JA, Petersen R, Spitz AM, et al. Violence and reproductive health: current knowledge and future research directions. Matern Child Health J 2000;4(2):79–84.

109. Meuleners LB, Lee AH, Janssen PA, et al. Maternal and foetal outcomes among pregnant women hospitalised due to interpersonal violence: a population based study in Western Australia, 2002-2008. BMC Pregnancy Childbirth 2011;11:70.

110. Quinlivan JA, Evans SF. A prospective cohort study of the impact of domestic violence on young teenage pregnancy outcomes. J Pediatr Adolesc Gynecol 2001;14(1):17–23.

111. Njoku OI, Joannes UO, Christian MC, et al. Trauma during pregnancy in a Nigerian setting: patterns of presentation and pregnancy outcome. Int J Crit Illn Inj Sci 2013;3(4):269–73.

112. Maghsoudi H, Samnia R, Garadaghi A, et al. Burns in pregnancy. Burns 2006;32(2):246–50.

113. Subrahmanyam M. Burns during pregnancy: effect on maternal and foetal outcomes. Ann Burns Fire Disasters 2006;19(4):177–9.

114. Rezavand N, Seyedzadeh A. Maternal and foetal outcome of burns during pregnancy in Kermanshah, Iran. Ann Burns Fire Disasters 2006;19(4):174–6.

115. Parikh P, Sunesara I, Lutz E, et al. Burns during pregnancy: implications for maternal-perinatal providers and guidelines for practice. Obstet Gynecol Surv 2015;70(10):633–43.

116. Jain M, Garg AK. Burns with pregnancy: a review of 25 cases. Burns 1993;19(2):166–7.

117. Chama CM, Na'Aya HU. Severe burn injury in pregnancy in Northern Nigeria. J Obstet Gynaecol 2002;22(1):20–2.

Cardiovascular Emergencies in Pregnancy

Joelle Borhart, MD[a,]*, Jessica Palmer, MD[b]

KEYWORDS

- Pregnancy • Deep vein thrombosis • Pulmonary embolism • D-dimer
- Aortic dissection • Myocardial infarction • Peripartum cardiomyopathy

KEY POINTS

- The physiologic changes of pregnancy place patients at increased risk for developing a cardiovascular emergency.
- Overall the management of cardiovascular emergencies in pregnant patients is similar to that of nonpregnant patients.
- The risk of venous thromboembolism is elevated at all stages of pregnancy and is highest in the first weeks postpartum.
- CT pulmonary angiography or ventilation/perfusion scan are both acceptable choices for diagnosing pulmonary embolism in pregnancy.
- When managing any critically ill pregnant patient, maternal well-being takes precedence because the best chance for fetal survival is maternal survival.

INTRODUCTION

Cardiovascular disease has overtaken all other causes of maternal death in the United States, accounting for 15.5% of pregnancy-related deaths between 2011 and 2013.[1] The physiologic changes of pregnancy place a significant amount of stress on the cardiovascular system and put pregnant women at risk for potentially catastrophic complications, such as pulmonary embolism (PE), aortic or coronary artery dissection, acute myocardial infarction (AMI), and peripartum cardiomyopathy (PPCM). The diagnosis of these conditions is challenging because the signs and symptoms overlap with each other and can mimic those experienced in normal pregnancies. There are subtle differences in the diagnosis and treatment of cardiovascular emergencies in pregnant patients that clinicians must be aware of; however, the overall management goals are similar to nonpregnant patients. When managing any critically ill pregnant patient,

No disclosures.
[a] Department of Emergency Medicine, MedStar Georgetown University Hospital & Washington Hospital Center, 3800 Reservoir Road, Washington, DC 20007, USA; [b] Department of Emergency Medicine, MedStar Southern Maryland Hospital Center, 7503 Surratts Road, Clinton, MD 20735, USA
* Corresponding author.
E-mail address: joelle.borhart@gmail.com

Emerg Med Clin N Am 37 (2019) 339–350
https://doi.org/10.1016/j.emc.2019.01.010
0733-8627/19/© 2019 Elsevier Inc. All rights reserved.

maternal well-being takes precedence as the best chance for fetal survival is maternal survival. A coordinated response by a team that includes emergency physicians, obstetricians, cardiologists, surgeons, and neonatologists is critical to ensuring a good outcome for both mother and fetus.

VENOUS THROMBOEMBOLISM IN PREGNANCY

Venous thromboembolism (VTE) includes both deep vein thrombosis (DVT) and PE. Pregnancy is a hypercoagulable state, and other physiologic and anatomic changes during pregnancy, such as increased venous stasis, decreased venous outflow, compression of the inferior vena cava and pelvic veins by the uterus, and decreased mobility, further increase the risk of developing VTE.[2] Women at all stages of pregnancy are at higher risk for developing VTE compared with nonpregnant women, but the rates of VTE are highest in the second half of pregnancy. The rates of VTE sharply increase again in the postpartum period, with first postpartum week particularly high risk. Incidence rates of DVT and PE are 25-fold higher during the first week postpartum than in the last trimester of pregnancy.[3]

Deep Vein Thrombosis

In pregnancy, DVT occurs more frequently in the left leg (likely due to compression of the left iliac vein by the right iliac vein and uterus) and tends to be proximal.[4] As with nonpregnant patients, compression ultrasonography of the proximal veins is the recommended initial diagnostic test when DVT is suspected. Iliac vein thrombosis is more common in pregnancy, however, and can be missed on ultrasound. If the ultrasound is negative or equivocal and iliac vein thrombosis is suspected, additional imaging with noncontrast MR imaging is recommended.[2] If the ultrasound is positive, treatment can begin even if PE is a concern, negating the need for additional testing, such as CT pulmonary angiography (CTPA) or ventilation/perfusion (V/Q) scan.

Pulmonary Embolism

The diagnosis of PE in pregnancy continues to pose challenges to clinicians. Signs and symptoms of PE (tachycardia, tachypnea, dyspnea, and lower extremity edema) can occur as part of the normal, physiologic changes of pregnancy. Commonly used pretest probability tools, such as the modified Wells and revised Geneva scores, have not been validated in pregnant patients. Diagnostic tools, such as the D-dimer, can be unreliable because levels steadily rise throughout normal pregnancies.[5] Imaging studies carry risks of ionizing radiation exposure to mother and fetus. Yet the stakes are so high—PE remains a leading cause of maternal mortality, resulting in up to 200 deaths per day worldwide.[1,6] Therefore, physicians tend to have lower thresholds for testing for PE in pregnant patients compared with nonpregnant patients, even though most pregnant patients selected for PE work-up have a low clinical probability.[7] In multiple studies of pregnant patients with suspected PE, the incidence of VTE is 5% or less compared with 20% to 25% in nonpregnant patients.[5] A clear, safe strategy for ruling out PE in pregnant patients, ideally without the use of radiologic imaging studies, is desperately needed.

D-dimer Test in Pregnant Patients with Suspected Pulmonary Embolism

The D-dimer is a fibrin degradation product present in the blood after a blood clot is broken down by fibrinolysis. It is a commonly used test with high sensitivity for ruling out VTE in nonpregnant patients. The results can be confounded, however, in the pregnant patient. Multiple studies have shown that D-dimer levels rise steadily throughout pregnancy, and few, if any, pregnant women have a normal D-dimer level using standard thresholds in the third trimester.[8–12] Other studies have attempted to identify alternative, trimester-specific D-dimer thresholds for pregnancy, but study methods and results have been inconsistent.[8–10,13–15] Importantly, even if a consensus were reached on normal pregnancy D-dimer levels, the threshold to safely exclude VTE would still need to be established. For these reasons, some investigators and society guidelines do not recommend the testing of D-dimer levels in pregnant patients to assess for VTE.[16–20] Other investigators and guidelines, including the authors of this article, believe that a negative D-dimer using standard thresholds is still reliably negative in pregnant patients with low pretest probability, especially in the first trimester.[21–24]

Clinical Decision Rules

Emergency physicians frequently use clinical decision rules, such as the modified Wells and revised Geneva scores, when evaluating nonpregnant patients for PE (**Table 1**). Neither of these decision rules has been validated in pregnant patients.

Table 1 Clinical decision rules	
Wells Score for Pulmonary Embolism	**Points**
Clinical signs/symptoms of DVT	3
Other diagnosis less likely than PE	3
Heart rate >100	1.5
Immobilization of major surgery in previous 4 wk	1.5
Previous PE or DVT	1.5
Hemoptysis	1
Malignancy (current or within the last 6 mo)	1
Scoring system	
Low probability	0–1
Moderate probability	2–6
High probability	>6
Revised Geneva Score for Pulmonary Embolism	**Points**
Age >65 y	1
Previous PE or DVT	3
Surgery (under general anesthesia) or lower limb fracture within 1 mo	2
Malignancy (active or within 1 y)	2
Unilateral lower limb pain	3
Hemoptysis	2
Heart rate 75–94 beats per minute	3
Heart rate ≥95 beats per minute	5
Pain on deep palpation of lower limb or unilateral edema	4
Scoring system	
Low probability	<3
Moderate probability	4–10
High probability	>10

Data from Touhami O, Marzouk SB, Bennasr L, et al. Are the wells score and revised Geneva score valuable for the diagnosis of pulmonary embolism in pregnancy? Eur J Obstet Gynecol Reprod Biol 2018;221:166–71.

Recently, there have been studies on the application of these rules in pregnant patients and results have been mixed. One study of 103 pregnant patients by O'Connor and colleagues[25] found a Wells score less than 6 had a 100% negative predictive value (NPV) for PE. Cutts and colleagues[26] also found an NPV of 100% for PE in a group of 183 pregnant patients with Wells score less than 4. A 2018 retrospective review by Touhami and colleagues,[27] however, calculated modified Wells and revised Geneva scores for 103 pregnant and postpartum women who presented to an emergency department (ED) with suspected PE. The investigators found that even for the patients with a low probability Wells score (modified Wells score <2) the prevalence of PE was 20.5%. The revised Geneva score also performed poorly in this population, with the prevalence of PE 17% in the low probability test group (Geneva score <3). Other investigators have proposed various combinations of clinical decision rules and trimester-adjusted D-dimer levels to evaluate for PE in pregnant patients, but the various combination of clinical decision rules plus trimester adjusted D-dimer levels has not been validated.[14,28]

Imaging Studies

Currently, imaging tests are the mainstay of diagnosis of PE in pregnant patients. The 2 most commonly used studies are CTPA and V/Q scan. Both studies have been shown to have similar NPVs (99%–100%) for the diagnosis of PE in pregnancy[29] CTPA confers a higher maternal radiation dose to the breast tissue compared with V/Q scan, although using bismuth breast shields can reduce radiation exposure.[30] V/Q scan confers slightly higher radiation dose to the fetus compared with CTPA, although the radiation dose for both studies is well below the threshold associated with pregnancy loss and teratogenesis.[16] CTPA may identify other clinically significant abnormalities, such as aortic dissection, and is often more readily available than V/Q scan. Some investigators have suggested that CTPA is more often nondiagnostic because pregnancy-related physiologic changes can result in decreased contrast enhancement.[31] A recent systematic review of 22 studies with 2391 scans (1165 V/Q scans and 1226 CTPAs), however, showed that number of nondiagnostic studies in pregnancy is similar between V/Q scans and CTPAs.[32] A 2017 Cochrane review concluded that CTPA and V/Q scan are both reasonable imaging choices for excluding PE in pregnancy, although the investigators noted that the quality of evidence was low.[33] A commonly proposed algorithm recommended by the American Thoracic Society and the Society of Thoracic Radiology is to begin by ordering a chest radiograph (CXR).[20] If the CXR is normal, proceed with V/Q scan. If the CXR is abnormal, proceed with CTPA. Other algorithms for pregnant patients recommend beginning with bilateral lower extremity ultrasounds when either DVT or PE is suspected, because many women with PE have evidence of DVT.[28] **Fig. 1** shows a suggested diagnostic algorithm for suspected PE in pregnancy. The investigators recommend beginning with bilateral lower ultrasound if a patient has leg signs or symptoms suggestive of DVT. In the absence of leg symptoms, and if V/Q scan is readily available, evaluation for PE can begin with a CXR. The authors believe that either CTPA or V/Q scan is an acceptable choice for evaluation of suspected PE in pregnancy; they prefer CTPA for its ability to identify alternate pathology and because the test is more readily available at their institutions.

Treatment

Treatment of DVT or PE in pregnant and postpartum patients usually involves either unfractionated heparin or low-molecular-weight heparin. Neither drug crosses the

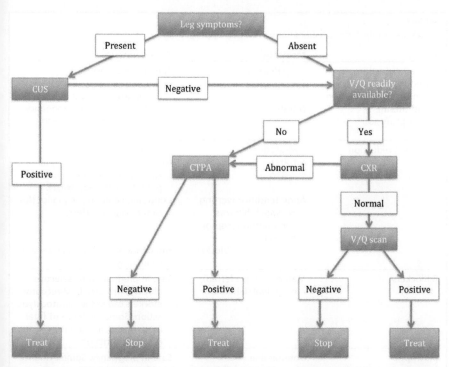

Fig. 1. Diagnostic algorithm for suspected PE in pregnancy. CUS, compression ultrasound.

placenta or enters breast milk. Unfractionated heparin is preferred in situations where urgent delivery or surgery may be necessary or in patients with glomerular filtration rate of less than 30 mL/min.[34] Warfarin in associated with birth defects and is contraindicated in pregnancy. Data are limited regarding the use of oral novel anticoagulants, such as dabigatran and rivaroxaban, and their use should be avoided in pregnancy[16] (**Table 2**). Thrombolytic therapy should be considered in cases of massive PE causing hemodynamic compromise.[17] Catheter-directed thrombolytic therapy can be used for limb-threatening DVT.[16] In cases of fatal PE, a majority of deaths occur in the first hour after onset of symptoms.[35] Treatment should not be delayed for diagnostic testing in unstable patients.

AORTIC DISSECTION

Aortic dissection, albeit rare, can be catastrophic for both mother and fetus.[36] Aortic dissection occurs when there is a tear in the intima of the aortic wall, leading to the creation of a second (false) lumen through the media of the wall.

Approximately one-half of aortic dissections in women under age 40 occur during pregnancy.[37] Aortic dissection typically occurs in the third trimester or postpartum, but risk factors, such as connective tissue disorders (Ehlers-Danlos and Marfan syndromes), aortic valve abnormalities, increased aortic root diameters, coarctation, and hypertension, can predispose pregnant patients to dissection earlier in pregnancy.[36] There is a lower incidence of hypertension in patients with aortic dissection in pregnancy compared with nonpregnant patients with dissection, which suggests pregnancy alone may lead to increased risk.[36] The physiologic changes during

Table 2
Common cardiovascular medications used during pregnancy

Action	Medication	Considerations
Preload reduction (reducing preload can cause hypotension and uterine hypoprofusion	Loop diuretics	Safe in pregnancy
	Spironolactone	Avoid in pregnancy due to antiandrogen effects.
	Nitrates	Nitroglycerine safe in pregnancy. Avoid nitroprusside due to potential cyanide toxicity.
Afterload reduction	Hydralazine	Safe in pregnancy
	Nitrates	Nitroglycerine safe in pregnancy. Avoid nitroprusside due to potential cyanide toxicity.
	Angiotensin-converting enzyme inhibitors/ angiotensin-receptor blockers	Contraindicated in pregnancy due to teratogenic effects
	Calcium channel blockers	Nifedipine safe in pregnancy and commonly used
β-Blockers	Metoprolol (preferred), carvedilol, labetalol	Safe in pregnancy; β1-selective blockers preferred; β2-receptor blockers can induce antitocolytic action. Some evidence of fetal bradycardia, intrauterine growth restriction
Inotropes	Dobutamine	Safe in pregnancy. Some evidence of worse outcomes when used for PPCM
	Milrinone	Safe in pregnancy
Antiplatelet	Aspirin	Low dose is safe in pregnancy (after first trimester). High doses may lead to premature closure of ductus arteriosis near term.
	Clopidogrel	Reserve for use after stenting procedures.
	Glycoprotein IIb/IIIa inhibitors	Avoid in pregnancy
Anticoagulants	Unfractionated heparin	Safe in pregnancy. Preferred if anticipate delivery or surgery or if glomerular filtration rate <30 mL/min
	Low-molecular-weight heparin	Safe in pregnancy
	Coumadin	Contraindicated in pregnancy
	Rivaroxaban, dabigatran	Avoid in pregnancy.

pregnancy can place increased stress on the aortic wall. By 32 weeks' gestation, intravascular volume increases by up to 50%, making the risk of dissection particularly high at this time.[37] Estrogen has been also shown to weaken the structural integrity of the aorta wall, making pregnant patients more susceptible to dissection.[37–39] The increase in afterload due to aortocaval compression in the second half of pregnancy also may play a role.[39–41]

Symptoms of aortic dissection include sudden-onset chest pain with radiation to the back, syncope, nausea, vomiting, sweating, and even bronchospasm due to irritation of the vagal nerve.[39] Pregnant patients tend to present with less specific symptoms compared with nonpregnant patients.[37] When they do present with classic symptoms, such as ripping chest or intrascapular pain, their complaints frequently are underestimated.[42]

The diagnosis of aortic dissection hinges on imaging studies. As in nonpregnant patients, CT angiography (CTA) may be used. The sensitivity of CTA for the diagnosis for aortic dissection approaches 100% whereas the specificity is 98% to 99%. Transesophageal echocardiography has a sensitivity and specificity approaching that of CTA and is an ideal test in pregnancy because it does not confer any ionizing radiation but is often unavailable in an ED.

Management depends on the location of the dissection. Aortic dissections are typically classified as those involving the ascending aorta (Stanford type A) or those not involving the ascending aorta (Stanford type B). Type A dissections almost always require immediate surgical intervention, whereas type B dissections typically are managed medically unless visceral ischemia or aortic rupture is involved. ED treatment includes lowering heart rate with β-blockade, followed by lowering blood pressure with vasodilators (see **Table 2**). Obstetric and surgical consults should be immediately obtained for any pregnant or postpartum patient with aortic dissection.

ACUTE MYOCARDIAL INFARCTION

AMI in women of childbearing age is rare, but a combination of factors, including advanced maternal age, obesity, and the hypercoagulable state occurring during pregnancy, increases the risk of AMI 3-fold to 4-fold.[43–46] The normal physiologic changes that occur during pregnancy also can contribute to cardiac events. Increased blood volume and resting heart rate and subsequently increased stroke volume increase myocardial oxygen demand. Physiologic anemia of pregnancy and decreased diastolic blood pressures lead to decreased myocardial oxygen delivery. Moreover, dyslipidemia is worsened during pregnancy because high-density lipoprotein levels are decreased.[45] In pregnancy, AMI tends to occur in the third trimester and most often involves the anterior wall.[45] Symptoms include chest pain, dyspnea, sweating, nausea, and vomiting.

The diagnostic criteria for women with AMI in pregnancy are the same as for nonpregnant patients: abnormal ECG plus increased troponin level and/or increased creatinine kinase from myocardium. A few pregnancy-specific changes to these diagnostic tests, however, should be noted. As the fetus grows, the diaphragm is displaced upward, which can result in left axis deviation on ECG.[47] Creatinine kinase from myocardium has been shown to be elevated with uterine contraction. Troponin levels tend to be unaffected by uterine contraction but may be elevated in cases of preeclampsia and gestational hypertension.[44,47]

Treatment of AMI in pregnant women is also similar to that in nonpregnant patients. Many of the usual medications (nitrates, aspirin, and β-blockers) are considered safe in pregnancy (see **Table 2**). Percutaneous coronary intervention (PCI) is the preferred treatment option for ST-segment elevation myocardial infarction. Proper shielding, using a brachial or radial approach, and reducing the length of fluoroscopy times can minimize fetal radiation. Thrombolysis is an alternative to PCI. The major risk with thrombolysis is maternal hemorrhage. Because streptokinase and tissue plasminogen activator have little placental transfer, hemorrhagic and teratogenic effects on the fetus are minimal. Thrombolysis is recommended only if PCI is not immediately available.[47]

Spontaneous Coronary Artery Dissection

Spontaneous coronary artery dissection (SCAD) makes up 40% of AMIs in pregnancy.[48] Most pregnancy-related cases occur near term or within the first 3 weeks after delivery.[49,50] Risk factors include multiparity and advanced maternal age, but the hormones associated with pregnancy itself are believed to weaken the vessel walls, making pregnant patients more susceptible.[48] Locations of SCAD tend to be anterior and anterolateral in pregnancy, with one-third of cases in a retrospective chart review involving the left main artery.[51]

Diagnosis of SCAD, as in other causes of AMI, includes abnormal ECG changes, elevated troponin levels, and regional wall motion abnormalities on echocardiography.[52] The definitive diagnosis of SCAD is by coronary angiography, but CT may detect some cases.[53] Treatment tends to be conservative. This includes blood pressure management and initiation of antiplatelet medications, such as aspirin and clopidogrel. Glycoprotein IIb/IIIa inhibitors are contraindicated due to increased bleeding risks and subsequent increased risk of dissection[52] (see **Table 2**). In cases of hemodynamic compromise or advanced lesions, patients may require procedural intervention—PCI or coronary bypass grafting.[49] Thrombolytic therapy can be harmful to patients with SCAD, because it can potentially propagate the false lumen. Therefore, a patient should be transferred to a center with cardiac catheterization capabilities if possible.[51]

Coronary Artery Spasm

Coronary spasm in pregnancy typically is due to dysregulation of the endothelium in addition to vasospasm due to pregnancy-induced hypertension and preeclampsia. Medications, such as ergotamines and bromocriptine, which are commonly used to treat postpartum hemorrhage and suppress lactation, also can lead to coronary vasospasm. Because of the fleeting nature of coronary vasospasm, it is difficult to diagnose. Patients seem to respond well to nitroglycerin, which allows for relaxation of the blood vessel.[45,52]

PERIPARTUM CARDIOMYOPATHY

PPCM is defined as cardiomyopathy with left heart failure due to left ventricular systolic dysfunction that occurs in late pregnancy or in the first few months postpartum that cannot be attributed to another cause.[54–56] The exact etiology of PPCM is unclear. Environmental factors, such as diet, viruses, and inflammation, have been linked to development of PPCM. Risk factors for PPCM, similar to many of the other cardiovascular emergencies discussed in this article, include advanced maternal age, multigravida patients, preeclampsia, hypertension, and African American race.[54]

Signs and symptoms of PPCM are the same as those of typical heart failure and include orthopnea, paroxysmal nocturnal dyspnea, pedal edema, chest pain, abdominal pain from hepatic congestion, persistent cough, palpitations, and dyspnea on exertion. Jugular venous distension, tachycardia, and a third heart sound are frequently present.[54] Differentiating PPCM from other cardiovascular emergencies, such as AMI and PE as well as preeclampsia, can be challenging. Like PE, AMI, and aortic dissection, the symptoms of PPCM also overlap significantly with the physiologic changes of pregnancy.

ED evaluation includes ECG, blood tests including N-terminal probrain natriuretic peptide measurement, CXR, and echocardiogram. Common ECG findings include sinus tachycardia, left ventricular hypertrophy, and ST-T wave abnormalities.[54–57] CXR may show pulmonary congestion. On echocardiogram, the left ventricle may be dilated and ejection fraction reduced. Mitral regurgitation and left ventricular thrombus also can be seen. Approximately 6% of cases of PPCM are associated with thrombo-embolic events, such as DVT, stroke, and PE.[54] Thromboembolic events is not only due to the hypercoaguable state of pregnancy but also because of ventricular dilatation, endothelial injury, venous stasis, and patient immobility.[55,56]

ED management of patients with PPCM is similar to that of nonpregnant patients. A patient's volume status should be determined and either fluids or diuretics should be administered to optimize preload. If the patient is still pregnant, diuresis may lead to decreased placental blood flow. Blood pressure should be controlled, but hypotension should be avoided because this may compromise placental perfusion.[54,55] Noninvasive forms of ventilatory support may be considered for patients with hypoxia or significant increased work of breathing. Critically ill patients may require intubation. If needed, inotropes can be used, but those with catecholamines should be avoided. Worse outcomes have been reported in patients receiving dobutamine for PPCM. Milrinone tends to be the preferred inotrope[54,56] (see **Table 2**). Left ventricular assist devices are required in approximately 5% of patients with PPCM population. Cardiac transplantation tends to be less successful in this population, with higher rates of rejection and complications.[54]

SUMMARY

Cardiovascular emergencies in pregnancy are rare but when they occur can have devastating consequences for both mother and fetus. Overall the management of cardiovascular emergencies in pregnant patients is similar to that of nonpregnant patients. The risk of VTE is elevated at all stages of pregnancy and is highest in the first weeks postpartum. CTPA and V/Q scan are both acceptable choices for diagnosing PE in pregnancy. ED management of pregnant patients with aortic dissection involves decreasing heart rate and then blood pressure. Pregnant patients with AMI are candidates for PCI, similar to nonpregnant patients. Signs and symptoms of PPCM are the same as of typical heart failure. When managing any critically ill pregnant patient, maternal well-being takes precedence because the best chance for fetal survival is maternal survival. Prompt recognition, resuscitation, and coordination of obstetric, cardiovascular, and surgical consultation are the cornerstones of ED care.

REFERENCES

1. Available at: https://www.cdc.gov/reproductivehealth/maternalinfanthealth/pmss. html. Accessed June 3, 2018.

2. James A. The Committee on practice bulletins. Practice bulletin no. 123: thromboembolism in pregnancy. Obstet Gynecol 2011;118:718–29.

3. Heit JA, Kobbervig CE, James AH, et al. Trends in the incidence of venous thromboembolism during pregnancy and postpartum: A 30-year population-based study. Ann Intern Med 2005;143:697–706.

4. Bourjeily G, Paidas M, Khalil H, et al. Pulmonary embolism in pregnancy. Lancet 2010;375:500–12.

5. Van der Pol LM, Mairuhu ATA, Tromeur C, et al. Use of clinical prediction rules and D-dimer tests in the diagnostic management of pregnant patients with suspected acute pulmonary embolism. Blood Rev 2017;31:31–6.

6. Say L, Chou D, Gemmill A, et al. Global causes of maternal death: a WHO systematic analysis. Lancet Glob Health 2014;2:323–33.

7. Kline JA, Richardson DM, Than MP, et al. Systematic review and meta-analysis of pregnant patients investigated for suspected pulmonary embolism in the emergency department. Acad Emerg Med 2014;21:949–59.

8. Kline JA, Williams GW, Hernandez-Nino J. D-dimer concentrations in normal pregnancy: new diagnostic thresholds are needed. Clin Chem 2005;51:825–9.

9. Kovac M, Mikovic Z, Rakicevic L, et al. The use of D-dimer with new cutoff can be useful in diagnosis of venous thromboembolism in pregnancy. Eur J Obstet Gynecol Reprod Biol 2010;148:27–30.

10. Wang M, Lu SM, Li S, et al. Reference intervals of D-dimer during the pregnancy and puerperium period on the STA-R evolution coagulation analyzer. Clin Chim Acta 2013;425:176–80.

11. Padgett J, Gough J, DeVente J, et al. The effects of childbirth on D-dimer levels. Acad Emerg Med 2015;S314.

12. Nishii A, Noda Y, Nemoto R, et al. Evaluation of Ddimer during pregnancy. J Obstet Gynaecol Res 2009;35:689–93.

13. Ercan S, Ozkan S, Yucel N, et al. Establishing reference intervals for D-dimer to trimesters. J Matern Fetal Neonatal Med 2015;28:983–7.

14. Parilla BV, Fournogerakis R, Archer A, et al. Diagnosing pulmonary embolism in pregnancy: are biomarkers and clinical predictive models useful? AJP Rep 2016;6:160–4.

15. Morse M. Establishing a normal range for D-dimer levels through pregnancy to aid in the diagnosis of pulmonary embolism and deep vein thrombosis. J Thromb Haemost 2004;2:1202–4.

16. Greer IA. Pregnancy complicated by venous thrombosis. N Engl J Med 2015;373: 540–7.

17. Guntupalli KK, Karnad DR, Bandi V, et al. Critical illness in pregnancy part II: Common medical conditions complicating pregnancy and puerperium. Chest 2015;148:1333–45.

18. Society of Obstetricians and Gynecologist of Canada. Venous thromboembolism and antithrombotic therapy in pregnancy. J Obstet Gynaecol Can 2014;36(6): 527–53.

19. Royal College of Obstetricians & Gynaecologists. Thromboembolic disease in pregnancy and the puerperium: acute management. London UK: Royal College of Obstetricians & Gynaecologists; 2015. p. 1–32. Green-top Guideline, No. 37b.

20. Leung AN, Bull TM, Jaeschke R, et al, ATS/STR Committee on Pulmonary Embolism in Pregnancy. American Thoracic Society documents: an official American Thoracic Society/Society of Thoracic Radiology Clinical Practice Guideline– evaluation of suspect pulmonary embolism in pregnancy. Radiology 2012; 262(2):635–46.

21. Chan WS, Chunilal S, Lee A, et al. A red blood cell agguluntiation D-dimer test to exclude deep vein thrombosis in pregnancy. Ann Intern Med 2007;147:65–170.

22. Sommerkamp SK, Gibson A. Cardiovascular disasters in pregnancy. Emerg Med Clin North Am 2012;30:949–59.

23. Working Group in Women's Health of the Society of Thrombosis and Hemostasis. Treatment of pregnancy-associated venous thromboembolism – position paper from the Working Group in Women's Health of the Society of Thrombosis and Hemostasis. Vasa 2016;45(2):103–18.

24. The Task Force for the Diagnosis and Management of Acute Pulmonary Embolism of the European Society of Cardiology (ESC). 2014 ESC guideline on the diagnosis and management of acute pulmonary embolism. Eur Heart J 2014;25: 3033–80.

25. O'Connor C, Moriarty J, Walsh J, et al. The application of a clinical risk stratification score may reduce unnecessary investigations for pulmonary embolism in pregnancy. J Matern Fetal Neonatal Med 2011;24:1461–4.

26. Cutts BA, Tran HA, Merriman E, et al. The utility of the Wells clinical prediction model and ventilation-perfusion scanning for pulmonary embolism in pregnancy. Blood Coagul Fibrinolysis 2014; 25:375–8.

27. Touhami O, Marzouk SB, Bennasr L, et al. Are the wells score and revised geneva score valuable for the diagnosis of pulmonary embolism in pregnancy? Eur J Obstet Gynecol Reprod Biol 2018;221:166–71.

28. Kline JA, Kabrhel C. Emergency evaluation for pulmonary embolism, part 2: Diagnostic approach. J Emerg Med 2015;49:104–17.

29. Shahir K, Goodman LR, Tali A, et al. Pulmonary embolism in pregnancy: CT pulmonary angiography versus perfusion scanning. Am J Roentgenol 2010;195: 214–20.

30. Hurwitz LM, Yoshizumi TT, Goodman PC, et al. Radiation dose savings for adult pulmonary embolus 64-MDCT using bismuth breast shields, lower peak kilovoltage, and automatic tube current modulation. AJR Am J Roentgenol 2009;192: 244–53.

31. Cahill AG, Stout MJ, Macones GA, et al. Diag- nosing pulmonary embolism in pregnancy using computed-tomographic angiography or ventila- tion-perfusion. Obstet Gynecol 2009;114:124–9.

32. Parker A, Alotaibi G, Wu C, et al. The proportion of nondiagnostic computed tomographic pulmonary angiography and ventilation/perfusion lung scans in pregnant women with suspected pulmonary embolism: a systematic review. Int Soc Thromb Haemost 2015;13(Suppl. 2).

33. van Mens TE, Scheres LJ, de Jong PG, et al. Imaging for the exclusion of pulmonary embolism in pregnancy. Cochrane Database Syst Rev 2017;(1):CD011053.

34. Bates SM, Middeldorp S, Rodger M, et al. Guidance for the treatment and prevention of obstetric-associated venous thromboembolism. J Thromb Thrombolysis 2016;41:92–128.

35. Brennan MC, Moore LE. Pulmonary embolism and amniotic fluid embolism in pregnancy. Obstet Gynecol Clin North Am 2013;40:27–35.

36. Zhu J-M, Ma W-G, Peterss S, et al. Aortic dissection in pregnancy: management strategy and outcomes. Ann Thorac Surg 2017;103:1199–206.

37. Ch'ng S, Cochrane A, Goldstein J, et al. Stanford type A dissection in pregnancy: a diagnostic and management challenge. Heart Lung Circ 2013;22:12–8.

38. Kamel H, Roman M, Pitcher A, et al. Pregnancy and the risk of aortic dissection or rupture: a cohort-crossover analysis. Circulation 2016;134(7):527–33.

39. Lee SH, Ryu S, Choi SW, et al. Acute type A aortic dissection in a 37-week pregnant patient: an unusual clinical presentation. J Emerg Med 2017;52(7):565–86.

40. Rajagopalan S, Nwazota N, Chandra S. Outcomes in pregnant women with acute aortic dissections a review of the literature from 2003 to 2013. Int J Obstet Anesth 2014;23:348–56.

41. Immer F, Bansi A, Immer-Bansi A, et al. Aortic dissection in pregnancy: analysis of risk factors and outcomes. Ann Thorac Surg 2003;76:309–14.

42. La Chapelle CF, Schutte JM, Schuitemaker NW, et al. Maternal mortality attributable to vascular dissection and rupture in the Netherlands: a nationwide confidential enquiry. BJOG 2012;119:86–93.

43. Pacheco L, Saade G, Hankins G. Acute myocardial infarction during pregnancy. Clin Obstet Gynecol 2014;57(4):835–43.

44. Roth A, Elkayam U. Acute myocardial infarction associated with pregnancy. J Am Coll Cardiol 2008;52:171–80.
45. Kealey AJ. Coronary artery disease and myocardial infarction in pregnancy: a review of epidemiology, diagnosis, and medical and surgical management. Can J Cardiol 2010;26(6):e185–9.
46. Sahni G. Chest pain syndromes in pregnancy. Cardiol Clin 2012;30:343–67.
47. Poh C-L, Lee C-H. Acute myocardial infarction in pregnant women. Ann Acad Med Singapore 2010;39:247–53.
48. Saw J. Pregnancy-associated spontaneous coronary artery dissection represents an exceptionally high-risk spontaneous coronary artery dissection cohort. Circ Cardiovasc Interv. 2017;10. pii:e005119.
49. Pabla JS, John L, McCrea WA. Spontaneous coronary artery dissection as a cause of sudden cardiac death in the peripartum period. BMJ Case Rep 2010. https://doi.org/10.1136/bcr.05.2010.2994.
50. Bezgin T, Gecmen C, Erden I, et al. Pregnancy-associated myocardial infarction. Herz 2014;39:530–3.
51. Havakuk O, Goland S, Mehra A, et al. Pregnancy and the risk of spontaneous coronary artery dissection an analysis of 120 contemporary cases. Circ Cardiovasc Interv 2017;10:e004941.
52. Lee R, Carr D. Pregnancy-associated spontaneous coronary artery dissection (PASCAD): an etiology for chest pain in the young peripartum patient. CJEM 2018;20(S2):S64–9.
53. Sharma N, Seevanayagam S, Rayoo R, et al. Spontaneous left main coronary artery dissection in pregnancy. Int J Cardiol 2012;159:e11–3.
54. Jackson AM, Dalzell JR, Walker NL, et al. Peripartum cardiomyopathy: diagnosis and management. Heart 2018;104:779–86.
55. Arany Z, Elkayam U. Peripartum cardiomyopathy. Circulation 2016;133:1397–409.
56. Goland S, Elkayam U. Peripartum cardiomyopathy: approach to management. Curr Opin Cardiol 2018;33:347–53.
57. Bhattacharyya A, Basra SS, Sen P, et al. Peripartum cardiomyopathy: a review. Tex Heart Inst J 2012;39:8–16.

Resuscitation of the Pregnant Patient

Philippa N. Soskin, MD, MPP[a], Jennifer Yu, MD[b,*]

KEYWORDS

- Pregnancy • Resuscitation of pregnant patient • Cardiac arrest in pregnancy
- Resuscitative hysterotomy • Perimortem cesarean section • Amniotic fluid embolism

KEY POINTS

- Maternal physiology and anatomy change throughout pregnancy.
- Resuscitation and airway management in the pregnant patient present unique challenges.
- CPR and resuscitation should follow standard AHA ACLS guidelines with minor modifications.
- Resuscitative hysterotomy or perimortem cesarean section is used to eliminate aortocaval compression in an attempt to restore perfusion to both mother and fetus.
- Amniotic fluid embolism is characterized by the triad of cardiovascular collapse, hypoxic respiratory failure, and coagulopathy.

INTRODUCTION

Resuscitation of the pregnant patient presents unique challenges. Many health care providers lack familiarity with maternal physiologic changes and the distinctive underlying etiology of cardiac arrest in pregnancy. Knowledge of what changes are expected in pregnancy and an understanding of how to adapt clinical practice accordingly is essential for the care of the pregnant woman in the emergency department.

PHYSIOLOGIC CHANGES IN PREGNANCY
Cardiovascular

During pregnancy there is an overall increase in blood volume producing an increase in preload.[1–4] The circulation of additional progesterone, estrogen, and prostaglandins

Disclosure Statement: No disclosures.
[a] Department of Emergency Medicine, MedStar Georgetown University Hospital, MedStar Washington Hospital Center, Georgetown University School of Medicine, 3800 Reservoir Road Northwest, Ground Floor CCC Building, Washington, DC 20007, USA; [b] Department of Critical Care Medicine, MedStar Washington Hospital Center, Georgetown University School of Medicine, 110 Irving Street Northwest, Suite 4B-42, Washington, DC 20010, USA
* Corresponding author.
E-mail address: Jennifer.Yu@medstar.net

Emerg Med Clin N Am 37 (2019) 351–363
https://doi.org/10.1016/j.emc.2019.01.011
0733-8627/19/© 2019 Elsevier Inc. All rights reserved.

generates increased vascular smooth muscle relaxation, reducing systemic and peripheral vascular resistance.[2,4,5] The resulting vasodilation reduces afterload and thereby increases stroke volume.[1,5] In pregnancy, heart rate increases and in turn cardiac output is increased.[1–3,5] This increase in cardiac output contributes to ventricular hypertrophy and increased end-diastolic volume.[2] The increase in cardiac output is not enough to compensate for the decrease in systemic vascular resistance, and blood pressure starts to decrease in the first trimester, reaching its lowest level in the 24th week and increasing back to normal by term.[2,6] Although there are many changes to the cardiovascular system in pregnancy, myocardial contractility and ejection fraction do not seem to be affected.[1,6] The increase in cardiac output also increases the pulmonary circulation while pulmonary capillary wedge pressure is maintained.[1,4] The overall smooth muscle relaxation is also manifested by a decrease in pulmonary vascular resistance. The resulting decrease in oncotic pressure increases the risk of edema.[1,3,4]

Changes to maternal cardiovascular physiology have several manifestations on clinical examination. New murmurs, common in pregnant women, can be attributed to both flow murmurs (caused by increased cardiac output) and regurgitant murmurs (caused by dilatation of the cardiac valves).[1] Peripheral edema, mild tachycardia, jugular venous distention, and lateral displacement of left ventricular apex may also be observed.[1,7] As pregnancy progresses, elevation of the diaphragm pushes the heart upward and to the left. This can translate to changes on the electrocardiogram including left axis deviation, prominent Q waves in II, III, and aVF, and flattened or inverted T waves in leads III and V1 to V3.[4,5]

After about 20 weeks the gravid uterus can produce aortocaval compression, which impedes venous return to the heart, resulting in hypotension in the supine position.[1,4,7,8] Compression of the inferior vena cava (IVC) reduces preload, which in turn decreases cardiac output and reduces overall perfusion to both the uterus and fetus. Reduction of aortocaval pressure and improvement of blood pressure may be achieved by laying the patient in the left lateral tilt position or by manual displacement of the uterus.[1,3] In cases of cardiac arrest, uterine emptying by resuscitative hysterotomy may be required to achieve return of spontaneous circulation (ROSC).[4,7,8]

Clinical Pearls

- Blood pressure is expected to decrease in pregnancy until the 24th week.
- Peripheral edema, mild tachycardia, jugular venous distention, and lateral displacement of the left ventricular apex are expected in pregnancy.
- After 20 weeks, aortocaval compression by the uterus can cause hypotension.
- Left lateral tilt position and manual displacement of the uterus may improve aortocaval compression.
- Resuscitative hysterotomy may be required to achieve ROSC in the case of cardiac arrest.

Pulmonary

Elevation of progesterone during pregnancy stimulates the respiratory center, thereby increasing tidal volume and respiratory depth and resulting in increased minute ventilation and oxygen consumption.[3,4,7] The respiratory rate is relatively unchanged.[3,4] These changes manifest clinically in the first trimester as dyspnea and increase throughout gestation as the enlarging uterus presses upward on the diaphragm.[4] In pregnancy partial pressure of oxygen (Pao_2) is high, which facilitates transfer of oxygen from maternal to fetal circulation, whereas a low partial pressure of arterial carbon dioxide ($Paco_2$) facilitates transfer of CO_2 from fetal to maternal circulation.[1,7] The low $Paco_2$ yields a respiratory alkalosis, which is partially compensated by an increase in bicarbonate excretion in order to maintain pH.[1–3] The low bicarbonate in pregnancy shifts the dissociation curve to the right, facilitating the release of oxygen from maternal hemoglobin into the fetal circulation.[1]

The gravid uterus elevates the diaphragm and increases abdominal pressure.[4] The chest wall circumference enlarges while the chest wall compliance decreases,[1,2,4] consequently decreasing total lung capacity, expiratory reserve volume, and functional residual capacity (FRC).[1–4] The combination of increased oxygen consumption and decreased FRC puts pregnant patients at higher risk for desaturation events, particularly in the setting of intubation. Intubation may be further challenged by increased nasal congestion and progesterone-mediated increases in hyperemia and mucosal edema.[1,4]

Clinical Pearls

- Dyspnea on exertion is common by the third trimester.
- Pregnant patients are more prone to desaturation.
- Consider a smaller endotracheal tube, as pregnant patients have more mucosal edema.

Hematologic

In pregnancy, increases in erythropoietin stimulates red blood cell production while rising aldosterone levels contribute to higher total body water and plasma volume.[1,2,7] The increase in red blood cells is disproportionate to the increase in plasma volume resulting in dilutional anemia or the relative anemia of pregnancy.[1,2,4] Platelet production also increases in pregnancy, but the overall platelet count decreases as a result of increased plasma volume as well as consumption.[1,2]

Pregnancy is considered to be a prothrombotic state.[2,3] Coagulation is enhanced because of an increase in clotting factors VII, VIII, IX, XII, fibrinogen, and von Willebrand factor (vWF), and elevated levels of plasminogen activator inhibitors promote fibrinolysis.[1–3,9] This state may be protective in incidents of postpartum hemorrhage but increases the overall risk of thromboembolism in pregnancy.

Renal

Increased cardiac output and systemic vasodilation in pregnancy increases renal flow and the glomerular filtration rate, thereby lowering serum creatinine levels.[2–4,7] There is an increase in urinary excretion of protein, albumin, and glucose.[1,2] Renal clearance of medications may also be affected.[1,3] Smooth muscle relaxation can lead to urinary stasis and increased risk of urinary tract infections, pyelonephritis, and kidney stones.[1,7] Progesterone dilates the renal calyx, pelvis, and ureters.[1,2] This dilatation along with the mechanical compression on the ureters by the enlarging uterus results in hydronephrosis, which is more prevalent on the right.[1,2]

Gastrointestinal

The placenta stimulates gastrin production, resulting in increased gastric acidity. Combined with loss of lower esophageal sphincter tone from smooth muscle relaxation and upward displacement of the stomach by the uterus, this contributes to increased gastroesophageal reflux, esophagitis, and aspiration.[1,2,4,7] Smooth muscle relaxation also decreases gallbladder contractility, which can yield biliary stasis and increase the risk of gallstone production.[7] Cholecystitis is the second most common nonobstetric surgical emergency during pregnancy after appendicitis.[4] Progesterone slows gastric emptying while increasing gastric transit times.[1–3] This process may result in nausea, vomiting, bloating, and constipation. The displacement of abdominal organs and stretching of the peritoneum caused by the gravid uterus may alter the abdominal examination.[1] Liver enzymes (alanine aminotransferase [ALT] and aspartate aminotransferase [AST]) are unaltered or decreased in pregnancy, whereas alkaline phosphatase increases[1,3,4] (**Table 1**).

Table 1 Physiologic changes to systems during pregnancy	
System	**Expected Change in Pregnancy**
Cardiovascular	
Heart rate	↑
Stroke volume	↑
Cardiac output	↑
Blood pressure	↓
Systemic vascular resistance	↓
Peripheral vascular resistance	↓
Pulmonary	
Respiratory rate	Unchanged
Tidal volume	↑
Minute ventilation	↑
Expiratory reserve volume	↓
Functional residual capacity	↓
pH	Unchanged
Pao_2	↑
$Paco_2$	↓
HCO_3	↓
Hematologic	
Blood volume	↑
Red blood cells	↓
Platelets	↓
White blood cells	↑
Factors VII, VIII, IX, XII, fibrinogen, vWF	↑
Plasminogen inhibitor factors	↑
Renal	
Renal blood flow	↑
Glomerular filtration rate	↑
Serum creatinine	↓
Gastrointestinal	
AST/ALT	↓ or unchanged
Alkaline phosphatase	↑

CARDIAC ARREST IN PREGNANCY

Though rare, cardiac arrest in pregnancy deserves special attention during resuscitation because there are two patients—mother and fetus—who require consideration. Owing to medical advances allowing for older maternal age with increasing comorbidities, women are at higher risk for cardiopulmonary events leading to cardiac arrest, which occurs in up to 1 in 12,000 pregnancies.[10–12]

Etiology

Causes of maternal circulatory collapse can be divided into obstetric-related or other medical conditions. Obstetric-related causes include hypertensive disorders (preeclampsia, eclampsia, HELLP syndrome [Hemolysis, Elevated Liver enzyme level, Low Platelet level]), obstetric or surgical hemorrhage, sepsis or infection, embolic causes (amniotic fluid embolism, pulmonary embolus, air embolism), and anesthetic or drug-induced cause. Preexisting conditions such as cardiac/valvular disease, cardiomyopathy, asthma, and thromboembolism are also major causes.[13,14] The 2015 American Heart Association (AHA) Scientific Statement regarding cardiac arrest in pregnancy offers an easy A-to-H list of the differential diagnoses to consider.[10]

Cardiopulmonary Resuscitation

Cardiopulmonary resuscitation (CPR) should be initiated immediately and should follow the standard AHA Advanced Cardiovascular Life Support (ACLS) guidelines for adult CPR. Continuous chest compressions should be performed at a rate of 100 per minute to a depth of 2.5 cm, allowing for full chest wall recoil. Hand placement should be in the center of the chest, similar to that in nonpregnant patients. For those patients in the third trimester, hand placement 2 to 3 cm higher on the sternum is recommended. Interruptions should be limited to less than 10 seconds with the exception of placement of an advanced airway.[10,15]

If a shockable rhythm is present, immediate defibrillation with biphasic shock (120 to 200 J) is recommended. Defibrillation should not be delayed if fetal monitoring is present.[10] There is a theoretic risk of electrical burns or arcing; however, the risk of delaying intervention outweighs this risk.[15] Compressions should be resumed immediately following shock delivery.

Current ACLS drug doses and intervals are recommended, and no modifications are necessary in pregnancy. The fear of medication teratogenicity should not prevent the administration of life-saving ACLS medications.

Clinical Pearls

- In cardiac arrest in pregnancy, CPR and resuscitation should follow the AHA ACLS guidelines.
- For shockable rhythms, biphasic shock with 120 to 200 J is recommended.
- Perimortem cesarean section/resuscitative hysterotomy may be required in an attempt to achieve ROSC in the case of cardiac arrest.

Airway Management

Upper airway changes include hyperemia, edema, and increased secretions can lead to an increased risk of bleeding and poor visualization. Mallampati scores and neck circumference both increase during pregnancy, and there is an increase in airway collapsibility.[16] Lung volumes such as the FRC decrease by 20% to 30%, with another decrease in 25% in the supine position in comparison with upright. Diminished FRC, increased minute ventilation, and increased oxygen consumption during pregnancy all lead to poor reserve and faster desaturation. These factors contribute to a significantly higher rate of failed intubation in obstetrics, occurring 8-times more frequently in pregnant compared with nonpregnant patients.[13,16,17] The most experienced provider should provide the first intubation attempt while minimizing interruptions to chest compressions. A smaller endotracheal tube (6.0–7.0 mm diameter) is recommended.[10]

In the case of an upper airway obstruction by a foreign body, the Heimlich maneuver should be avoided in advanced gestational age (exceeding 24 weeks) or maternal obesity because uterine rupture may occur. In these patients, chest thrusts may be attempted.[13,14]

In the absence of an advanced airway, ventilation should occur with 2 breaths every 30 compressions; with an advanced airway 8 to 10 breaths per minute. Hyperventilation should be avoided because this decreases venous return and increases vasoconstriction, thereby decreasing blood flow to the uterus and brain.[13,17] Use of continuous capnography is recommended to assess the quality of CPR, verify endotracheal tube placement, and evaluate for ROSC, targeting an increasing end-tidal CO_2 (P_{ETCO2}) or levels greater than 10 mm Hg.

Clinical Pearls

- Avoid hyperventilation, which can lead to decreased uterine blood flow.
- A smaller endotracheal tube (6.0–7.0 mm diameter) is recommended for intubation.
- The Heimlich maneuver should be avoided after gestational age 24 weeks or in cases of maternal obesity; chest thrusts may be attempted as an alternative.

Morbidity and Mortality

Maternal survival is estimated at between 15% and 59%, which remains higher than that in other cardiac arrest populations.[10–12,18] Complications of CPR such as rib fractures, ruptured abdominal organs, and fetal injuries may occur.

Resuscitative Hysterotomy

Resuscitative hysterotomy, also known as perimortem cesarean section, is an important option in the resuscitation of the mother and should not be considered only as a heroic effort to save the fetus. Increasing perfusion to the mother through increased cardiac output can best be achieved by relieving the pressure on the IVC by emptying the uterus. Less invasive methods such as left lateral tilt positioning and manual displacement of the uterus should be attempted first but may not be sufficient. Delivery of the fetus may also improve compliance of the thoracic wall for more effective chest compressions and lung ventilation.[15,19] Resuscitative hysterotomy is indicated in cardiac arrest of a pregnant patient at 20 weeks or later with the fundus palpated at or above the umbilicus and ROSC not achieved by usual resuscitative measures, left lateral tilt positioning, and manual displacement of the uterus.[10] CPR should continue throughout and following the procedure. Supine positioning with manual displacement of the uterus is recommended for high-quality chest compressions.[20] To be most effective, resuscitative hysterotomy should be initiated by 4 minutes following arrest. The goal is to complete the procedure within 5 minutes of arrest to minimize hypoxia and improve neurologic outcomes of both mother and fetus.[15,21–23] There may still be a benefit to resuscitative hysterotomy when initiated after 5 minutes, particularly for later term patients (30 to 38 weeks).[20] The procedure should be performed in as sterile manner as possible without causing delays.[10]

Resuscitative Hysterotomy: Supplies[24–26]

- #10 blade scalpel
- Sterile scissors
- Sterile gloves
- Sterile blue towels
- Chlorhexidine swab or betadine
- Umbilical clamps

Resuscitative Hysterotomy: Steps[24–26]

- Make a vertical midline incision through all layers of the abdominal wall from the uterine fundus to the pubic symphysis.
- Expose the anterior surface of the uterus and retract the bladder inferiorly.
- Make a small vertical incision through the lower uterine segment of the uterus.
- Lift the uterine wall away from the fetus and use scissors to extend the incision to the fundus.
- Deliver the infant, clamp and cut the cord, and hand off for neonatal resuscitation.
- Deliver the placenta.
- Pack the abdomen with sterile blue towels.
- Consider antibiotics and oxytocin.

Postarrest Management

Therapeutic hypothermia versus targeted temperature management (TTM), aiming for a temperature between 32°C and 36°C, may improve neurologically intact survival. The current (2015) AHA guidelines recommend consideration of TTM in pregnancy on an individual basis. If used, hypothermia protocols should be followed in a fashion similar to that for nonpregnant patients.[10] In the past 5 years there have been 3 case reports of therapeutic hypothermia showing effectiveness in both neurologic recovery and mortality.[27,28]

Oxygenation and ventilation goals of oxygen saturation (SpO_2) 94% to 98% and normocapnia ($PaCO_2$ 40–45 mm Hg) should be targeted. Hyperoxia can worsen ischemic reperfusion injury to the brain. Avoid prolonged hyperventilation or hypocapnia, which may cause decreased cerebral blood flow.[13,29,30]

Mean arterial pressure of greater than 65 mm Hg is ideal with avoidance of excessive fluid administration, which may require vasopressors. Because hyperglycemia and hypoglycemia may worsen morbidity, glycemic control targeting glucose levels of 140 to 180 mg/dL should be used.[13,29,30]

Clinical Pearls

- Consider therapeutic hypothermia or TTM to improve neurologically intact survival.
- Goals of gas exchange: SpO_2 94% to 98%, $PaCO_2$ 40 to 45 mm Hg.

AMNIOTIC FLUID EMBOLISM

One rare cause of cardiac arrest in pregnancy is amniotic fluid embolism (AFE), an obstetric condition characterized by the triad of cardiovascular collapse, hypoxic respiratory failure, and coagulopathy. It is also commonly associated with neurologic symptoms (encephalopathy/coma/seizures) with persistent neurologic deficits in survivors.

Incidence

The incidence of AFE varies between 1 in 8000 and 1 in 80,000.[31–34] In the United States and North America, it occurs in 1 in approximately 12,000 to 15,000 pregnancies.[29] The low frequency of AFE may be due in part to underestimation of the syndrome because it is a diagnosis of exclusion, and also from underreporting of nonfatal cases. Despite the low incidence, there is significant maternal and fetal morbidity and mortality, and resuscitation considerations differ slightly from other causes of cardiopulmonary collapse.

Risk factors associated with increased risk of AFE include advanced maternal age (35 years or older), placental abnormalities (previa, accreta, abruption, rupture), medical induction of labor, operative deliveries (cesarean delivery, forceps-assisted delivery, vacuum-assisted delivery, termination of pregnancy), amniocentesis, trauma, eclampsia, cervical lacerations, prolonged gestation, male fetus, and multiple gestations.[29,31,32,34–36]

Pathogenesis

A sentinel event occurs when there is a breach in the physical barriers between mother and fetus, with amniotic fluid entering the maternal circulation.[29] The exact mechanism is disputed. The traditional understanding of AFE describes amniotic fluid embolization into the pulmonary vasculature, resulting in mechanical obstruction of pulmonary capillaries, but this is not reliably observed in all cases of AFE nor in multiple animal studies.[33] Those opposed to the traditional view argue that the clinical syndrome of coagulopathy, cardiovascular collapse, and hypoxic respiratory failure are not typically seen in pulmonary thromboembolism. More recent studies suggest that amniotic fluid initiates an abnormal immunologic response with complement activation and release of endogenous proinflammatory mediators. This abnormal host response is similar to those found in anaphylactic shock or endotoxin-mediated septic shock.[32,37–40] Thus the term "anaphylactoid syndrome of pregnancy" has been used by some experts to more accurately describe the physiologic diagnosis, although it has not been widely adopted.[32,39–41]

Timing and Clinical Presentation

Analysis of the national registry reveals that 70% of AFE occur during labor, but may occur in the immediate postpartum period and has been reported to occur as late as 48 hours postpartum.[29,39]

Cardiovascular Collapse

The hemodynamic response in AFE is biphasic (**Fig. 1**). The initial response to hypoxia is pulmonary vasoconstriction, which leads to severe pulmonary arterial hypertension and right ventricular (RV) failure (cor pulmonale). Echocardiographic evidence of RV strain and leftward deviation of the intraventricular septum may be present. Hypoxia, acidosis, and hypercapnia may further worsen pulmonary vasoconstriction and should be avoided. Specific treatments for pulmonary hypertension (sildenafil, inhaled nitric

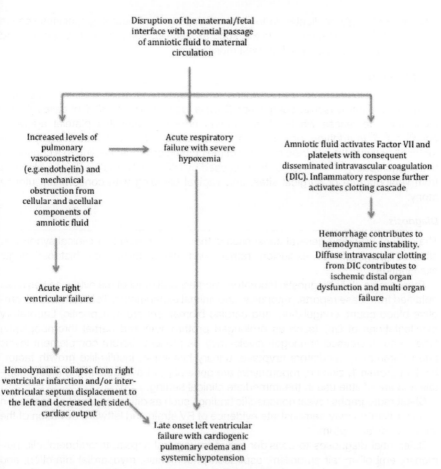

Fig. 1. Proposed pathophysiology of amniotic fluid embolism. DIC, disseminated intravascular coagulation. (*From* Society for Maternal-Fetal Medicine (SMFM), Pacheco LD, Saade G, Hankins GD, et al. Amniotic fluid embolism: diagnosis and management. Am J Obstet Gynecol 2016;215(2):B17; with permission.)

oxide, and inhaled or intravenous prostacyclin) and RV support with inotropes (dobutamine, milrinone) are effective. Next, increased RV distention may obliterate the left ventricular (LV) cavity and thus decrease cardiac output. LV failure follows, either as a result of RV failure or as the direct effect from amniotic fluid or other mediators.[29,32,35,40] Hallmarks of LV failure may include hypotension and pulmonary edema, which can be treated with vasopressors and diuretics, respectively, along with inotropes for increased cardiac contractility.

Hypoxic Respiratory Failure

Hypoxia is an early finding and presents in up to 93% of patients.[33,39] Early hypoxia is due to a severe ventilation and perfusion mismatch from the initial embolism and cardiogenic pulmonary edema. Later hypoxia may be due to noncardiogenic pulmonary edema from alveolar capillary leakage of a proteinaceous exudative edema containing amniotic fluid debris, consistent with acute respiratory distress syndrome. This hypoxia is strongly implicated in the encephalopathy and neurologic injuries seen in survivors.[32,33,39] Evidence of hypoxia such as decelerations, loss of variability, and bradycardia may be observed on fetal monitoring.

Coagulopathy

The exact mechanism for AFE-induced coagulopathy is most likely multifactorial. Disseminated intravascular coagulation (DIC) is present in up to 83% of cases.[39] Amniotic fluid decreases whole blood clotting time and activates platelet aggregation.[28,32,35,39] In addition, procoagulant components of amniotic fluid (namely tissue factor III) activate the extrinsic pathway of the clotting cascade, leading to a consumptive coagulopathy.[35,39,42] Hemorrhage caused by DIC may be manifested by bleeding from venipuncture or surgical sites, and vaginal bleeding with concomitant uterine atony.

Diagnosis

The current view and general consensus is that AFE represents a clinical syndrome, albeit a diagnosis of exclusion rather than being based on histopathologic examination.

There are no clear diagnostic laboratory markers and most of the evidence has been obtained from case reports, autopsies, and animal experiments. Tests such as a complete blood count, coagulation, and cardiac biomarkers are nonspecific. Laboratory manifestations of DIC (such as prolonged prothrombin and partial thromboplastin times, and decreased fibrinogen levels) may be present. Serum complement levels and inflammatory mediators (tryptase, urinary histamine, insulin-like growth factor-binding protein 1, zinc coproporphyrin) are generally not available in the most hospitals and are of little use in the immediate clinical setting.

Chest radiographs reveal nonspecific findings such as diffuse bilateral opacities. An echocardiogram may demonstrate evidence of RV strain and leftward deviation of the intraventricular septum.[29]

Differential diagnoses to consider include puerperal sepsis, thromboembolic pulmonary embolism, air embolism, aspiration pneumonitis, myocardial infarction, and eclampsia.

Management

Treatment is supportive and should take place in the intensive care unit with a multidisciplinary team including maternal-fetal medicine, critical care, anesthesia, and respiratory therapy.[35] Critical care management is focused on hemodynamic support (mechanical ventilation, vasopressors, and inotropes). Excessive crystalloid fluid administration should be avoided.

In the case of cardiac arrest, a presumptive diagnosis of AFE does not preclude standard high-quality CPR with ACLS protocols. Possible use of venoarterial extracorporeal membrane oxygenation has been described, but may exacerbate existing coagulopathy and bleeding and thus is not routinely recommended in the management of AFE.[35]

AFE coagulopathy may require both medical and surgical management. Medical management includes transfusion strategies to maintain a platelet count greater than 50,000/mm^3, a normal activated partial thromboplastin time and international normalized ratio, and a fibrinogen level greater than 200 mg/dL. Early and aggressive transfusion, including activation of a massive transfusion protocol (hemostatic resuscitation in a 1:1:1 ratio) in severe hemorrhage could improve outcomes. Other pharmacologic therapies such as recombinant factor VIIa, fibrinogen concentrates, tranexamic acid, and prothrombin complex concentrates can also be considered.[32,43] Massive crystalloid resuscitation may result in a dilutional coagulopathy and increased intravascular hydrostatic pressures, which could worsen bleeding.

Mortality and Outcome

Death usually results from multiorgan failure, massive hemorrhage, or cardiac arrest.[31,39] Maternal mortality is estimated to be 0.5 to 1.7 deaths per 100,000 live births, with a mortality rate of 60% to 85% in the most severe form or classic AFE syndrome.[29,31,39,40] AFE accounted for 5.0% to 15.0% of all maternal deaths in developed countries, and is the second leading cause of maternal death in the United States.[29,44–47] Perinatal mortality is estimated to be 9% to 44%.[29] Both maternal and perinatal mortality have decreased thanks to improvements in the recognition and early delivery of critical care. The recurrence rate is unknown, but likely low.

SUMMARY

Resuscitation of the pregnant patient presents unique challenges. Being knowledgeable about maternal physiologic changes and the distinctive underlying etiology of cardiac arrest in pregnancy is essential in providing high-quality and potentially life-saving care for both mother and fetus.

REFERENCES

1. Tan EK, Tan EL. Alterations in physiology and anatomy during pregnancy. Best Pract Res Clin Obstet Gynaecol 2013;27(6):791–802.
2. Carlin A, Alfirvic Z. Physiologic changes of pregnancy and monitoring. Best Pract Res Clin Obstet Gynaecol 2008;22(5):801–23.
3. Yeomens ER, Gilstrap LC. Physiologic change in pregnancy and their impact on critical care. Crit Care Med 2005;33(10 suppl):S256–8.
4. Chestnutt AN. Physiology of normal pregnancy. Crit Care Clin 2004;20(4):609–15.
5. Sunitha M, Chandrasekharappa S, Brid SV. Electrocardiographic QRS axis, Q wave, and T wave changes in 2nd and 3rd trimester of normal pregnancy. J Clin Diagn Res 2014;8(9):BC17–21.
6. Sanghavi M, Rutherford JD. Cardiovascular physiology of pregnancy. Circulation 2014;130(12):1003–8.
7. Talbot L, Maclennan K. Physiology of pregnancy. Anaesth Intens Care Med 2016; 17(7):341–5.
8. Katz VL. Perimortem caesarean delivery: its role in maternal mortality. Semin Perinatol 2012;36(1):68–72.
9. Hellgren M. Hemostasis during normal pregnancy and puerperium. Semin Thromb Hemost 2003;29(2):125–39.
10. Jeejeebhoy FM, Zelop CM, Lipman S, et al. Cardiac arrest in pregnancy: a scientific statement from the American Heart Association. Circulation 2015;132(18): 1747–973.
11. Mhyre JM, Tsen LC, Einav S, et al. Cardiac arrest during hospitalization for delivery in the United States, 1998-2011. Anesthesiology 2014;120(4):810–8.
12. Einav S, Kaufman N, Sela HY. Maternal cardiac arrest and perimortem cesarean delivery: evidence or expert-based? Resuscitation 2012;83(10):1191–200.
13. Montufar-Rueda C, Gei A. Cardiac arrest during pregnancy. Clin Obstet Gynecol 2014;57(4):871–81.
14. Farinelli CK, Hameed AB. Cardiopulmonary resuscitation in pregnancy. Cardiol Clin 2012;30(3):453–61.

15. Lipman S, Cohen S, Einav S, et al. The Society for Obstetric Anesthesia and Perinatology consensus statement on the management of cardiac arrest in pregnancy. Anesth Analg 2014;118(5):1003–16.
16. Hegewald MJ, Crapo RO. Respiratory physiology in pregnancy. Clin Chest Med 2011;32(1):1–13.
17. Lapinsky SE. Cardiopulmonary complications of pregnancy. Crit Care Med 2005; 33(7):1616–22.
18. Cobb B, Lipman S. Cardiac arrest: obstetric CPR/ACLS. Clin Obstet Gynecol 2017;60(2):426–30.
19. Morris S, Stacey M. Resuscitation in pregnancy. BMJ 2003;327(7426):1277–9.
20. Jeejeebhoy FM, Zelop CM, Windrim R, et al. Management of cardiac arrest in pregnancy: a systematic review. Resuscitation 2011;82(7):801–9.
21. Whitten M, Irvine LM. Postmortem and perimortem caesarean section: what are the indications? J R Soc Med 2000;93(1):6–9.
22. Katz VL, Dotters DJ, Droegemueller W. Perimortem cesarean delivery. Obstet Gynecol 1986;68(4):571–6.
23. Katz V, Balderston K, DeFreest M. Perimortem cesarean delivery: were our assumptions correct? Am J Obstet Gynecol 2005;192(6):1916–20.
24. AirCare Series: Resuscitative hysterotomy. In: Taming the SRU. Available at: http://www.tamingthesru.com/blog/air-care-orientation-curriculum/resuscitative-hysterotomy. Accessed June 20, 2018.
25. Parry R, Asmussen T, Smith JE. Perimortem caesarean section. Emerg Med J 2016;33(3):224–9.
26. Vora S, Dobiesz VA. Emergency childbirth. In: Roberts and Hedges' clinical procedures in emergency medicine and acute care. 7th edition. Philadelphia: Elsevier Inc; 2019. p. 1186–210.
27. Chauhan A, Musunuru H, Donnino M, et al. The use of therapeutic hypothermia after cardiac arrest in a pregnant patient. Ann Emerg Med 2012;60(6):786–9.
28. Oguayo KN, Oyetayo OO, Stewart D, et al. Successful use of therapeutic hypothermia in a pregnant patient. Tex Heart Inst J 2015;42(4):367–71.
29. Conde-Agudelo A, Romero R. Amniotic fluid embolism: an evidence-based review. Am J Obstet Gynecol 2009;201(5):445.e1-13.
30. Steiner PE, Lushbaugh CC. Maternal pulmonary embolism by amniotic fluid as a cause of obstetric shock and unexpected deaths in obstetrics. JAMA 1941; 117(15):1245–54, 1340-45.
31. Neligan PJ, Laffey JG. Clinical review: special populations—critical illness and pregnancy. Crit Care 2011;15(4):227.
32. Clark SL. Amniotic fluid embolism. Obstet Gynecol 2014;123(2):337–48.
33. Moore J, Baldisseri MR. Amniotic fluid embolism. Crit Care Med 2005;33(10): S279–85.
34. Abenhaim HA, Azoulay L, Kramer MS, et al. Incidence and risk factors of amniotic fluid embolisms: a population-based study of 3 million births in the United States. Am J Obstet Gynecol 2008;199(1):49.
35. Pacheco LD, Saade G, Hankins GD, et al. Amniotic fluid embolism: diagnosis and management. Am J Obstet Gynecol 2016;215(2):B16–24.
36. Meyer JR. Embolia pulmonary amnio caseosa. J Bras Med 1926;1:301–3.
37. Benson MD. Current concepts of immunology and diagnosis in amniotic fluid embolism. Clin Dev Immunol 2012;2012:946576.
38. Benson MD, Kobayashi H, Silver RK, et al. Immunologic studies in presumed amniotic fluid embolism. Obstet Gynecol 2001;97(4):510–4.

39. Clark SL, Hankins GD, Dudley DA, et al. Amniotic fluid embolism: analysis of the national registry. Am J Obstet Gynecol 1995;172(4):1158–67.
40. Shamshirsaz AA, Clark SL. Amniotic fluid embolism. Obstet Gynecol Clin North Am 2016;43(4):779–90.
41. Tamura N, Farhana M, Oda T, et al. Amniotic fluid embolism: pathophysiology from the perspective of pathology. J Obstet Gynaecol Res 2017;43(4):627–32.
42. Rudra A, Chatterjee S, Sengupta S, et al. Amniotic fluid embolism. Indian J Crit Care Med 2009;13(3):129–35.
43. Pacheco LD, Saade GR, Costantine MM, et al. An update on the use of massive transfusion protocols in obstetrics. Am J Obstet Gynecol 2016;214(3):340–4.
44. Brennan MC, Moore LE. Pulmonary embolism and amniotic fluid embolism in pregnancy. Obstet Gynecol Clin North Am 2013;40(1):27–35.
45. Clark SL. Amniotic fluid embolism. Clin Obstet Gynecol 2010;53(2):322–8.
46. Rittenberger JC, Kelly E, Jang D, et al. Successful outcome utilizing hypothermia after cardiac arrest in pregnancy: a case report. Crit Care Med 2008;36(4):1354–6.
47. Bennett TA, Katz VL, Zelop CM. Cardiac arrest and resuscitation unique to pregnancy. Obstet Gynecol Clin North Am 2016;43(4):809–19.

Moving?

Make sure your subscription moves with you!

To notify us of your new address, find your **Clinics Account Number** (located on your mailing label above your name), and contact customer service at:

Email: **journalscustomerservice-usa@elsevier.com**

800-654-2452 (subscribers in the U.S. & Canada)
314-447-8871 (subscribers outside of the U.S. & Canada)

Fax number: **314-447-8029**

Elsevier Health Sciences Division
Subscription Customer Service
3251 Riverport Lane
Maryland Heights, MO 63043

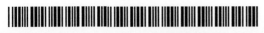